D0027046

LUNCH WARS

JEREMY P. TARCHER/PENGUIN

a member of Penguin Group (USA) Inc.

New York

LUNCH WARS

How to Start a
School Food Revolution
and Win the Battle
for Our Children's Health

AMY KALAFA

WESTPORT PUBLIC LIBRARY
WESTPORT, CT
203-291-4800

JEREMY P. TARCHER/PENGUIN
Published by the Penguin Group
Penguin Group (USA) Inc., 375 Hudson Street, New York, New York 10014, USA • Penguin Group
(Canada), 90 Eglinton Avenue East, Suite 700, Toronto, Ontario M4P 2Y3, Canada (a division of Pearson
Penguin Canada Inc.) • Penguin Books Ltd, 80 Strand, London WC2R 0RL, England • Penguin Ireland,
25 St Stephen's Green, Dublin 2, Ireland (a division of Penguin Books Ltd) • Penguin Group (Australia),
250 Camberwell Road, Camberwell, Victoria 3124, Australia (a division of Pearson Australia Group Pty Ltd) •
Penguin Books India Pvt Ltd, 11 Community Centre, Panchsheel Park, New Delhi–110 017, India •
Penguin Group (NZ), 67 Apollo Drive, Rosedale, North Shore 0632, New Zealand (a division
of Pearson New Zealand Ltd) • Penguin Books (South Africa) (Pty) Ltd,
24 Sturdee Avenue, Rosebank, Johannesburg 2196, South Africa

Penguin Books Ltd, Registered Offices: 80 Strand, London WC2R 0RL, England

Copyright © 2011 by Amy Kalafa
All rights reserved. No part of this book may be reproduced, scanned, or distributed in any
printed or electronic form without permission. Please do not participate in or encourage piracy of
copyrighted materials in violation of the author's rights. Purchase only authorized editions.
Published simultaneously in Canada

Most Tarcher/Penguin books are available at special quantity discounts for bulk purchase for sales promotions,
premiums, fund-raising, and educational needs. Special books or book excerpts also can be created to fit specific
needs. For details, write Penguin Group (USA) Inc. Special Markets, 375 Hudson Street, New York, NY 10014.

Library of Congress Cataloging-in-Publication Data

Kalafa, Amy.
Lunch wars : how to start a school food revolution and win the battle
for our children's health / Amy Kalafa.
p.   cm.
ISBN 978-1-58542-862-5
1. National school lunch program.   2. School children—Food—United States.
3. School children—Nutrition—United States.   4. Education—Parent participation—
United States.   5. Educational change—United States.   I. Title.
LB3479 U6K35   2011   2011018962
371.7'16—dc23

Printed in the United States of America
1   3   5   7   9   10   8   6   4   2

BOOK DESIGN BY MEIGHAN CAVANAUGH

Neither the publisher nor the author is engaged in rendering professional advice or services to the
individual reader. The ideas, procedures, and suggestions contained in this book are not intended as
a substitute for consulting with your physician. All matters regarding your health require
medical supervision. Neither the author nor the publisher shall be liable or responsible for
any loss or damage allegedly arising from any information or suggestion in this book.

While the author has made every effort to provide accurate telephone numbers and Internet addresses
at the time of publication, neither the publisher nor the author assumes any responsibility for
errors, or for changes that occur after publication. Further, the publisher does not have any control over
and does not assume any responsibility for author or third-party websites or their content.

34015070284292

CONTENTS

You have much more power when you are working for the right thing than when you are working against the wrong thing.

—Mildred Lisette Norman, aka Peace Pilgrim

PREFACE

When I'm interviewed, I'm often asked to share my story. Why did I become so passionate about school food? I've had to think long and hard to answer this question, because now that I'm so involved in the school food movement, it's difficult to remember the "before"!

Like most members of my generation, I grew up on a typical American diet of soda, chips, pizza, Velveeta cheese, steak, chicken, potatoes, and peas. Not nearly as much fast food as today's kids, but Burger King, McDonald's, Kentucky Fried Chicken, and others were a new, cool phenomenon in the sixties and early seventies, and we ate our fair share. In elementary school, we never questioned the food in the cafeteria line. There wasn't a choice of menu items beyond substituting a PB and J for the hot lunch. I recall referring to the meatloaf as "barf loaf," and looking forward to a dessert of frosted white cake about one inch square in size. Our simple school meals were cooked by lunch ladies in hairnets, most of whom were related to someone in the lunch line.

I was and still am a highly sensitive person. As a child I was diagnosed with allergies to trees, grass, pollen, synthetic clothing, and other chemicals. I considered myself a closet hypochondriac, never wanting anyone to know how lousy I felt much of the time. Sinus infections, skin eruptions, menstrual cramps, migraine headaches, and fatigue were medicated with progressively stronger tablets and elixirs. My eccentric temperament caused me to believe that I could never have a "normal" career, so I joined the ranks of the self-employed long before such status became fashionable. As a film and video editor and later as a producer, I was able to hide behind the scenes, creating an alternate reality that did not have to take place in real time. Thus, I could work around my schedule of symptoms.

On this path, I met and married a fellow filmmaker who took me home to meet his family in France. On first impression, I was amazed and somewhat appalled by their apparent obsession with food and drink. Each extended visit required hours around the table several times a day, an experience that made me long for sandwiches chewed over the kitchen sink with my dad when my mother wasn't home.

I had experimented with health food in college; a housemate shared with me during his macrobiotic phase, but in those days, "organic" was often synonymous with "deformed" and all that tofu made me gassy. Over time, though, I began to realize that I felt better when I ate my husband's French food (which was also quite delicious). I enjoyed following his mom to the market—a huge open-air plaza with dozens of vendors selling scores of species of seafood, an entire aisle of stalls featuring locally made cheeses, aisles of vivid fruits and exotic vegetables I'd never seen before and pastries that were delicate beyond any I'd ever tasted in America. Curious, I began learning more about the connection between whole, unprocessed food and health (mine in particular). I also discovered the politics of food in America. I learned that our food system is one of the major causes of global warming. I realized that farm-fresh, chemical-free, whole, unprocessed food was not only good for me, it was healthier for the planet, and probably better for lots of other people as well.

Eventually, my husband's "gourmet" obsession merged with my awakening "sustainability" obsession. In 1985, with a friend, we purchased a defunct dairy farm in Bovina, New York, and soon launched the first certified organic poultry and game bird operation on the East Coast, while maintaining our other life as filmmakers in New York City. Then along came the kids; our two girls were raised on mostly organic and homegrown whole foods. My husband packed the girls a homemade lunch for school most days, and neither of us gave much thought to the food served in the school cafeteria. Periodically, I would try to sell my various television network employers and friends on the idea of a program on food, the environment, health, and politics. "It's just not sexy" was the typical refrain.

My food world and my film world intersected but never meshed until December 2004, when an assignment for *Martha Stewart Living* sent me to the exclusive Ross School in Easthampton, Long Island. At the Ross School I met chef Ann Cooper, who had been lured from a "white tablecloth" restaurant in Vermont to run the school's wellness program. Ann coined an acronym for the school's food: Regional, Organic, Seasonal, and Sustainable (ROSS). Meeting Ann Cooper was an epiphany for me. The day of our interview I told her I'd be back to make a documentary about school food.

I spent many months researching the chemistry, sociology, and politics of industrialized food. I learned how dramatically our food supply has changed in the past fifty years. The processing and commodification of food in America have resulted in abundance and affordability, but like a balloon squeezed at one end, there's an opposite impact at the other. American kids are often overfed, yet undernourished. Studies, books, articles, and my own experience convinced me irrefutably that there is a link between childhood consumption of junk food not only with obesity and diabetes, but also with other health, learning, and behavioral disorders in children. My passion became more than a personal interest; I felt strongly that the American system of food production and distribution was a political issue affecting every child in America, and that schools *had* to play an important role in it.

School food is a reflection of American food policy and food culture in general. Since school is where we teach our kids what we think they need to know to be prepared for the future, I felt there was a huge missed opportunity to include real food education in the curriculum as well as in the cafeteria. I wanted to reach as large an audience as possible with my message that we need to examine our food culture, that this isn't just about cupcakes and childhood obesity. Every controversy has a bad guy, and the food industry

PR firms had been quick to point fingers at parents. I wanted to counter the spin and point a finger back at the industry. I felt powerless as a parent to have any impact locally or nationally, and I wanted to know what I could do. I wanted to find out what was being done, and what could be done, to change policies and implement programs that provide better food and better food education for children.

I hadn't actually been in a public school lunchroom in years, so one of the first places I filmed was my daughter's middle school cafeteria. Reading the labels on the many packaged products for sale confirmed my worst suspicions: the school cafeteria was a microcosm of American fake food culture. Healthy-sounding products like Nutri-Grain bars had high fructose corn syrup listed as one of the first ingredients (well hidden under a foil flap that you had to fold down to read the tiny print!). The low-fat yogurt also had high fructose corn syrup, aspartame (artificial sweetener), artificial flavoring, and coloring. I asked the food service representative to show me how the computerized checkout system worked. She produced a readout of my daughter's purchases over the year and that's how I became an "angry mom." We had put money on account in the cafeteria for days when our daughter might forget her lunch, or when we might be running too late to pack one for her. I was truly shocked to discover that she had been purchasing fries, Rice Krispies Treats, Pop-Tarts, and soft drinks on a daily basis. No wonder her lunches often came home half-eaten.

I felt isolated in my community and wondered if we were the only parents in our school district who believed our efforts to feed our kids well at home were actually being undermined by the food offered in school. *Two Angry Moms* became the story of my quest to learn what parents like me needed to know, and do, in order to change the food environment of our children's schools.

Searching for someone who was leading the charge, I found and interviewed many moms (and one very angry dad) who had sat on food committees, nutrition committees, and wellness committees, and valiantly tried, and failed, to get better food into their schools. Criticized as nutrition Nazis and food police, they were often ostracized, banished from school cafeterias,

and occasionally even run out of town. It was a greater effort to find successful models to document, but I was eventually led to many.

The frustrated parents I met advised me to steer clear of attempting to create change in my own school district while I was making the movie. These
moms suggested I would get so bogged down in local politics that I would
never have time to produce the film. They were right. After a few thwarted
local interactions, I heeded their counsel and stayed under the radar in my
hometown, choosing instead to travel the country with my camera, following
the revolution fomenting on a national scale. I also documented the crusade
of Dr. Susan Rubin, her organization Better School Food, and its impact on
one suburban school district over the course of a school year.

Just a couple of weeks into the project I read a quote from then–secretary
of agriculture of Texas Susan Combs, who said, "It's going to take two million angry moms to change school food." I figured if we could grow from
two to two million, we could impact policy both locally and nationally. I
realized that this was a movement as well as a movie. Along with making
the film, I built a website, angrymoms.org, where parents, teachers, administrators, school food service workers, health professionals, and students can
download information, sign up to host screenings of the movie, and find
each other to form local networks.

I found model school food programs in the rarefied halls of Yale University, in a largely Hispanic desert community in California, in the urban
streets of Harlem, in the chilly mountains of New Hampshire, and in a community just a few miles from my home. By the time I caught up again with
chef Ann Cooper (my original inspiration from the Ross School), she had
been hired by Alice Waters, owner of the famous Chez Panisse Restaurant
in Berkeley, California, whom I consider to be the fairy godmother of school
food. Each example shows how the efforts of parents and community leaders
have led to the implementation of new policies and programs. Many of these
programs, if adopted on a large scale, would go a long way toward reversing
the ominous statistics on declining children's health. Due at least in small
part to *Two Angry Moms*, the controversy over school food is now part of a
national conversation, and that's a step in the right direction.

Since the film's release, I've been traveling with the movie, speaking at libraries, school auditoriums, movie theaters, and conferences. Wherever I go, the questions I'm asked most are "How can we get more information about this?" and "How do we begin in our school district?" What follows is a hard drive's worth of research compiled into a manifesto that can be used as a guide to school food activism. There's no one-size-fits-all solution, so I've highlighted lots of examples from people I've met and places I've been to over the past few years. I've tried to give you the information you need to get acquainted with the issues surrounding school food so you can immediately start making a difference in your own community.

INTRODUCTION

DON'T POISON THE KIDS!

Our kids might be the first generation in history on track to lead shorter lives than their parents.

—MICHELLE OBAMA

Why is the subject of better school food so controversial, so political? Why do we need to gather two million angry moms in a movement for change? In 2004, when I began research for my documentary *Two Angry Moms*, mass media coverage of America's food supply focused mostly on mad cow disease and the occasional *E. coli* panic. Nonprofit watchdog groups were producing much of the information I could find on the Web. A few years earlier, Eric Schlosser's book *Fast Food Nation* had topped the bestseller list and several other journalists and renowned professors (Kelly Brownell, Michael Pollan, Marion Nestle) were weighing in with highly rated volumes of their own. These researchers warned that the American agricultural policies that had successfully led to the production of abundant, cheap food were in fact sacrificing food quality and moreover sacrificing our nation's health. Added to this was an emerging discussion about the impact of our fossil fuel–dependent agricultural system on global warming. Although the connection was intentionally muddied by food industry propaganda, it was also at this time that our national media was beginning to sound the alarm about a crisis of obesity and diabetes among America's children.

Food industry public relations firms were quick to spin the story toward lack of exercise. These companies campaigned for children's physical fitness, giving away pedometers at "Get Moving" and other industry-sponsored events. McDonald's, Coke, and Pepsi all initiated in-school fitness programs and some even "donated" branded playground equipment. The big food corporations continued to make nutritional claims on their highly processed products, initiating a check-mark system for products deemed healthy because they had reduced fat or calories. Parents, school food service directors, and dieticians were counseled to follow government nutrition guidelines that claimed, "There are no bad foods; all foods are fine in moderation." It comes as no surprise that the food industry has lobbied hard to influence policies that establish those government guidelines.

Yet despite the upbeat campaign by the food industry, America's children continue getting fatter and sicker. Today, newspapers, radio programs, bloggers, and TV news all run daily stories about the connection between our food supply and our nation's health. Exposés about factory farming and feel-good pieces about Michelle Obama's organic garden are run as featured items. Many more movies, both documentary and fictional, have been released, depicting a food system where quantity trumps quality and government subsidies make the least healthy foods also the least expensive.

Now there's a PR war being waged for control of our school food programs with the marketers and lobbyists of highly processed, branded junk food on one side and the bloggers, critics, and children's health advocates on the other. Advertisers spend $10 to $15 billion annually on ads targeted specifically to children and those ads have migrated from TV, coloring books, and fast-food outlets directly into schoolbooks and school cafeterias. I recall when one of my daughters brought home a math practice sheet with a word problem that read something like, "If Julio has 24 Skittles and Kim has 8 M&Ms, how many more candies does Julio have than Kim?" Here the author had taken pains to replace the Jane and Johnny of my schoolbook memories with multicultural-sounding names for the kids, but had either intentionally or inadvertently also replaced the apples and oranges of yesteryear with junk food.

As a television producer, I was taught to be careful not to show brands when filming for network television shows—the networks take precautions not to offend current sponsors by showing competitive products, and not to promote a brand unless they've been paid for product placement. When I began filming in school cafeterias, I had to throw my network-induced caution to the wind. Everywhere I turned, my camera lens focused on a brand. Drinks of all kinds were sold out of refrigerators wrapped in images of giant Snapple or Pepsi bottles. Baskets of Lay's potato chips were strategically placed on counters where the hot food and sandwiches were sold. And bushel barrels filled with Welch's Fruit Snacks and Kellogg's Pop-Tarts beckoned at the checkout counters.

Research shows that repeated brand exposure works. The Campaign For a Commercial-Free Childhood reports: "About 98 percent of all televised food ads seen by children are for foods high in sugar, fat, or sodium. One thirty-second commercial can influence the brand preferences of children as young as two. In a 2007 study, preschool children reported that food in McDonald's wrappers tasted better than the same food in plain wrappers, suggesting that branding can even trump sensory input." A 2010 Yale University study found that "children significantly preferred the taste of foods that had popular cartoon characters on the packaging, compared with the same foods without characters. The majority of children selected the food sample with a licensed character on it for their snack, but the effects were weaker for carrots than for gummy fruit snacks and graham crackers." The weaker effect for carrots suggests that these kids were already habituated to the connection between cartoon characters and processed foods. The study concludes: "Branding food packages with licensed characters substantially influences young children's taste preferences and snack selection and does so most strongly for energy-dense, nutrient-poor foods. These findings suggest that the use of licensed characters to advertise junk food to children should be restricted."

Marion Nestle, NYU's Goddard Professor of Nutrition, Food Studies, and Public Health, says that for the food industry, "Number one is to get kids to pester their parents.... what you really want to do is convince kids that they have to have their own special foods, in special packages with special colors and designs . . . and not eat adult food regardless of the quality of the food."

And in fact, the advertisers proudly point to this strategy.

"We're relying on the kid to pester the mom to buy the product, rather than going straight to the mom."

—Barbara A. Martino, advertising executive

"Brand marketing must begin with children. Even if a child does not buy the product and will not for many years . . . the marketing must begin in childhood."

—James McNeal, The Kids Market

"The school system is where you build brand loyalty."

—John Alm, president and chief operating officer, Coca-Cola Enterprises

Coca-Cola, PepsiCo, and other members of the American Beverage Association have consistently lobbied against state and local legislation that would restrict marketing of unhealthy foods and beverages in schools. Yet as I write this, the ABA today expressed public support for reauthorization of the Child Nutrition Act. Susan K. Neely, ABA president and CEO, said, "Reauthorizing the Child Nutrition Act this year is critical, and our industry is proud to be working with members of Congress on this important issue."

Behind the scenes, ABA lobbyists have cleverly negotiated the removal of full-calorie soft drinks and replaced them with diet beverages. Could this obsequiousness have anything to do with the fact that artificial sweeteners cost less to produce than old-fashioned sugar? Or perhaps with their campaign to make these proposed federal guidelines take precedence over any state or local mandates? "Our industry continues to welcome opportunities to work alongside Congress to improve nutritional standards set for children in schools. We urge our elected officials to vote on the Child Nutrition Act this year," Neely goes on to say.

Studies link the colorings, preservatives, and artificial sweeteners in these beverages to behavior and health issues in humans, particularly children. A recent study published by the American Psychological Association found that no-calorie sweeteners in foods might actually make it more difficult for people to control their food intake and body weight. The no-calorie sweeteners trick the metabolism, which expects an influx of calories when sweets are consumed. Those calories normally trigger a feeling of satiety. The study showed that rats fed diet sweeteners "later consumed more calories, gained more weight, put on more body fat, and didn't make up for it by cutting back later."

Kelly Brownell from Yale's Rudd Center supports legislation to place stiff taxes on soda because "you can never compete with the amount of marketing money that the industry spends to educate people to consume these beverages."

The ironies abound. Lovable animated character Shrek appeared in public service ads (PSAs) as part of President George W. Bush's Healthier US Initiative. In the PSAs, the pudgy ogre urges kids to "get up and play an hour a day." At the same time, Shrek's green grin adorned the packaging of Twinkies, Snickers, Pop-Tarts, Pez, M&M's, Frosted Flakes, McDonald's Happy Meals, and Keebler E.L. Fudge Double Stuffed cookies. Senator Tom Harkin criticized this monstrous scam, saying, "Shrek now becomes a bad guy, trying to get our kids to eat unhealthy food. Shame on the advertisers taking a likeable, lovable character . . . and now using Shrek to poison our kids. I use the word 'poison' because that's what this food does, it poisons our kids."

Humans are the only species on earth that aren't born with an instinct to discern good foods from bad. We have to learn which foods are safe and which are dangerous. I meet many parents and kids who wonder what's really okay to eat. I've heard the four food groups for children referred to as "Soda, Chips, Nuggets, and Dessert." No wonder parents are confused! Our media, our role models, our entertainers, and even our schools are all encouraging us to consume, consume, consume. Dr. Stephen Cowan, a developmental pediatrician, insists that the rise in chronic and acute childhood disorders he sees is provoked by diet and lifestyle. Dr. Cowan says, "In the U.S. we view our children as consumers, and when they consume, we blame them for consuming."

For years, I lived in denial, thinking that my kids were immune to all the advertising and promotion because we ate well at home. When I went to the middle school cafeteria to film there and learned that my daughter had been eating junk food nearly every day, I realized that the school was actually encouraging this behavior, making junk food socially acceptable. Although they were teaching so-called proper nutrition in health class, the message in the cafeteria was "anything goes." A conversation with the school's then-superintendent confirmed that indeed, he found no contradiction in the messaging because, he insisted, it was not the school district's responsibility to feed the kids, just to educate them.

Not an Educational Issue?

We're now into a third fast-food generation. The effect of poor nutrition in the form of highly processed food on successive generations is a controversial topic, but one that was well documented by Dr. Weston A. Price back in the 1920s and 1930s. At that time, there were still numerous isolated cultures on earth, and he and his wife traveled the world, photographing generations of these people before and after they adopted a diet of what he called "the displacing foods of modern commerce." Price, who was a dentist, found severe jaw and facial deformations, as well as cavities, in the offspring of parents who had perfectly developed jaws and teeth. He also documented degenerative diseases and immune disorders among those exposed to the "modern" diet. While Dr. Price's research has led to a current controversy over his advocacy of a diet rich in fatty acids, there's not much dispute over the degenerative effect of the modern American diet.

Today, nearly a century after Dr. Price's research, we see successive generations eating not only a diet of highly processed foods, but also a diet polluted by chemical residues from our industrial food system. Airborne pollution and our children's sedentary lifestyle are unhealthful stressors, but the fact is that 80 percent of the toxins our children are exposed to come through the food and water they ingest. Our country uses 15 trillion pounds a year of over 80,000 different industrial chemicals, tested only by the manufacturers.

Pesticides account for 4.4 billion pounds of those chemicals annually. Many of the chemicals intentionally or inadvertently found in today's foods actually block the natural processes of digestion and assimilation of nutrients, and a child's growing body may be permanently affected by such disturbances. For this generation of America's children the results of this cumulative decline in nutrition are dire. The issues kids face today go way beyond obesity: physicians report soaring rates of asthma, autism, ADHD, anorexia, and clogged arteries—and that's just the A's! Bipolar disorder, bone weakness, bulimia . . . and the alphabetical list of increasing diet-related childhood epidemics could fill pages. Our children's life expectancy is now shorter than our own and we can expect them to be plagued with worse health than our own as well.

Of course it's an educational issue! As Yale's Dr. Kelly Brownell tells me in the movie, "There's a lot of nutrition education going on for our children, but it's done by the food industry." Our schools teach kids in health class that smoking cigarettes is bad. Wouldn't parents be up in arms if they knew that cigarettes were sold in vending machines in high school cafeterias? The food manufacturers argue that kids need choices. Dr. Brownell says, "I don't see any rationale for offering unhealthy choices in school just for the sake of having choices. You don't have unhealthy reading for the kids. You don't have an unhealthy playground that has toxic substances on it. Why do you want to have unhealthy food?"

There's a frequent argument made that food is different, food is personal. And unlike smoking, there's no secondhand heart disease—or is there? A 2007 *New England Journal of Medicine* study found that among friends, overeating and obesity does appear to be contagious. Researchers studied a social network of 12,000 people over a period of more than thirty years. They found a 57 percent increase in the likelihood of an individual becoming obese when a friend became obese.

And, like smokers of a generation ago, people who know they should be eating better are often defensive about their habits. Dr. David Kessler, former head of the Food and Drug Administration, is well known for exposing the tobacco industry's intentional manipulation of nicotine and other chemicals in cigarettes to make them more addictive. His recent research concludes that the food industry has done something similar by manipulating the sugar, fat, and salt content of foods to hit our taste buds at the "bliss point" that makes them irresistible. Dr. Kessler believes that our "brains have been captured" by these manufactured foods. Addiction, whether to foods or cigarettes or drugs, certainly is a personal issue, but it's also a matter of public health . . . which is why we teach kids about it in school and make every effort to avoid exposing them to addictive substances at school (as long as it's not food!).

Research shows that in obese individuals, the brain's reward circuitry becomes less responsive to food stimuli in the same way an addict builds up a tolerance to drugs. In both cases, it takes more and more of the substance to produce the same satiety, which is now thought to explain why obese children tend to become obese adults, even when they are put on a normal diet. This research supports the importance of forming healthy eating behaviors early in life when the brain is still growing, adapting, and patterning what will become lifelong habits.

The tobacco wars were won with media exposés, lawsuits, public health campaigns, changes in public opinion, and finally legislation on both the local and national levels. Advocacy groups fought long and hard against industry lobbyists paid to obfuscate the issues. Despite what most of us considered common knowledge, the tobacco industry insisted there just wasn't enough compelling evidence linking cigarettes with cancer and death. Eventually, numerous judges and juries found that there was clear evidence that proved the connection, awarding large settlements for individual and class action lawsuits against the cigarette manufacturers. Similarly, I often heard that there just isn't enough good research linking junk food to declining children's health. As a filmmaker, I needed to back up my research with irrefutable statistics. I began digging through general statistics about America's health and the health of our children. What I found adds up to far more than a headline. America's third generation of fast-food babies has produced some stunning results.

What follows is a list of fearsome facts and scary statistics that reveal the shortcomings of American food policy as it relates to disease prevention. I often review this list before I go to meetings to help me remember some of the scary numbers, and to remind myself why I remain involved in the school food movement now that my kids are older. We must change the way we nourish and feed the generation of children currently in school in order to stem the tide of declining children's health.

- Americans spend $200 billion per year in diet-related health care costs; twice as much per person than any other developed nation.
- The estimated annual cost of obesity is $123 billion—half of which is paid for by Medicare and Medicaid.
- Fifty percent of all cancer could be prevented through healthy diet and exercise.
- Over 95 percent of America's health care dollars is spent on disease treatment; less than 5 percent is spent on prevention.
- The average American life expectancy ranks 46th in the world.
- The cost of fresh fruits and vegetables has risen 40 percent in the past twenty years.
- The cost of soda, sweets, meat, dairy, fats, and oils has decreased by as much as 20 percent in that same time.
- Americans spend less than 10 percent of their income on food, but 17 percent of our GDP (Gross Domestic Product—our national income) is spent on health care.
- Europeans spend 17 percent of their earnings on food, but less than 10 percent of their GDP on health care.
- In 1960, Americans spent 17.5 percent of their income on food and 5.2 percent on health care.
- Only 2 percent of school-age children eat the USDA's serving recommendations for all five major food groups. Half of America's school-children eat less than one serving of fruit a day.
- Nearly 30 percent of American children eat less than one serving a day of vegetables that are not fried.
- According to the Institute of Medicine, "at least 30 percent of the calories in the average child's diet derive from sweets, soft drinks, salty snacks, and fast food."

- Over two-thirds of all foods consumed by schoolchildren are foods that are recommended for occasional intake.
- Children's sodium intake is 214 percent above recommended levels.
- Children two to eighteen years old consumed an average of 118 more calories per day in 1996 than children did in 1978. That's equal to 12 pounds of weight gain annually.
- In 2009 Americans consumed 63 percent of their calories from processed foods high in added sugars and fats. Another 25 percent of calories were consumed as meat and animal products, with just 12 percent of calories consumed as fruits and vegetables, an estimated half of which were in the form of candy bars or desserts.
- Eleven percent of the calories consumed by adolescents come from soda and other soft drinks.
- Since the 1970s obesity rates have tripled among children ages six to nineteen.
- Twelve percent of American children currently have type 2 (adult-onset) diabetes and rates are increasing annually. The CDC reports that one in three children born in 2000 (30 percent of boys and 40 percent of girls) will develop type 2 diabetes.
- Nineteen percent of American children are obese and 35 percent are overweight and the trend is increasing. The prevalence of overweight or obesity in children will nearly double by 2030.
- One quarter of children ages five to ten have elevated blood cholesterol or high blood pressure—early warning signs of heart disease.
- One in four children take prescription medication on a daily basis for chronic illness.
- Childhood asthma rates have more than doubled in the past thirty years and autism rates have increased by 57 percent. Now autism affects one in 110 children, one in 60 boys.
- There's been a 700 percent increase in amphetamine prescriptions for children since 1990.
- Between 1995 and 1999, antidepressant use increased 74 percent among children under eighteen, 151 percent among children from seven to

twelve, and 580 percent among children under six years of age. The use
of mood stabilizers increased by 4,000 percent among children under
eighteen, and use of new antipsychotic medications increased 300 percent among the same age group.

- American girls are beginning puberty one to two years earlier than they
  were a generation ago.
- The United States ranks near the bottom of the world's thirty most-
  developed countries in math (25th) and science (21st).

New studies are appearing clearly linking childhood obesity and learning
and behavior problems to junk food, and even specifically to school food. I'll
report on some of them in the following chapters. I expect the lawsuits will
soon follow.

Despite the nationwide epidemic of childhood obesity, one in ten households in the United States is food insecure, meaning some 16.7 million children in the United States go to bed hungry, and the numbers are on the
increase. America's children are both overfed and undernourished. Why
have we allowed this crisis to spin so dangerously out of control?

> A 2008 study found that children who bought lunch at school were at an
> increased risk for being overweight. The study also found that students with
> a higher consumption of foods rich in omega-3 fatty acids, fruits, and veg-
> etables performed better on a standardized literacy assessment, independent
> of socioeconomic factors. The researchers report that there was an association
> between overall diet quality and academic performance.

School food is certainly an economic and social justice issue, but it also
cuts across the social classes. I found equally poor quality food and toxic food
environments in both wealthy and poor school districts. One important distinction is that for many kids in poor districts, school food may be the only
food they eat all day. In my comfortable suburban enclave, it's easy to ignore

the health problems our children face. We don't see as much obesity, which is highly correlated with the lower end of the socioeconomic spectrum in America. Yet the incidence of less visible afflictions such as ADHD, autism, anxiety, and depression among kids in the burbs is reportedly higher than in less affluent, more ethnically diverse populations. Several years ago I filmed at a summer camp catering to mostly suburban kids. One still frame continues to haunt me. A group of about a dozen kids six to ten years old was lined up against a fence. At first I smiled back at the portrait of grinning kids, their spindly arms and legs sticking out of tie-dyed T-shirts and shorts. Suddenly the photograph morphed as my attention was drawn to their narrow faces and rounded bellies protruding from the colorful T-shirts. The appearance of this group of campers reminded me of photos of hungry children in Biafra, India, Haiti, and the United States, during the Great Depression. According to the World Health Organization, physical findings associated with "protein-energy malnutrition" include "decreased subcutaneous tissue: Areas that are most affected are the legs, arms, buttocks, and face. Abdominal distension secondary to poor abdominal musculature." It's often said in medicine that a doctor will tend to find what she's looking for and overlook that which she isn't. Could these suburban kids be exhibiting signs of something we only look for in the Third World?

Westchester, New York–based health and lifestyle counselor Gerri Brewster says, "They're all running around at recess and everybody looks just fine, but they're all leaving school and going to their allergists and immunologists and pulmonologists and gastroenterologists. And then they're getting a whole host of support services to help with visual processing problems and auditory processing problems and sensory integration issues. So why are we so sensitized and over the top? Our bodies, our immune systems are just so overly reactive right now."

In aggregate, the scary statistics on children's health, diet, and hunger make a pretty good argument for a complete overhaul of our agro-industrial food and health care system. That's a mighty overwhelming job. When looked at on the local level, school district by school district, the task seems a bit more possible. Traveling around making the film, I saw that the greatest changes were taking place at the local level, sometimes in a single school, sometimes across a district. Big projects always look easier when you break them down into small steps, and that's what I hope this book will help you do.

Change in America has a long tradition of growing from these small steps, the grassroots. As we grow our movement, we need to incorporate our efforts into permanent programs, and create policies that institutionalize the processes that are getting positive results. Food policies currently in place both locally and nationally are woefully inadequate to reverse the avalanche of declining children's health, and changing those policies is now becoming a national priority. The food industry's blatant exploitation of our children, according to NYU's Marion Nestle, is actually the impetus for many of the policy changes taking place. Dr. Nestle says that "marketing to kids is the food industry's big point of vulnerability."

As a result of the burgeoning school food movement and all the media attention it has cast upon Big Food, we are now beginning to see some reform coming from the top. Federal, state, and local policies have begun to address some of the most egregious sins of the food industry and those policies and new opportunities are discussed in chapters three and four. But regulation will never be enough without educated parents, teachers, school staff, and students willing to create, interpret, and implement those policies.

Marion Nestle was one of the people who inspired me to believe that parents do have the power to influence policy, but she also says, "If there aren't angry moms pushing for it, it's not going to happen."

A 2008 study of 1,349 students in grades four through six from ten schools, in an unnamed U.S. city with a high proportion of children eligible for free and reduced-price school meals, participated in a multi-component School Nutrition Policy Initiative. The study reports that the intervention resulted in a 50 percent reduction in the incidence of overweight. Significantly fewer children in the intervention schools (7.5 percent) than in the control schools (14.9 percent) became overweight after two years.

There are model school food programs that work—in our own country and in others around the world. We can draw many lessons and inspiration from the programs and leadership examples I've documented in the following chapters.

You don't have to quit your job or neglect your children to become a school food advocate. There are many ways in. The advice and practical suggestions in the following chapters all come from people and programs I've met, seen, or learned about because they were featured as a success story. Each suggestion or case history serves as a model and contains some small, manageable steps you can take. So feel free to peek around in the chapters and find something that resonates with you!

These examples are the positive ammunition you'll need to share with your community, along with some nutrition information that isn't funded by the food industry. The effort to get better food into the schools has not only engendered policy changes on a national scale, it has won lots of popular support in school districts around America and around the world. You can be the driving force behind your own local movement, using this book to guide your way. Amazing things will happen once you make that leap.

ONE

LET'S DO LUNCH

One should not have to be a superhero, a magician, or a saint to get healthy, tasty food into the school cafeteria.

—JANET POPPENDIECK

Whether your child brings lunch or buys it, you need to know what your school's food environment is like. The cafeteria, the classrooms, the hallways, the playgrounds, the athletic fields, and the buses are all part of a school's food environment. The food itself and the messages about food, whether overtly taught or insidious, dictate the school's food culture and will have a great influence on your child over the course of 180 days a year for twelve years.

The typical American child eats less than one serving of fruit a day and anywhere from 30 to 156 pounds of sugar per year, depending upon which statistics you read. Is your school system reinforcing this diet by handing out candy in class and selling junk food in the cafeteria? I didn't think much about the school food environment when my daughters were young. I figured since we ate well at home and sent them to school with a packed lunch, they were immune to the school's food culture. I thought school food was a missed opportunity to educate children about food, but I didn't realize that the school system was actually undermining our family's healthy food habits until I went to my daughter's middle school to investigate the lunch program. Learning that she had been purchasing Pop-Tarts, Rice Krispies treats, french fries, and soft drinks on a daily basis became the focal point for a movie and a movement.

Since that time, I've been on a quest to learn what parents need to know and do to get better food into their children's schools. I've met hundreds of other parents who describe themselves as Angry Moms, but we're also less affectionately known as the Food Police or Nutrition Nazis. Really we are all just parents trying to take back the school food environment from the Junk Food Bullies. It's a tough job, and everyone wants to know what to do first. The Web abounds with articles promising "Five Ways Parents Can Reform School Food," "Seven Tips for Better School Food," and "Three Simple Steps to Clean Up the Cafeteria." These magic lists are filled with good ideas, but the *one* piece of advice that every list has in common is *go have lunch with your child*. In fact, the USDA (United States Department of Agriculture), the agency that oversees the school meals programs, in their "Ten Steps for Parents," counsels as step 1, "*Do lunch with the kids.* Eat breakfast or lunch at school with your kids. See what the meals are like. Notice the atmosphere. If you don't like what you see, *do something*." Indeed, one of the first things every parent should do, skeptics and advocates alike, is make a date for lunch. Let the folks at the front office know you're there. Most schools will require you to wear a visitor's badge. Some schools may try to keep you out. I hear stories of parents being banned from the cafeteria but it's your right to visit there with your child—the USDA says so!

Most kids will be proud to have Mom, Dad, or Grandma join them for lunch. Some might be a bit embarrassed. If that's the case, you can plan your lunch date as a group event with several other parents, so that your child won't feel singled out. If you're ready to draw some attention to the school food issue in your district, organize a Lunch-In—a day or week when lots of parents join their children for breakfast or lunch. Notify your school's food service director ahead of time so he or she can plan ahead for some extra meals. Let the food service director know that you are an ally, not an adversary, and that your intention is to bring attention to the importance of the school food environment and gather resources and support for making improvements.

There's a trade group for everything, and school food is no exception. Largely supported by contributions from the food industry its members purchase from, the School Nutrition Association (SNA) represents school food service workers. The organization promotes a National School Lunch Week each year in late October. Since the release of *Two Angry Moms*, we have encouraged parents to attend a school Lunch-In during the SNA's National School Lunch Week. The goal for the SNA is to bring awareness to the school meals program. Our goal is to up the ante by examining the quality of the food and the school food environment.

Most schools publish their weekly or monthly menus online. I've got a Connecticut middle school menu in front of me with a Wednesday entrée seductively called Love at First Delight. It's described as a roasted turkey breast sandwich with American cheese, lettuce, tomato, and Russian dressing on a kaiser roll. I might have named it Détente, but the description does make it sound like a yummy lunch. A menu from Birmingham, Alabama, simply describes Wednesday's meal as "Lasagna, green beans, corn on the cob, tossed salad, orange wedges, sugar cookie, roll, and milk." Sounds like good, filling comfort food. So what's the reality for these two meals? Are they tasty and healthy? Or are they nasty, greasy, soggy, and full of chemicals? You don't need a nutrition degree to conduct a good investigation, but you do need to look beyond the menu.

What's in the Food?

The menu may sound great, the food may look fine, and even taste decent, but it's not time to leave the cafeteria. You need to know what's in the food. My list of the Scary Six substances to watch out for includes some things that are just plain bad for all kids, some items that are known to cause problems for some kids, and some things that we just don't know enough about because they're too new. These false foods can play havoc on a child's immune system and nervous system, causing repeated illnesses, behavioral problems, and long-term chronic sickness. Note that a number of the chemicals described below are on the Food and Drug Administration's (FDA's) Generally Recognized as Safe (GRAS) list. Countless additives that were once also on that list were subsequently found to cause organ damage, cancer, and other toxic reactions.

1. Residues—pesticides, herbicides, hormones, and antibiotics
2. Flavorings—MSG, autolyzed yeast extract, hydrolyzed protein
3. Additives—preservatives and artificial colorings
4. Hydrogenated oils
5. Sugar and artificial sweeteners
6. Genetically engineered foods

RESIDUES

In Europe, the policy toward pesticides, herbicides, and other chemical pollutants requires that the burden of proof of safety fall on the manufacturer. In the United States, the Environmental Protection Agency is charged with the burden of proving a pesticide does not meet acceptable risk standards before regulatory action can be taken. The EPA, however, does not have adequate resources to follow through on many of the cases it investigates. Furthermore, the agency's mission seems a bit muddled. A 1970s Environmental Protection Agency document on pesticide regulation states, "EPA has the complex task of making difficult trade-offs between the often conflicting objectives of protecting man and the environment from pesticide hazards and realizing the economic advantages afforded by pesticide use." Which leaves us, as parents in America, to bear the burden of protecting our children.

Some of the countries from which we import our food have even more lax pesticide and herbicide regulations than we do. These chemicals are dangerous for the workers in the field, and they're dangerous for our kids. In fact, American manufacturers are known to export chemicals banned for use in agriculture in the United States to countries from which we later import fruits and vegetables. Some pesticides are known to disrupt a child's normal hormonal balance and are believed to be contributing factors for the declining puberty age of girls, rising rates of sterility in young men and increasing rates of childhood cancers. There are many good reasons to ask your school's food service director to purchase produce from a local vendor. One of the most important reasons is to reduce your child's exposure to residues from these agricultural chemicals. Ask where the produce comes from. If the answer is "I don't know," or "It comes from the big truck," it's time to dig deeper.

Hormones and antibiotics are used in the production of industrially farmed beef and other livestock. Livestock consumes over 70 percent of all the antibiotics used in the United States. Most of the animal food we humans consume is from ruminants—cows' and other animals that thrive when allowed to graze on pastures of grasses and herbs. When forced to live in overcrowded, filthy conditions and fed grains that their digestive systems cannot handle, these confined animals are also fed antibiotics to prevent bacterial infections that would otherwise cause them to sicken and die. The USDA, which supplies surplus American beef and poultry free as commodity items to our school systems, has lower standards than many fast-food chains. In the past decade, the USDA paid $145 million for pet-food grade "spent-hen meat" that went into the school meals program.

In February 2008, 143 million pounds of ground beef was recalled in the wake of a hidden camera exposé of battered, sick, and crippled cattle on the killing floor of a California meat packer. Because of the way ground beef is produced in America, what the public soon learned was that meat from a handful of sick cattle could contaminate 143 million pounds of product. A reported 37 million pounds of that beef had been delivered to schools across the United States. Nearly all of it had already been consumed by the time of the recall.

So ask your food service director where the meat comes from and how it was raised. Many students are asking these kinds of questions too (that video exposé went viral on YouTube). These sorts of questions are empowering for kids and help them begin to understand the food web that they are part of. We have a local grocery store that buys beef from one specific ranch; the owner has been to visit the ranch and can personally vouch for the ethics and practices of the ranchers. His ground beef costs a bit more than the factory farmed brands. In our family that translates into less beef, more beans. This is great food for thought for a school district wellness committee.

VIRGINIA: NINA GONZALEZ

Nina Gonzalez started thinking about her food at a very early age. When she learned that bacon came from pigs, she gave it up. She couldn't bear the thought of eating Mr. Pig, her favorite fuzzy stuffed animal. As a teenager, Nina learned about factory farming. "I couldn't believe that they didn't teach us about this at school. How could animals live in such horrible conditions? That couldn't be healthy for me," Nina realized. "I thought my best option was to cut out meat altogether. As a young person with no money, that was a way I could make an impact. A lot of people make an argument that vegetarianism is a cover-up for anorexia or strange eating disorders but it made me get really educated about my food and where it was coming from. I became more aware of the nutritional value of things. Before that I would eat a lot of junk food."

Nina's mom had diabetes so she was really happy to cut up carrots for Nina's snacks instead of supplying her with Fruit Roll-Ups and chips. But at school Nina found it harder. "The only vegetarian options were fries and greasy pizza. I sat at a table with a lot of athletes. We would talk about the food and a lot of other people didn't like it. We talked about how the bad food affected them in class and then at the track meet after school or at the wrestling match that evening. I looked at a lot of different food service websites and then found one that had a file for vegetarian options in the school cafeteria. It suggested that you get the kids to petition the school. I started walking around and talking to people at different tables. I found some friends who were really excited about the idea. We went and asked the lunch ladies who were in charge. They sent me to the school nutrition director. He called me in for a meeting! I had printed out menus from schools that were successful. I showed him the things they had offered and how they labeled them on their menus. I also read the nutrition requirements for protein and fat. I put all my information in a little folder and told him I was speaking on behalf of a lot of other students."

With so much careful preparation, Nina made an impression on the nutrition director. "A couple of months later the head lunch lady came by and told me that the nutrition director was really excited about adding some new options. They made a taste-testing and we gave them a lot of ideas of how they could add signs that would say what options were available for the day so that students wouldn't have to stand in line to find out. The food service director was really excited to see that lots of guys were involved too, not only girls, and they were all athletes."

Student athletes are often admired as leaders in high school, so Nina's group was in a position to have some positive influence. Nina proudly told me, "Every day there would be at least a vegetarian option and once a week the main meal would be vegetarian. I didn't try to change the other students, but what I did inspired them. I know of about six other people who became vegetarian because of what I did. The way I would explain it made eating more exciting and interesting. It's strange today that fresh food is more expensive than chips. I can't understand why. A pound of potatoes is more expensive than a pound of chips? The media tells us what they think we shouldn't eat but I say you have to listen to your body. You have to look at food in a way that is positive and fun."

Her philosophy about food stems from another childhood memory: "I remember when we went to restaurants, my dad always made me order for myself. I was really excited to be able to make my own choices. Usually as kids our parents make so many choices for us. School food is one of the first times you are making choices over what you eat. You learn about good choices in health class and if you have the desire to make healthy choices you need options available. If those healthy options aren't there you don't have the power to exercise those good choices. The choices that you make about friends or classes are choices you make once in a while but the choices that you make eating, you make every day, several times a day. What you eat now is going to make an impact on your whole life."

Nina's success didn't end at her high school. She testified before Congress for the Healthy Meals Act and is now working with her college's food service to get them to label the food better. "I didn't think I would be able to make a big difference because I was just one person."

Sustainable Table, an organization that has been at the forefront of exposing some of the unsavory practices of factory farms, surmises that about two-
thirds of America's beef cattle are injected with synthetic hormones to make
them grow faster. This faster growth is important to the industry, because
not only does it save money on feed, it increases the chances that the animals
will stay alive long enough to bring to slaughter. Along with pesticide residues, hormone residues in beef are believed to be another culprit for early
onset of puberty in girls. The hormones are excreted in cow manure, which
is either recycled as fertilizer or pooled into lagoons where it leaches into
groundwater. Aquatic life is also vulnerable to these endocrine disrupters;
certain species of fish and frogs have suffered gender and reproductive aberrations from exposure to hormones, pesticides, and other environmental
contaminants. The use of growth-promoting hormones is banned by the
European Union, and for that reason the EU also prohibits the import of
hormone-raised beef products from the United States.

The USDA does not permit the injection of hormones in hogs, chickens,
or turkeys, but they can be fed chemical growth enhancers. If we want to
ensure that our schoolchildren are not ingesting meat from animals that have
eaten these growth accelerants, we need to ask our schools to purchase certified organic products. Organic certification requires that meat and poultry
are not given hormones or growth enhancers. Organic usually costs more,
so that's asking a great deal from our cash-strapped public schools, but with
committed leadership and proper management, it can happen.

An injectable bovine growth hormone called rBGH (aka BST) was developed in the mid-1990s by agrichemical giant Monsanto to increase milk
yields in lactating cows. Research has shown serious health problems among
treated cows and it too is prohibited in Europe, Japan, Australia, and Canada. While the FDA insists that drinking milk from rBGH-treated cows
has no impact on children's health, many parents remain skeptical. In 1998,
Monsanto quashed a story by a pair of veteran Fox TV reporters that would
have exposed a potential link between rBGH and human cancer. Though
the two reporters lost their jobs and the story never aired, the incident and

ensuing lawsuit made public the amount of power Monsanto has over the media and our legal system. Monsanto and other members of the dairy industry have lobbied hard to prevent producers of non-rBGH milk from labeling their cartons as "rBGH-free." A 2010 ruling from the U.S. Court of Appeals for the Sixth Circuit in Ohio ruled in favor of the Organic Trade Association's appeal to allow continued use of the "rBGH-free" labeling. Due at least in part to the large public outcry against the hormone, farmers are cutting back on its use and Monsanto has sold the patent to another company. Many schools have already made the switch to rBGH-free milk as a first step toward sourcing better-quality food.

FLAVORINGS

The chemical structure of MSG actually occurs naturally in some substances, like aged cheese and kelp. The synthetic version is highly concentrated, which is why it's used as a flavoring to cover up the bland cardboard taste of many processed foods. When you eat out, there's usually MSG hiding in the coating on your curly fries, in the sauce on your barbecued wings, and in the dressing on your side salad. I have a pet peeve against MSG because it gives me migraines. It's known to cause many other reactions including confusion, diarrhea, heart irregularities, asthma, and mood swings. These reactions can occur anytime from immediately upon ingestion up to forty-eight hours later, so it's very hard to pin them to a single food item. The worst thing about MSG is that the active chemical, processed free glutamic acid, is hidden in dozens of other food additives, including many described as "natural flavorings."

Federal law requires that all processed foods be labeled with a list of all ingredients in descending order by weight. In the case of a child with documented food allergies, the school is required to provide parents with ingredients lists for all the foods they serve. Many parents have told me that they've had trouble getting these lists from the school's food service providers. Even if your child doesn't have a documented food allergy, you can inquire on behalf of a child that does. Like everything else in the world of public school, the parent that persists most often prevails. My school's food service provider is a company named Chartwells. They're one of the biggest in the business. I recently asked their dietician for a list of ingredients in all the foods in our cafeteria. She quickly responded with an e-mail link (www.westonk12-ct. org/page.cfm?p=3621) that brings you to a page listing foods by category: beverages, cereals and grains, dairy, dry goods, snacks, condiments, frozen foods, soups, meats, and so on. Each category links to a page of label photos. It doesn't seem like every food in the cafeteria made it to the list, and some of the labels weren't complete, but I did find plenty of unpronounceable ingredients that are known code names for MSG. The Truth in Labeling campaign has crafted this list of the many ingredients that may contain processed free glutamic acid:

Glutamic acid

Glutamate

Monosodium glutamate

Monopotassium glutamate

Calcium glutamate

Monoammonium glutamate

Magnesium glutamate

Natrium glutamate

Yeast extract

Autolyzed yeast

Hydrolized protein

Calcium caseinate

Sodium caseinate

Yeast food, Yeast nutrient

Gelatin

Textured protein

Textured vegetable protein

Vetsin

Ajinomoto

Many other food additives may also contain the MSG compound. When you read the labels in the cafeteria, look out for the ingredients on this list from Truth in Labeling as well:

Carrageenan
Bouillon and broth
Stock—unless it's made from scratch
Whey protein
Whey protein concentrate
Whey protein isolate
Any "flavors" or "flavoring"
Maltodextrin
Citric acid
Anything "ultra-pasteurized"
Barley malt
Pectin
Protease
Anything "enzyme modified"
Anything containing "enzymes"
Malt extract
Soy sauce
Soy sauce extract
Soy protein
Soy protein concentrate
Soy protein isolate
Anything "protein fortified"
Anything "fermented"
Seasonings
Modified food starch

That's a long list. I found many of these sneaky ingredients on the labels of Chartwells dairy foods, snack foods, condiments, chicken products, soup bases, frozen egg rolls, and french fries. Printed on the box of egg rolls were

the words "NO MSG ADDED*." I couldn't find the footnote for the aster-
isk, but it was probably a disclaimer of some sort. You will hear the argument
that "these things are safe for kids because they're in such small amounts."
When you start adding up those small amounts in every item, every day, the
picture changes.

NEW YORK: THE TSE FAMILY

Autism rates (now estimated at around one out of every 110 children in the
United States) have increased so dramatically in the past few decades that
probably everyone reading this will find Beth's a familiar story. Her son
Josh was a happy baby; he seemed to be developing normally until sometime
around two years old his behavior began to change. He became uncommuni-
cative, couldn't make eye contact, and he often had such violent outbursts that
Beth could no longer take him to playdates, birthday parties, or family events.
Josh was diagnosed with autism and thus began a battery of therapies and
interventions. As moms will do, Beth tried everything to find a cure for her
son. She came across a book that suggested making some dietary changes that
specifically eliminated all food additives as well as gluten and dairy because
these proteins appear to trigger allergic reactions in some sensitive children.
Beth was amazed at the almost instant change in her son. "People don't
believe me. We don't have the before and after videos. I was too caught up in
the day to day. I could tell you what he looked like the week before the diet
and the week after. His stomach was distended, he had constant diarrhea." As
they tweaked his diet and put him on a vitamin and detoxification regimen
under the guidance of an experienced medical doctor, Josh responded and
began to thrive. I met Josh when he was six years old. His pediatrician, Dr.
Stephen Cowan, suggested that the story would be a good one for my film.
"When I first met him, he was in trouble," says Dr. Cowan. "PDD—Pervasive
Developmental Disorder. He was locked out; he couldn't engage." I filmed
Josh with his younger sister playing on the patio, making gluten-free, sugar-
free cookies with their mom, and at his karate class. He laughed easily and
chatted freely with his family and his concentration was focused in the class.

Beth and her husband had recently started Josh in a new school because his old school refused to remove his earlier diagnosis of autism.

When I included their story in an early preview version of the movie *Two Angry Moms*, focus groups reported that Josh's tale wasn't credible—no one would believe a truly autistic child could be cured this way, and the movie would lose credibility if I included it. We deleted the scene. Due in large part to the recent book and publicity for pop culture icon Jenny McCarthy, who used a similar diet to reverse her own son's autism, this story is now accepted as plausible. "I know what I know; I'm a mom," says Beth. "It's true, some kids just grow out of it. And not every kid will respond the way Joshua did." I spoke with Beth recently and she reports, "He's in middle school now and he's still doing well. We tried reintroducing wheat in the fourth grade but noticed he was getting distracted so he still eats no wheat but he does drink raw milk. He's more aware of the food than I am now. He looks things up and tells me if they're okay." I asked Beth for her advice to other parents trying to modify their children's diets. "At my daughter's gymnastics studio they gave her a lollipop two weeks in a row. I had to talk to them. They vilify the role of the mom, say you're being too tough. You've got to spend the time with your kid. Go back to the basics. We live this fast-paced life and everyone's running from activity to activity. Plan your meals; think about what you're cooking. Don't just grab your pizza on the run. You know those studies that say kids who sit at the dinner table with their families are smarter? They say it's the social interaction, but what about what the kids are eating?" And Dr. Cowan adds, "Nobody makes money on diets; there's a lot more money in pharmaceuticals than natural food."

ADDITIVES

A 2007 study published in the British medical journal *The Lancet* reports, "Artificial food colour and additives commonly found in children's food exacerbate hyperactive behaviours in children. . . ." The researchers found that even among children who normally did not exhibit hyperactive behavior, a combination of the widely used food preservative sodium benzoate and some FDA-approved food dyes (think soda and sports drinks) triggered "behavior that was significantly more hyperactive."

On an after-school visit to our local high school, I witnessed a scene in the hallway: a bright red pond of liquid spreading on the floor, an over-turned bottle, the vice principal hollering at a group of boys—the boys, most clutching their own red bottles, all with cheeks as red as the spilled beverage, yelling back. No one was in control. Not the kids, not the VP. These kids probably would have been expelled for that behavior if it were a result of smoking crack. Yet the drinks were purchased in a vending machine down the hall, with money that will mostly contribute to the marketing budget of the beverage industry.

Many school systems have now eliminated the worst of these artificially colored and preserved beverages, although many still contain some "natural flavorings and preservatives." You really have to read labels on all the beverages, because some of the most healthy-sounding names belong to the most chemically laden bottles, and some of the all-natural ice teas are laden with naturally occurring caffeine—not something young kids should be getting dosed with.

Plastic bottles themselves are a source of concern. While there is still debate as to whether plastic compounds can leach into the beverage, the negative environmental impact of billions of disposable plastic bottles is indisputable.

Colorings and preservatives are found in many baked goods, snack foods, and frozen entrées that may be served in your school's cafeteria and vending machines. Preservatives, whether natural or synthetic, are compounds that prevent food from breaking down as part of the normal process of decay or digestion. Children who eat a lot of foods containing preservatives may not be able to properly digest whatever nutrients are contained in those foods because the preservatives are doing their job, preventing digestion. One famous example of the power of food preservatives is filmmaker Morgan Spurlock's (*Super Size Me*) experiment with french fries from a local restaurant and french fries from McDonald's. After eight weeks the fries from the local restaurant were black and so putridly decayed that he had to toss them out. After ten weeks, the McDonald's fries looked like they had just come out of the deep fryer. Along with the MSG family, I found preservatives such as calcium propionate, sodium acid pyrophosphate, sodium nitrate, disodium dihydrogen pyrophosphate, and calcium pyrophosphate on the ingredients labels of the frozen foods in my school district.

HYDROGENATED OILS

These artificial fats are made by combining hydrogen gas with oil. They are often also known as trans fats. This is actually a misnomer, since there are some naturally occurring trans fats that provide health protective benefits, whereas hydrogenated oils are generally recognized as unhealthy. Hydrogenated or interesterified oils are solid at room temperature. Food manufacturers love them because they help prolong a product's shelf life. They usually appear in baked goods such as crackers, cookies, and snack foods. Because these fats have received so much bad press, many schools have already made efforts to eliminate them. I read the ingredients on my district's baked goods list and it looks like most of the hydrogenated oils have been replaced by soybean or cottonseed oils. Soybean and cotton crops are some of the most heavily treated with chemicals. Both oils are inexpensively produced using hexane and other chemical solvents. In other words, junk food is still junk food!

FOOD ADDICTIVES

My daughter once referred to all the artificial and chemical ingredients in junk food as "food addictives." I started to correct her but then realized that she was right. Recently there have been many studies published about the addictive nature of fast food with its combination of salty, sugary, and fatty flavorings. Humans are programmed to crave sugar. It's one of the main components of breast milk, which is twice as sweet as cow's milk. Milk sugar—lactose—helps a baby's developing digestive system maximize absorption of critical minerals and other nutrients. Only in recent human history has sugar in its many forms been so readily available after weaning. A French study found that sugar was a more powerful choice than cocaine, even for a rat population addicted to cocaine. We have so many sources now of inexpensive sugar and sweeteners that nearly every processed food item contains some form of sugar. If you went through your school's cafeteria and eliminated all the foods that contain sugar, you would probably not find much left to eat.

A cheaper sugar substitute, high fructose corn syrup (HFCS), has really taken a beating in the media lately, and for good reason. While the manufacturers claim it's all natural and made from corn, they decline to mention the complicated chemical process by which it's extracted. A 2010 Princeton study finds that consumption of HFCS causes significant weight gain in lab animals, as well as abnormal increases in body fat and triglyceride levels. There's a strong correlation between America's type 2 diabetes crisis and the widespread introduction of HFCS in 1980.

Another 2010 study reports that cancer cells proliferate when fed the type of sugar in HFCS, which is about 50 percent fructose. The tumor cells were able to metabolize the HFCS much more readily than plain glucose. The food industry loves HFCS because, as the Corn Refiner's Association literature says, "It keeps food fresh, enhances fruit and spice flavors, retains moisture in bran cereals, helps keep breakfast and energy bars moist, maintains consistent flavors in beverages, and keeps ingredients evenly dispersed in condiments." HFCS has been banned from many school cafeterias, although again, it's important to check those labels because it somehow seems to creep back in if parents aren't vigilant.

In 2010, the New York State legislature introduced a bill that would tax all beverages sweetened with sugar or high fructose corn syrup. The bill was narrowly defeated, but other similar bills are under consideration. While the beverage industry lobbied against the bill, they are working diligently to create a new line of products using a host of noncaloric sweeteners. Most of these sweeteners are less costly to produce than real sugar, so the industry stands to gain by their introduction. Consumers may stand to gain more weight as the sweet taste without the satiety that a caloric sweetener provides confuses their metabolism.

These new sweeteners have names like Naturlose, sucralose (Splenda), and neotame. A few that have been around for a while are saccharin, acesulfame, and aspartame, which is sold under the brand names Equal and NutraSweet. Like MSG, aspartame, while generally recognized as safe by the FDA, is also known as an "excitotoxin," a type of chemical that reacts with receptors in the brain that cause destruction of certain types of brain cells. Dr. Russell L. Blaylock, author of the book *Excitotoxins: The Taste That Kills*, reports that "these substances play a critical role in the development of several neurological disorders, including migraines, seizures, infections, abnormal neural development, certain endocrine disorders, specific types of obesity, and especially the neurodegenerative diseases, a group of diseases that includes: ALS, Parkinson's disease, Alzheimer's disease, Huntington's disease, and olivopontocerebellar degeneration."

Professor of nutrition Karen Siclare works with children and families, retraining their taste buds and getting them unhooked from sugar and junk food. Karen says, "To say that 'my kid is fine eating chicken nuggets,' well, if you really looked at that child from a biochemical point of view, and looked at their B vitamin content and the health of their GI tract and inflammation markers, you might see a different story. All the diseases that are plaguing the United States right now and causing so many older people to be on medications actually began in their childhood."

While you're in the school cafeteria, check to see if there are artificial sweeteners in the yogurt, like I found at my daughter's middle school. Maybe this stuff is perfectly safe, but those degenerative diseases take some time to develop, and we shouldn't allow our kids to be used as guinea pigs.

A 2010 study from the Australian Telethon Institute for Child Health Research shows "an association between ADHD and a 'Western-style' diet in adolescents." Researchers found that a diet high in take-out foods, processed meats, dairy, and sweets and low in omega-3 fatty acids, fresh fruits and vegetables, whole grains, and fish more than doubled the risk of an ADHD diagnosis.

GMOs

The final category in the Scary Six is genetically modified organisms (GMOs). These foods, affectionately nicknamed "Frankenfoods," are produced through genetic engineering, a sophisticated process of inserting a gene for a specific trait from one organism into a different species in order to produce that desired trait in the target organism. Currently in the United States about 89 percent of soy, 83 percent of cotton, 75 percent of canola, and 50 percent of corn is grown from genetically modified seed. There's no way to know if the foods served in your school cafeteria are made from GM ingredients, because government policy considers them identical to other foods and therefore labeling is not required. GMOs are awash in controversy. The giant agro-industrial firms that hold power over federal legislators have forced their creations upon us. Manufacturers claim that the foods have been thoroughly tested for safety, but the government doesn't require independent testing so the manufacturers themselves do the testing. Consumer groups fear that new allergens, toxins, and bacteria may be introduced into our food. It's reported that animals fed GMOs have exhibited a variety of strange symptoms and people living in proximity to GMO fields have developed skin, intestinal, and respiratory reactions during pollination periods. In addition, the developers of the GM foods hold patents on the genetic material—a situation that has put many unsuspecting farmers out of business. These GMO seed companies have a history of suing farmers who may unintentionally have GM crops growing in their fields, a phenomenon that may occur via cross-pollination or when seeds from intentionally cultivated GM crops drift into neighboring fields.

One type of genetic engineering creates strains of plants that are engineered to withstand herbicide applications that will kill every other type of plant. Monsanto's "Roundup Ready" soybeans, sugar beets, and alfalfa will survive application of the herbicide Roundup (active ingredient glyphosate). The manufacturer claims that Roundup breaks down rapidly in the environment. However, these genetically modified herbicide-resistant plants may absorb the herbicide into their tissue prior to being consumed by animals or humans.

In 2010, a genetically modified salmon was introduced that grows at least twice as fast as its non-GMO relatives. To date, no special labeling will be required for the "Frankenfish." Michael Hansen, a senior scientist at the U.S. Consumers Union, says, "It is essential to label a genetically engineered animal so that any unexpected effects will be recognized and consumer health protected." For now, the only way to ensure our food isn't from a genetically modified organism is to purchase certified organic foods, which cannot be grown from GM seeds or raised from a genetically modified animal. Lobbyists are currently working on allowing GM foods to qualify for the certified organic label.

Talk to the Teachers

While you're visiting the cafeteria, if there's a teacher on duty, strike up a conversation. Ask her or him if they notice a difference in their students' behavior after lunch. When I filmed a group of Harlem elementary school students on a field trip, their teacher told me that she had to do all of her instruction before lunch because after lunch the kids were too wild. The group we took on the field trip accidentally gave us a clear illustration of that phenomenon. The day of the field trip, our group only had six children, because, I was told, none of the other kids in the class were well behaved enough to leave the building. Our group however, was delightful and interested in the tour of the vegetable aisle of the grocery store we visited. They were excited but focused and engaged when they got to sample fresh coconut milk from a sidewalk fruit vendor. When we stopped for lunch at a community garden, the kids ate their sandwiches and then the gardener handed out sugary Capri Sun drinks, cookies, and chips. Suddenly and dramatically, the kids all went bonkers. They began poking one another, yelling, tugging on their clothes and were unable to pay attention to the teachers in the garden. We captured this behavior on film. The teachers were very apologetic for the kids, until we all realized what had happened. The teacher pointed out that the kids buy "icies" (frozen, flavored, colored sugar) every day at lunchtime from a vendor at the school fence. The kids admitted that they eat two or three icies before heading back to class.

On your visit to the cafeteria, find out who's minding the store. Some schools require teachers and administrators to take a tour of duty in the cafeteria, others solicit parent volunteers, and still others allow the kids free rein at lunchtime. I've witnessed countless kids making a meal of fries and a chocolate chip cookie. The model school food programs I visited had staff or parents helping kids make choices based on completing a colorful plate, or sending kids back to take a piece of fruit. A recent Yale University Rudd Center for Food Policy Study reports that in schools where a cafeteria worker suggested that students take a piece of fruit, 30 percent more students decided to take the fruit. Independent of whether or not they had been encouraged to take the fruit, 80 percent of students ate the fruit if they had it on their tray. Not all schools condone this type of encouragement, however. I recently spoke with a mom who was expelled from the cafeteria for making suggestions to the students. She was told it was against school lunch policy. National guidelines do state that a teacher may not insist a child take a specific menu item, but I have never seen a regulation that prohibits encouragement! What happens in the lunchroom should be a reflection of the school's wellness policy—something we'll explore in depth in chapter four.

Liquid Assets

What are the kids drinking in your school? Sodas, sugared juices, and sports drinks have been banned from many school cafeterias during the lunch hour. The American College of Sports Medicine states, "During exercise lasting less than one hour, there is little evidence of physiological or physical performance differences between consuming a carbohydrate-electrolyte drink and plain water." These drinks are just salty sugared water disguised by clever marketing, and most contain artificial flavors and colors. Some schools allow the drinks to be sold after school hours—that was the case when I witnessed the shouting teens at our high school. The default work-around for many schools is 100 percent fruit juice and artificially sweetened electrolyte replacement beverages. Also beware of the suspiciously neon-colored ubiquitous fruit juice slushies. In the effort to fight childhood obesity, our nation is on high alert against sugar, and many parents question the wisdom of fruit juice, which has as much sugar and calories as soda. When you go down this road, people tend to throw their hands in the air and ask, "So what's left to drink?!"

Got Milk?

The eight-ounce carton of school milk is the icon of school lunch, but school milk isn't what it used to be. Chocolate, strawberry, and even coffee-flavored milk far surpass the white stuff in popularity. The flavored milks generally have as much sugar as soda, often in the form of high fructose corn syrup. They also often contain ingredients like starch, dextrose, caramel coloring, artificial flavoring, salt, and carrageenan. There's a common argument that kids won't drink their milk if the only option is the white stuff. The School Nutrition Association is touting a study by MilkPEP, an industry trade group, that states that milk consumption in schools dropped by 35 percent when chocolate and other flavored milks were removed from the lunch line. Because the milk is fortified with vitamin D and vitamin A, dieticians worry that kids won't get these essential nutrients if they don't drink their milk.

Compounding the milk issue is the commonly held belief that eating (or in this case drinking) fat makes you fat. The federal government now requires that schools sell only 1 percent or fat-free milk to children over two years old. Studies show that America's kids eat too much unhealthy fat, but most of that is consumed in the form of hydrogenated oils or other fats in junk food. It's highly unlikely that the naturally occurring fat in milk is the cause of childhood obesity. In fact, several studies have found an association between low-fat and nonfat milk consumption and weight gain in children, but no association with consumption of full fat milk and weight gain in kids. Nutritionists point out that the fat in milk is necessary for proper uptake of milk protein, calcium, and the fat-soluble vitamins A and D. Full-fat milk is more flavorful as well. In our efforts to reverse childhood obesity, we may be contributing to other more subtle health problems. A child's brain consists of over 60 percent fat cells and our children need good fat for their brains to develop properly. On the other hand, fat is where most of the toxins in animal products are stored, so it's important to ask where the school's milk comes from. Milk from cows allowed to graze on fresh pasture and fed organic hay will have fewer toxic residues than milk from conventionally raised grain-fed cows, and the fat will have a much healthier essential fatty acid profile.

In addition to being the icon of school lunch, milk is probably one of the most controversial lunchroom subjects. The USDA is working on adding substitutions for milk in their guidelines to accommodate the estimated 80 percent of ethnic Asians, Hispanics, African-Americans, Jews, and Native American kids who are lactose intolerant. (Non-Jewish children of European descent have only a 2 percent incidence of lactose intolerance.)

Both beef and milk production are a major source of global warming gases, accounting for 37 percent of global methane production. Grain-fed cattle excrete methane from both ends because they have constant indigestion. Stonyfield Farms, the New Hampshire–based yogurt manufacturer, is conducting a pilot program that feeds cows a diet that their multiple stomachs are better able to digest. This diet of alfalfa, flax, and grasses is high in natural omega-3 sources, resulting in a 19 percent decrease in methane production and a 30 percent increase in the milk's omega-3 content with a corresponding decrease in the levels of saturated fats. In other words, healthier cows, healthier milk, healthier kids!

H_2O

One more thing to look for in your school cafeteria—water! A study in the journal *Current Opinion in Pediatrics* concluded that offering drinking water to students throughout the school day increased their consumption of water and was effective in the prevention of obesity for high-risk children. Most schools sell bottled water to bring in extra revenue for the lunch program. As a result, drinking fountains have fallen into disrepair, and the water in thousands of schools is no longer fit to drink. Many schools do not offer free water. New York City schools are asking parents to raise money (about $1,000 per school) to install Water Jets, similar to soda dispensers, in the cafeterias. I've seen schools with water filtration systems connected between a tap and a large dispensing tank in the cafeteria. Pure water is an essential nutrient for our kids. In California, 40 percent of the schools have no water in the cafeteria. Legislation recently passed in that state requires all schools to provide clean drinking water in their dining areas, and new federal legislation that goes into effect for school year 2012–2013 requires all schools to provide access to drinking water during the lunch period.

Special Diets

Our children's developing brains and immune systems are normally quite resilient and most kids' bodies will manage to eliminate some amount of toxins without any sign of stress. In an environment that's laden with toxins, some children will react to excess toxins and stress more readily than others. Kids come in all shapes and sizes, from different ethnic backgrounds, with different activity levels, sensitivities, allergies, and tastes. Though the practice of dietetics seeks to make nutrition uniform and quantifiable, there really is no one-size-fits-all diet. The incidence of food allergies among schoolchildren—some life threatening—is on the rise. The Unquowa School, a private day school, has a certified nut-free kitchen that can accommodate children with special dietary needs. My daughter's elementary school has a nut-free table, and parents are provided with a list of nut-free snacks that are safe for the students at that table. Children with ADHD, autism, IBD, or Crohn's disease may be on a special diet free of grains, sugar, and food additives.

Does your school accommodate special needs diets or religious diets like kosher and halal? More kids are being brought up vegetarian or choosing to be vegan these days. Special diets are challenging to accommodate in a typical cafeteria filled with processed food. Schools that cook from scratch have more control over what's in the food because they use fewer ingredients. A trained chef can usually make an alternate version of a recipe that suits special needs by leaving out the meat or the grain.

How Are Most Schools Doing?

The preceding suggestions are all things to look for when judging the quality of the food in your school's cafeteria. The government uses a different set of standards, which are based on more traditional dietary notions of balancing the macronutrients—protein, fat, and carbohydrates—and limiting saturated fat and sodium. School dieticians are trained to analyze meal components in these terms, and they are required to design meals based on quantity, not quality. The USDA requirements for school meals state that the meals should comply with the most recent Dietary Guidelines for Americans that recommend "plenty of grain products, vegetables, and fruits; choose a diet moderate in sugars and salt; and choose a diet with 30 percent or less of calories from fat and less than 10 percent of calories from saturated fat. In addition, lunches must provide, on average over each school week, at least one-third of the daily Recommended Dietary Allowances for protein, iron, calcium, and vitamins A and C." Based on those standards, the USDA funds a periodic evaluation of the overall school nutrition program. Private research firms conduct these School Nutrition Dietary Assessments. The SNDA III, conducted in 2007 but never well publicized, concluded that the vast majority of schools in America exceed USDA guidelines for saturated fat, total fat, and sodium. By their own assessment, our government determined that American schools are flunking lunch.

The American Dietetics Association has recently released several reports on the impact school meals have on children's health. Among elementary school children, they reported, offering french fries, Tater Tots, and other potato products in school meals more than once per week and offering dessert more than once per week were each associated with a significantly higher likelihood of obesity.

Training and Tools

So who's planning the meals? Who's doing the cooking? Is the food coming preprocessed from far away, or does your school system have a trained culinary staff? What are the facilities and equipment like in your school? Some schools don't have kitchens at all, while others have underutilized facilities. Box cutters are the tools of choice for many kitchen workers. Their job is to heat and serve boxloads of frozen, precooked individual items, often in the same plastic wrap that they're shipped in. A stylish graphic poster listing all fifty-plus of its ingredients has immortalized one of these popular items, Hot Pockets.

Government grant money for new school kitchens and upgraded equipment was made available as part of the 2010 economic stimulus package. Schools that took advantage of these funds were able to install refrigeration, cooktops, ventilation, ovens, mixers, and other hardware necessary for scratch cooking. Larger school districts like New York City, Baltimore, and Washington, D.C., are all looking at moving toward a central kitchen, or commissary-style food service where the food is prepared in one or more centralized local facilities for same-day delivery to satellite school kitchens.

Food service directors complain that the School Nutrition Program is overregulated. We could be doing a better job with fewer regulations, they claim. They have a point. The website Oprah.com featured a series on school lunches around the world. In Finland, government regulations require meals to be "tasty, colorful, and well-balanced." According to the site, "Finnish regulations simply state that vegetables, cooked and raw, must cover half the plate (carrot and beet salads are popular), with proteins and starch taking up one-quarter plate each." Most schools in Finland offer a daily vegetarian option. A mandate like the Finns' would certainly make life less complicated for the lunch staff, and maybe free them up to spend more time cooking, less time calculating.

Talk to Your Food Service Director

Your school's food service director (aka director of nutrition services or food service manager) may be a registered dietician; he or she may have a background in nutrition, a culinary background, management, or food brokerage experience. You need to understand the role and responsibilities of your food service director and if possible make friends with this important person. He or she may be defensive when first approached, so make reassurances that you come in peace. Most food service directors see our children as their customers, and their job is to please those little customers. The prevailing model in school food service is choices, lots of choices. Switching to healthier, seasonal foods and scratch cooking necessitates limiting those choices, something most food service directors are loath to consider. John Turenne, former food service director at Yale University and now a private consultant, concurs. "I was a part of this. After twenty-five years in the food service business, we became our own worst enemy, and I'm talking about institutional food service. Over those years, as customers got more and more dissatisfied with the food, our knee-jerk reaction was to give 'em more choices, give 'em more options, add, add, add to the menu and the only way to do that without subsequently increasing labor was to buy more what we call value-added, heat-and-serve, readily prepared products."

Food service directors often complain they are stuck between a rock and a hard place. Their programs are underfunded, the kids complain about the food, and the parents and administrators generally look upon school food service as a necessary evil. Listen and learn about the challenges your food service director faces. He or she can help you understand the rules and regulations, and maybe suggest some ways that you can help improve the meal program in partnership.

Your school's kitchen must pass regular health inspections, which means one or more staffers must be certified in food safety and the school must have a Hazard Analysis Critical Control Point (HACCP) Food Safety Plan in place. The HACCP plan must address all stages of food production, from procurement and safe handling to proper processing, sanitation, and serving. Some school districts contract with unionized cafeteria workers. Some of these contracts don't permit workers to prepare food from raw ingredients. Ask your food service director if the staff has been trained in basic food prep skills, knife skills, and food safety. Ask her what she needs. A dad in my school district asked the middle school cook what she needed and was told that a spatula and a food processer would go a long way!

SARATOGA SPRINGS: MARGARET SULLIVAN

I first met Margaret in a panel at a screening of *Two Angry Moms* in New York City. Her comment was, "Parents never talk to me about what they want in my lunch program." She suggested that all the angry moms in the room talk to their schools' food service directors and ask what they can do to help get better food in schools.

Margaret's been in charge of the lunch program in Saratoga Springs, New York, for thirteen years. Over that time, she's been able to convince her board of education to support the lunch program. She now credits her board and the district superintendent with backing her up 100 percent. As a result, the district participates in a Farm to School program, and homemade entrées like vegetarian chili with bulgur, quinoa salad, and stir-fry with Asian veggies are now on the menu. "The district gave us $70,000 to improve the quality of the meals. Last year we took off those highly processed chicken products— the patties, nuggets, and the mozzarella sticks. These used to be our biggest-selling items. We lost so much money that we had to bring them back to the high school and middle school as an option every other week. I borrowed an idea from your film, a recipe for marinated chicken thighs. It's a delicious lunch and the adults love it but it's one of our lowest-number days. I am determined to keep it on the menu until the students like it. When sales drop I use that as an opportunity to go into class and meet with student nutrition councils."

(continued)

Margaret gets out of the kitchen and into the classroom to teach students about sustainable agriculture and to educate them about where their food comes from. She has interns from a local teacher's college come in to teach wellness and nutrition education in the cafeteria. The district also partners with the local agricultural cooperative extension. Several of the district's schools have vegetable gardens where kids grow produce that is used in the cafeteria. A winter farmers' market approached the superintendent to ask if they could rent space in the elementary school. Instead of paying a full rent for the location, the farmers donate produce to the school lunch program. Margaret incorporates the donations into her lunch menus. "I put kale and beans on the menu at the high school last week. The high school kids are more adventurous and willing to try new things. Those fresh greens on the salad bar are like a work of art, they're so beautiful."

She also speaks to PTAs and a superintendent's group and sits on panels at health conferences. "School lunch is so maligned for causing the problem with obesity. We don't have the ability to change the culture alone, but we do have a captive audience. People say, 'Nobody wants that healthy stuff you are peddling.' And I say, 'Check with me after you see your cardiologist.' Our culture is changing. I'm not going to give up. We have to stick with it." I asked Margaret if she serves chocolate milk to her students and she quickly replied, "I'd rather have them have chocolate milk than no milk. It's a long-range health issue, especially for girls, so it's not a battle that I choose to fight. The thing that needs to change is that students need to have a greater variety of whole foods prepared in healthier ways. If we can achieve those things, then we can go there with the milk."

It's slow but steady progress with the students, she tells me. As for the staff, she adds, "Going from convenience to scratch shakes up the whole system." Many of her staff had job descriptions that didn't allow them to handle raw food. Still, she says, "Job descriptions can be changed, and I'm lucky because I have some people who are really skilled and they are willing to do the work." Some much-needed confidence bolstering came when her program was covered in the *Wall Street Journal*. More recently a visit from a USDA undersecretary garnered a mention on *Good Morning America*. Margaret says the positive attention brought her staff together as a team and made them feel part of something good.

Margaret is pleased that the updated federal Child Nutrition Act reauthorization will require all schools to do what she is doing. "I'd like the USDA
to control all foods at school, not just the reimbursable meals. Fund-raisers,
vending—we need a level playing field so we're all giving the same message
at the same time. It would make our jobs a little easier."

It's challenging to get kids to participate in the program as the food gets
healthier, and Margaret's aim is to eliminate processed food entirely. How
will she bring in the diners? "More marketing, newsletters, get the parents
informed," she says. "And how great is it when parents call and say they are
happy that we're promoting beans!"

No Such Thing as a Free Lunch?

Your food service director can help you understand the economic constraints
of your district's school meal program. Most lunch programs are required by
the district to break even. That means food costs, staff, and other operating
expenses must all be covered by income from the lunch program. Ninety-
nine percent of public schools participate in the National School Lunch Program (NSLP). For each qualifying lunch they serve, the federal government
reimburses the school. For students eligible for free lunch, the school will be
reimbursed for the full meal at a rate of about $2.75. The school will receive
as little as 30 cents to subsidize a meal for a student who pays full fare.

Some states also provide a bit of additional reimbursement. For example, in my state, Connecticut, schools are encouraged to participate in the
Healthy Food Certification initiative with a ten-cent-per-meal incentive.
Unfortunately, many schools in more prosperous areas of the state have
opted out of the certification because it restricts the types of food that can be
sold in the cafeterias and vending machines. For most districts, even with
the reimbursements, after factoring in labor and other costs, schools have
less than $1 per student to spend on food for lunch. A board of education
that determines that school food is a priority for the district may also opt

to subsidize the meal program in some way, either by providing training, hiring a chef or wellness coordinator, or adding a stipend to the food costs. Most schools charge between $1.75 and $4 for a meal, and many food service directors have complained that they lose money on kids who pay full price. This can create a situation where the reimbursements for free meals are actually subsidizing the kids who pay for the meal! Schools with a very high proportion of students eligible for free lunch may offer universal free lunch and breakfast to all students in the school. This eliminates some of the complicated paperwork for your food service director.

I've met some very creative food service directors. They're finding ways to augment the food budget in order to provide better quality for their students. A friend recently told me about chef Paul Correnty, the food service director in her small Massachusetts town. Chef Paul's made-from-scratch soups were so popular with the students that he decided to offer them to patrons at the local farmers' market. Each week he brings a selection of seasonal soups to the market, using ingredients sourced from other market vendors. Proceeds from Chef Paul's stand benefit the town's school lunch program. Big city schools like New York City are also working with local vendors to procure quality products at bargain prices. At close to a million school meals a day, the city has a lot of purchasing power.

Ask your school food service director what her biggest challenges are and what parents can do to support her. Through our efforts as parents and advocates, we can help food service directors go from scapegoats to school food heroes like Chef Paul.

CHEF PAUL—TAKING RESPONSIBILITY

When all the stars are in alignment, fixing school food sounds almost easy. Well, not quite easy, says Chef Paul. "It's hard work. Restaurant work is hard work and that's what this is. I'm there at 4:30 a.m. because we've got kids coming at 6:30 a.m. for breakfast. Today for lunch we had fresh hake [a flaky white fish] with sautéed carrots, celery, onions, snow peas, and spinach topped with panko bread crumbs and baked with a little butter. The kids went nuts for it. My ladies made a fresh slaw and we had beautiful tangelos and mineolas. I only have a small refrigerator so I get deliveries three times a week. I spent my whole life in the restaurant business where you have to be innovative; you have to change. Schools don't encourage that. The system isn't set up for change. Teachers and administrators don't like change."

Although Paul is a hero in his hometown, he doesn't make the grade with the USDA. He proudly declares, "Every few years the USDA comes in and does an evaluation and I flunk it badly. If they can't count and measure then you don't meet the regulations. They ask for production records; I don't have them because we spend all our time cooking. They'd like to see canned pears all lined up in little plastic three-ounce cups. We serve family-style using real plates and cutlery and allow kids to take as much as they want. The system is designed to squash innovation and creativity."

With administrators resistant to change, and a system that doesn't value creativity, how did he manage to get the job? He tells me, "I started here twelve years ago with a superintendent who was an Armenian with family in the restaurant business. I knew nothing about the school food system, but I'm good out in front, I have a good personality, and I know how to cook, so he hired me. When I started the lunch program was losing money, and we were making $136,000 in sales. Now we're at $535,000 in sales. And we had $236 left over at the end of last year, which I'm very proud of, because all the money went into the food."

He's been able to get raises and Christmas bonuses for his staff of fifteen women, all of whom have benefits provided through the school system. And, he says, "They love coming to work. What you hear in the morning is rock-and-roll on the radio, people chatting, and the sound of knives chopping. The mentality really changed. Now they clip recipes and come in and test them out. We have fun. Not every dish is a success but that's how we learn and change."

Every day Chef Paul offers a vegetarian option, but he doesn't advertise it as such. That's part of his philosophy. "The vegan and vegetarian kids are

(continued)

comfortable—it's not just a cheese pizza—today it was a delicious ratatouille, and the meat eaters can have it on the side of their chicken breast filet [which is not a patty, but real chicken]. So we're educating them by offering them great choices. Every meal comes with soup, and all the vegetable sides and fruit sides they want."

His soups, now locally famous, grossed over $12,000 in seven Saturdays at the farmers' market. He tells me, "The kids helped me make it. I love soup—my mother was a great soup cook. We also do catering and all the profits go back to the lunch program. And now I get to cater weddings for kids I fed when they were little and I know I had a part in making those kids strong and healthy." Which is what it's all about for Chef Paul. "We see every kid every day. We have more responsibility than anybody else in the school system. The administration has to realize that we are as valuable as teachers and they have to realize what an opportunity they are missing. There are so many chefs in the restaurant business who get to be thirty or thirty-five and they miss their families because they're always working when the kids are home. And they'd love a steady job where you work during the week and are home with your family."

Paul's passion and creativity led to real transformation in his district. His bottom line, "Change is hard but if you're all on the same page you just do it. All it required was for people to care. Just hire a chef!"

The Commodity System

How do most schools serve lunch with only $1 for food? Depending on how you look at it, the commodity system is either a blessing or a curse. Commodities are foods that the government purchases from farmers and in turn donates to the National School Lunch Program. Commodity products are allocated to schools and comprise 15 to 20 percent of most schools' food sourcing. In addition to federal reimbursement dollars and based on previous year's reporting, food service directors are given a dollar amount with which they can purchase commodities each school year. States administer the distribution of the commodities, so schools must choose from a list of items offered by the state.

Primarily created to stabilize the American agricultural system and support farmers, the commodity system has evolved over the years into a free source of dubious quality, highly processed foods for schools. Some of the worst foods I've seen in schools are based on government commodities. Patties and crumbles filled with texturized vegetable protein and hydrolyzed soy protein fillers, stabilizing starches, color-enhancing sugars, and chemical flavor boosters are manipulated beyond recognition and offered along with processed cheese, beef and chicken nuggets, canned goods full of syrup, and preservatives and peanut butter blended with oil and sweetened with high fructose corn syrup.

School food experts say it doesn't have to be this way. Many of the basic commodity items begin their journey to the cafeteria relatively unadulterated. What's happened is that as fewer schools are capable of doing actual on-site cooking, the state distributors, on behalf of the schools, send the commodity items to large processors where they turn the commodities into the familiar popcorn chicken, Uncrustables, stuffed Pizza Rolls, French toast sticks, and Bacon and Cheese EggStravaganza. The processing of government commodity items for schools has been a boon to American food processors. Over 150 companies—Tyson, Land O'Lakes, Cargill, Schwan's, and so on—provide their branded products to the schools.

As the school food movement catches on, more food service directors are asking for unprocessed or less processed commodities. One challenge is that commodities need to be ordered a year in advance, so schools switching over to whole foods and scratch cooking are often stuck with an inventory of frozen dreck that they can't afford to discard. There's also a bonus commodity program that provides surplus items on a more casual basis. When I visited the St. Louis school system, they had just received a bumper crop of dried cherries—a gift that prompted local school chefs to bake some delicious breakfast muffins.

VERMONT: KATHY IRION

"I was a stay-at-home mom for twelve years. In 2005 Vermont passed some wellness policies aimed at curbing childhood obesity. I was the nutrition expert on our district's wellness committee, so they offered me the job." When Kathy Irion took on the job of food service director for the two schools in Arlington, Vermont, the schools were losing money on the lunch program and the kids were tossing most of the lunches, eating only the dessert. Her mission was to cook the way she would for her own kids and prepare as much from scratch as possible. She doesn't believe in offering unhealthy choices in the cafeteria. Kathy has managed to reduce food costs by using minimally processed government commodity items; she gets shredded cheeses, whole-grain or regular pasta, canned tomato sauce, unsweetened applesauce, roast turkey, and other meats from the USDA. Kathy turns down the junky processed foods and won't serve any foods that contain artificial colors, flavors, or preservatives. Every day there's a salad option and all meals are accompanied by a choice of several side options, including baby carrots, broccoli, celery, apples, grapes, melon, raisins, cucumber, dried cranberries, unsweetened applesauce, and tomatoes. Her produce is purchased locally whenever possible. A conversation with local restaurant owners led her to a small local distributor who advises her on the most economical offerings in season. Her menus are planned around seasonal items.

For six years Kathy has managed to break even on the lunch program. In addition to the federal reimbursement dollars she receives for students on the free or reduced price meal program, Kathy charges $2.50 for an elementary school lunch and $2.75 in the high school. Adults pay $3.25.

How does she get the kids to eat the new food? Simply by encouraging them to try it. She offers little tasting cups of each new item. When students give her the thumbs-up on an item, it gets added to the menu. So far, almost all of her recipes have met with approval. There's nothing too exotic on Kathy's menu; but Kathy's burgers, pasta with sauce, sandwiches, and salads aren't boring and the ingredients are much less toxic than what the kids were fed in the past.

Her lunchroom also models environmental awareness for the students.

Meals are served on washable melamine trays and the paper plates and utensils are compostable.

Despite the old kitchen and minimal staff (she has one assistant and two
part-timers) she inherited in Arlington, Kathy has managed to provide meals
cooked from scratch that are mostly free of dyes, flavorings, synthetic sweeteners, and preservatives. One exception is the chocolate milk—she's trying
to find a better version rather than attempting to wean her students off it
entirely.

À La Carte

It's a term borrowed from the French so it sounds like it should be good, and
many kids prefer the à la carte items to the USDA "Type A" complete lunch
menu. Also known as competitive foods, these items are sold in 90 percent
of U.S. schools as options alongside the subsidized school meal. Most school
districts rely heavily on the à la carte items to cover the school meals budget.
Competitive foods can be priced higher than the subsidized lunches. One
suburban middle school has a typical à la carte menu listed alongside the
main menu on its website. The à la carte items offered every day include
a cheeseburger for $3.50, curly fries for $3.00, a deli sandwich for $5.00,
chicken tenders for $3.50, a pizza pretzel for $2.25, and pizza for $2.50. That
surely is tough competition and it can create issues with stigmatization and
social justice.

Does your school have a separate line for à la carte and subsidized school
lunch? Some lunch directors may find the separate lines make it easier to
count the number of meals qualifying for reimbursement being sold. For
others, it's a response to regulations that prohibit à la carte items from being
sold in the same place as subsidized meals. The intent of such regulation is
to discourage à la carte and junk food, but some schools instead have created

a separate location for the à la carte goodies. While sorting meals by separating lunch lines this way may be a pragmatic response to various regulations, kids are going hungry rather than be seen in the subsidized lunch line. It's reported that as few as 35 percent of eligible high school students are utilizing the subsidized meal program, and even kids who pay might prefer the subsidized lunch, but they too don't want to be perceived as uncool.

Some school systems require students to purchase the subsidized lunch before they're allowed to buy any à la carte items. Other schools have instituted a system of debit cards so that no one knows who pays and who doesn't. The latest technology uses fingerprint biometrics in place of debit cards, which can get lost or stolen. In either instance, families with means are able to deposit funds on account for their kids. What I didn't know—and it wasn't much publicized in my district—is that these POS (point of sale) systems permit parents to restrict certain à la carte purchases. Score one for the "let the parents decide" movement. And good luck to the parents who use it!

Food service staff promote the sale of competitive à la carte food items in the belief that they will bring in extra revenue to make up for financial shortfalls. This practice not only undermines consumption of complete meals but, research shows, may actually result in overall loss of revenue through decreased reimbursement dollars from the federal government. Recent federal legislation requires competitive foods to meet the same USDA nutritional guidelines as the subsidized meals, but don't hold your breath waiting for schools to comply. Several consecutive USDA studies found that most schools didn't meet the federal nutritional requirements for the subsidized meals, so what are the odds that the competitive foods will be better?

A typical student will consume over 3,000 school meals between kindergarten and twelfth grade.

Vending

Vending machines operate in 88 percent of high schools, 52 percent of middle schools, and 16 percent of elementary schools, according to a University of Michigan study. Vending machines in schools offer a fast-food alternative to the lunchroom fare, or a quick snack between classes or after school. What's in your school's vending machines? I've seen everything from soggy frosted pastry, sugary granola bars with healthy-sounding names, and countless varieties of chips and candy bars to bananas, yogurt, and trail mix. The food in the vending machines is another form of competitive foods, and until recently was not regulated by the USDA. The Child Nutrition Act of 2010 calls for new nutrition standards that will be applied to all food sold in schools, including vending machines, by 2012. The new regulations will not ban vending machines from schools, contrary to some publicity on the subject. Representatives from the National Automatic Merchandising Association actually claim to welcome uniform national standards, which will establish limits on calories, fat, sugar, and sodium. My guess is that those standards won't address the long lists of unpronounceable items that will no doubt substitute for the forbidden ingredients.

Until federal standards go into effect, and depending upon your current state and local regulations, your school vending machines may be selling soda, sports drinks, vitamin-enhanced waters (check the ingredients!), fruit juices, or bottled water. The giants of the beverage industry pay dearly for the right to place their machines in your district's schools. So called "exclusive pouring contracts" between a school and Coke, Pepsi, or one of their competitors can supply the schools with tens of thousands of dollars, into the millions for a larger district. As an incentive, your school may be given a branded scoreboard, gymnasium, or playground. Typically, the contract provides the school with 25 percent of sales.

Supporters claim the kids will buy the vended items anyway, so the school might as well make a profit. Opponents not only object to the commercialization of school resources; they also believe that the contracts create a conflict of interest by providing schools with an incentive to jack up the price of vended items in order to make more revenue. Many school superintendents find these contracts too lucrative to pass up. The Rudd Center's Kelly Brownell says, "I believe that one of the greatest myths that's been perpetuated mainly by the soft drink industry is that they're helping schools financially. But in fact who's putting money into those vending machines? It's the children and the parents giving the kids the money, so in some ways it's almost like a tax on the community."

Professor Marion Nestle from NYU agrees. "If I were czar, I would take the vending machines out of the schools. I had a student who did a calculation of how much money the schools actually got and it amounted to about $20 a student." An extra $20 per student that could just go directly into the lunch program, suggests Dr. Brownell. "Why not just increase the tax a little bit, fund the schools better, so you're not hurting the kids in the process?"

Sharon Lauer, head of the Unquowa School in Fairfield, Connecticut, puts it this way: "There's this notion that at lunchtime our children turn from being students into customers or patrons. With tight budgets and government regulations, administrators are tempted to make bad decisions because they see the children as a revenue stream. And it's shameful."

Studying Junk Food in Schools

As a filmmaker with a point of view, I've been careful to back up my claims with research. Research can sometimes refute beliefs long held to be true, and is also the basis for amazing scientific discoveries. Americans in particular seem to be easily swayed by research, especially when it comes to diet and nutrition. I have friends who send me articles on the latest discoveries about antioxidants, vitamin D, acai berries, and blue-green algae, always filled with studies and usually touting a new product. Another friend, a Fulbright scholar and a researcher himself, once explained to me that in sociology there are two types of studies. One type he called the "Duh" study—a report that proves something obvious. The other he called the "Huh" study—one that reveals something that is so arcane, contradictory, or inconsequential that you simply lift your eyebrows and say, "Huh, how about that?"

Several new studies specifically examining consumption of competitive foods in school fall into what I would consider to be the "Duh" category. The 2010 University of Michigan Medical School study that looked at foods sold in vending machines, school stores, snack bars, and other related sales that compete with USDA lunch program offerings finds that "Schoolchildren who consume foods purchased in vending machines are more likely to develop poor diet quality—and that may be associated with being overweight, obese, or at risk for chronic health problems such as diabetes and coronary artery disease. Usage was highest in high school, where competitive food and beverage consumers had significantly higher sugar intakes and lower dietary fiber, vitamin B levels and iron intakes than nonconsumers." An American Dietetics Association study informs us that, "among middle school children, the availability of low-nutrient, energy-dense foods in vending machines in or near the food service area was associated with a higher BMI (Body Mass Index—fat) score." Here's one from Lincoln, Nebraska: "Schools that ban all junk food from their lunch lines can reduce student obesity by 18 percent."

My nutrition education also taught me that when it comes to food studies, for every new finding, you could find a study that proves its opposite. In February 2009, the RAND Corporation published a study titled, "Junk Food in Schools and Childhood Obesity. Much Ado About Nothing?" This one gets a "Huh." The study, funded by the Robert Wood Johnson Foundation, reports, "There is a growing belief among policymakers and the general public that competitive foods in schools are a significant contributor to the childhood obesity epidemic. Numerous policy initiatives are underway at the local, state, and federal level to regulate the availability of competitive foods in schools. However, the existing empirical evidence motivating these efforts is limited. . . . We find that competitive food availability generates in-school purchases of junk foods, but contrary to common concerns, there is no significant effect on children's BMI. Nor do we observe significant changes in overall consumption of healthy and unhealthy foods, or in physical activity.

Finally, our results find no support for broader effects of junk foods in school on social/behavioral and academic outcomes."

One may draw several conclusions from the RAND study. The results seem to imply that junk food in schools has no impact. What I think they're really saying is that whether a child obtains his or her junk food from school, home, or elsewhere has no impact on BMI, academic or behavioral outcomes, because every child in the study is consuming junk food. And indeed, the report goes on to state, "The *total* amount of soda and fast food, consumed in- and out-of-school, is not significantly influenced by competitive food availability, which is consistent with substitution between in-school and out-of-school consumption." There's that argument that the kids are going to get it anyway. The authors of the study might have suggested a comparison of the effects of offering healthy food in school with those of the junk food. Oops, that's already been done. Haven't we've studied this enough? What about replacing the junk in the vending machines with better choices?

That's what several socially engaged entrepreneurs have begun to do.

YoNaturals, Stonyfield Farms, and h.u.m.a.n. Healthy Vending are now competing with Coke and Pepsi for your students' pocket change. These vendors offer some 100 percent organic options and "no added sugar" options. Most of their products are free of unpronounceable ingredients and schools are reporting that while some students complain about the change at first, they quickly adapt. H.u.m.a.n. is also paying attention to affordability. In the Miami school system, the snacks in their vending machines all sell for $1.

The financial impact has been monitored in districts that have made these types of changes. North Community High School in Minneapolis stocked vending machines with 100 percent fruit and vegetable juices and water. They priced the healthier beverages slightly less than the standard fare and found that sales of these items were strong and reported no loss in total vending revenues.

Vista Unified School District in California generated $200,000 more in sales than it had in the previous year by filling vending machines with yogurt and granola, fruit, cheese and crackers, bottled water, 100 percent juice, milk, and smoothies.

It's Not Just About the Food

We've looked at the *food* in the cafeteria, but what about the cafeteria itself? What's the food *culture* like at your school? What's the noise level when it's full of kids? A noisy environment can be a huge distraction for a child, and may be as much of a reason for your child not to eat as her opinion of the food. Is it reasonably comfortable? Do the kids have a place to sit and enough room at a table? What's the seating arrangement like? Do children get to choose whom they want to sit with? Are there cliques and loser/loner tables? Do teachers eat in the cafeteria? Are parents helping out as volunteers? How much time do the children have to purchase a lunch and eat it? Is recess before or after lunch?

When my younger daughter was in middle school, the district instituted a wellness policy that required students to have fifteen minutes of recess after lunch. My daughter complained that this meant they had just fifteen minutes for lunch. Even though she brought her lunch to school and didn't have to wait in line for a school meal, this just wasn't enough time for her to eat. For the first month of school, she and a group of other slow eaters were kicked out of the cafeteria each day with mouths still full of food, forced to abandon the uneaten part of their meals. Finally she and the other students took matters into their own hands. They went to see the principal, and after some back-and-forth debate were eventually allowed to finish eating before heading out for recess.

CONNECTICUT: THE UNQUOWA SCHOOL

At the Unquowa School in Fairfield, Connecticut, chef Peter Gorman and his apprentice chef (a recent graduate of the Italian Culinary Institute) prepare about 250 lunches a day for students and staff. Ingredients for the meals are all sourced from local farms, and Peter has recently started baking his own whole-grain breads with fresh ground spelt, barley, kamut, and amaranth

(continued)

flours. Students and teachers sit together at round tables, family-style. The seats are assigned and each group of ten or so has students of mixed ages. Since most families no longer have time to eat daily meals together, the school becomes the students' family—and you can't choose your family. Theirs is a small, close-knit community. Several years ago, at a conference for independent schools, the head of school, Sharon Lauer, attended a workshop on sustainability for schools. The workshop really resonated for Sharon, and she immediately began implementing many of its teachings. School gardens supplement the local produce and students learn to grow, harvest, and prepare their own food. They also help serve and clean up in the cafeteria. Early on, the individual, conventional eight-ounce milk cartons were jettisoned in favor of half-gallon cartons of certified organic milk. "We wanted to move to better products, less waste, without the backing of funds, and as much as we could using regional and seasonal products in our dining room," Sharon explains. "Not just because we didn't have additional funds, but because I really feel strongly that I want this program to be repeatable. The milk that we're using now costs twice as much as the milk we were using before. There have been lots of studies showing that hormones in milk are really not great for kids. And actually, we're spending less on milk now because before kids had milk cartons and you couldn't see inside it. A child might drink half of it and throw the rest away. Now we use half gallons and they're poured at the table in a glass. And so, because they're at the table every day with a faculty member, the teacher knows if today a child takes a full glass and doesn't drink the whole thing, they might say, 'Y'know, you might want to take a little less tomorrow.' So we've actually been tracking right on target."

Better by Design

There's been a flurry of articles lately about design and placement of healthy foods in the school cafeteria. When I filmed at our high school, there were attractive barrels of Welch's Fruit Snacks, Pop-Tarts and other sweets right where the students were waiting in line to pay. This is a standard marketing ploy akin to putting the gum and candy at children's eye level in the check-out line at the grocery store. A study out of Cornell University shows that when food service directors began spotlighting healthy choices by placing fresh fruit in attractive baskets at convenient locations, students passed up the junk and grabbed the fruit. Hiding the chocolate milk behind the plain milk produced similar results, as did putting salad bars next to the checkout registers. One school in upstate New York implemented this design change and increased salad sales by 300 percent! Some schools are now requiring students to purchase cookies with cash and they're reporting that kids are passing up the cookies and putting more fruit on their debit accounts. These marketing and design techniques are proving to be more effective than banning items outright. The changes cost next to nothing, and they have no impact on overall sales and participation in the lunch program. The USDA has recently commissioned a $2 million study to find more ways to use psychology and marketing techniques to improve kids' choices in the lunch line.

Absent

If you're child has been in school for more than a couple of months, you've probably noticed how quickly a stomach bug, strep throat, cold, or flu spreads through the school. I never took notice of the absence of hygiene in the lunchroom until, on a tour of an elementary school in Berkeley, California, my guide pointed out a line of kids entering the cafeteria. On the way into the dining area, each child paused at a little fountain to wash his hands. Witnessing this simple act was an epiphany for me. Back home I asked my children, "Have you ever been instructed to wash your hands before going to the cafeteria?" "No, we wouldn't have time to all do that and eat our lunch" was the response. Every doctor's office and health clinic, and many public schools have large posters emphasizing the importance of hand washing in

preventing contagious diseases. As parents, it's one of the basic rules we reinforce at home. Yet it seems that most schools can't afford the time to require
their students to perform this simple act of hygiene before a meal.

Children who are not getting adequate nutrients have lower test scores; even
transient hunger from missing a meal affects performance. The hidden cost
of hungry children includes extra staff time needed for students with low
academic performance or behavior problems caused by poor nutrition and
physical inactivity, as well as costs associated with time and staff necessary
to administer medications needed by students with associated health problems. In states that use attendance to help determine state funding, a single-
day absence by just one student can cost a school district anywhere from $9 to
$20. If each child misses just one day per month, this could cost a large school
district like New York about $28 million each year, while Chicago would for-
feit about $9 million each year in state funds. This type of absentee rate is
highly probable, and could cost an average-size school district from $95,000 to
$160,000 annually in important state aid.

The School Food Environment

Your school's food environment extends beyond the cafeteria. What types of
foods are offered or sold at athletic practices and events, school play rehears-
als, and music performances? Does your high school have an open campus
near fast-food outlets? Are the school's fund-raisers always candy and bake
sales? Would the PTO or PTA be willing to try one of the many alternative
fund-raisers?

Talk to your principal and find out his or her food principles. School food
may not be on their radar, but you might get them thinking.

GEORGIA: YVONNE SANDERS-BUTLER

Dr. Yvonne Sanders-Butler is an elementary school principal in rural Georgia. After suffering a near-stroke in her thirties, Dr. Butler cleaned up her own diet and returned to her district determined to put into practice all that she had learned about prevention. Not knowing that "it couldn't be done," she simply refused to allow the soda truck drivers to make their deliveries, insisting instead upon nothing but bottled water for the school's vending machines. Now her school is a sugar-free environment. She's banned high-fat, processed foods from the cafeteria. Several years of tracking have demonstrated dramatic improvements in students' test scores, behavior, and attendance. Standardized test scores went up 25 percent, discipline reports dropped by 25 percent, counseling referrals declined by 23 percent, and there was a 60 percent reduction in visits to the nurse's office. Dr. Sanders-Butler wrote a book on nutrition for families and now consults with other schools districts ready for change.

Check out the teacher's lounge. This inner sanctum may be the place where teachers hide foods that would be contraband in the cafeteria. Teacher's union rules prohibit regulating which foods are offered or sold in the teachers' lounge, but you might want to ask teachers to think about what kind of message they're sending when the kids get a peek at that big box of Dunkin' Donuts on the counter every morning.

What messages are students learning about food in the classroom? Do teachers receive any development training around teaching media literacy or how to incorporate food education in their lessons? How are classroom birthdays and celebrations handled? Are food rewards being used? Are branded candies and junk food incorporated into textbook word problems?

What happens on field trips? When I chaperoned my daughter's eighth-grade field trip from Connecticut to Washington, D.C., I was posted to the back of the bus, where, as expected, the unruly kids chose to sit. The bus pulled out of the school's driveway at 6 a.m. Bleary-eyed, the kids pulled bags of Doritos and Skittles out of their backpacks and breakfast commenced. What didn't end up on the floor of the bus was quickly consumed. Before long the kids started goofing around, laughing loudly. Soon the clamor turned into an argument, with kids jumping out of their seats and yelling at one another. The teachers repeatedly asked them to settle down but the requests were ignored. After several hours, I pulled an apple out of my bag. One of my agitated seatmates eyed it hungrily. I had brought along a big bag of apples just in case, and soon all of my neighbors were excitedly asking me to share them. When we finally got to the Baltimore rest area where the kids were released for lunch at the food court, the teachers apologized to me for the students' behavior. I asked them what the food policy was for the field trip. Were the students supposed to bring a bag breakfast? (My daughter had one.) The teachers, frustrated, explained that there was no food policy for field trips and the kids always brought all kinds of junk food for the bus.

Is Your School Food Green?

Does your school focus on sustainability? Are there school gardens, after-school cooking classes, and field trips to farms? What gets recycled? How is cafeteria waste managed? Annie Leonard, author of *The Story of Stuff*, suggests finding out what the school district is paying for waste disposal. She says, "Increasingly there are solutions out there that cost less money and are good for the health of the planet, good for the health of the kids, and good for the school's bottom line, so that makes it a lot easier." She advises researching some of these options and presenting them to the school. Certainly presenting your district with a plan to save money is a good way to start greening the school's food system.

Audit It

By now you've realized that your casual visit to the cafeteria could turn into a more in-depth investigation. In fact, the information you are gathering can be compiled into a school food audit. The word itself strikes fear in most tax-paying adults, so it's not surprising that many school boards express reluctance to perform a school food audit, but the results can benefit the lunch program and the district's bottom line. You and your wellness group (see chapter two) can do a school food audit, or a school sustainability audit yourselves, or there are professionals your district you can hire to perform a formal audit for you. These consultants can make recommendations based on the needs and wants of your school system. They'll come in and assess your resources and requirements. Does the school system have proper facilities to cook real food? Is there a central kitchen where meals could be prepared in bulk for efficiency? Is there adequate cold storage space for fresh ingredients? Is there a computerized system for ordering provisions, calculating recipes and nutrition requirements, monitoring food safety, reporting meal counts, and tracking supplies? If infrastructure is found lacking, there are federal, state, and local grant funds periodically available to fund capital expenses for school food service upgrades.

When I was filming, I spent a day following consultant Kate Adamick around the kitchens of several schools in Katonah-Lewisboro, New York. Her company, Food Systems Solutions, takes a clear-eyed look at what she calls the "simulated food" found in most school cafeterias, and offers a workable plan to replace the rubbish with real food. She identified lurid pink Trix yogurt with a curt, "Food doesn't come in that color, you know that!" and concluded her visit by telling the food service director, "The job at the local schools is to start demanding products that are not going to essentially poison our kids." As a parent advocate, you need to maintain a level of diplomacy with the school, which is a good reason to advocate for an independent audit. In Katonah-Lewisboro, Kate's take-no-prisoners approach led to major changes over the course of a single school year. It takes a strong stomach, and sometimes even stronger words, to expose the reality of school food, but when parents, administrators, and community leaders are all on the same page, changes get made.

WASHINGTON, D.C. — EXPOSED

Here's a case study that illustrates the adage "timing is everything." It also showcases one very talented writer, Ed Bruske. A reporter for *The Washington Post* in a previous life, Ed now tends his urban farm, teaches after-school food appreciation classes, and blogs. What got him started? "We were inspired by 9/11," Ed responds. "Like a lot of people, we took stock and decided we wanted Sunday suppers, more time with family and friends. My wife is a catering chef and we are both inspired by good food. I looked out at the yard one day and thought, Why don't we start growing our own? Over the course of a few years, I dug up our front yard and started turning it into a vegetable garden. I took a master gardening class and someone said I should write a blog," which led to the birth of his first blog, *The Slow Cook*. Ed's urban garden sits on a corner lot in Washington, D.C., about a mile from the White House. His project got a lot of attention. The D.C. Farm to School folks learned about Ed and asked him to sit on their advisory board. "Prior to that I had no interest in school food and had no idea what my daughter was eating in school," he says. "I paid no attention."

The food service in almost all of the D.C. schools was outsourced to Chartwells, a global giant in the world of food service management. "One of the Chartwells nutritionists was on the committee. She told me they were switching over to fresh cooked. We had just enrolled our daughter in a newly renovated local school. In a meeting at the school, to talk about installing a school garden, the vice principal bragged about their new kitchen." Ed asked if he could spend a week there to get an inside look at the switch to fresh cooking. The principal gave his consent and Ed showed up on a Monday with his notebook, ready to see the lunch ladies cook from scratch. "That's when I saw the baked ziti made with the infamous bag of frozen beef crumbles. That's when

I realized this was a very different story and actually more interesting than what I thought." The beef crumbles proved to be the tip of the iceberg for Ed's week of careful observations. Scrambled eggs came from a Minnesota factory and were shipped in plastic bags with a long ingredient list that included some decidedly un-eggy substances. Ed's exposé went viral via the Internet. He was asked to post on the online environmental news service Grist. He did an op-ed piece in *The Washington Post*. A couple of months later, he spent a week observing the in-house, self-operated sustainable school food service in Berkeley, California, after which he wrote a series that described a sharp contrast with the D.C. school kitchen. Through his blogging, Ed linked up with other groups in D.C. that were working to improve the food environment citywide. Parents United for Better D.C. School Food formed as an umbrella group, and the *Better D.C. School Food* blog became Ed's next media venture.

One of his early blogs for *Better D.C. School Food* was about a proposal for strong school food guidelines proposed by D.C. Councilmember Mary Cheh—the Healthy Schools Act. The school district had a new food service director in place, Jeff Mills, who also wanted to implement school gardens and scratch cooking. A result of strong leadership emboldened by a good dose of investigative reporting, the landmark Healthy Schools Act legislation, perhaps the strongest in the country, passed in May 2010. The act provides supplemental funding for the district's school food, and requires that all food offered in D.C.'s schools meets the new USDA Healthier Gold Level Standards.

By the autumn of 2010, Ed reported that the school food in the District of Columbia was not perfect, but vastly improved. Chartwells had gotten rid of a lot of the worst junk. Ed's daughter had transferred to a new elementary school and Ed says, "I'm there every day for breakfast and lunch. The approach is a lot more thoughtful than it was before. They've done an item-by-item overhaul." He says the Apple Jacks, chocolate Mini-Wheats, PopTarts, and Golden Grahams are gone. There's no more flavored milk. Instead, for breakfast there's cottage cheese, French toast from scratch, a scrambled egg pocket, pancakes with blueberries, and yogurt. "It's harder for me to get all of the ingredients. I was getting them mainly by dumpster diving for packaging. Under the city

(continued)

council Healthy Schools Act, they are supposed to publish all the ingredients for all of the foods." The management company expects to launch an interactive website with ingredients lists very soon. Ed explains that along with the legislation, the city added a five-cent per meal incentive for purchasing locally sourced fresh ingredients. He says you can see that incentive working "around the edges of the plate. There's local fruit, cucumber, and zucchini. The staff had quite a bit of training over the summer. They're learning to use steamers, convection ovens, and cook more things from scratch, like lasagna."

Most of the schools in D.C. are still outsourced to Chartwells. However, a couple of pilot projects have also taken root. Seven of the city's public schools now serve meals catered by a nonprofit organization, D.C. Central Kitchen. They are using a commissary model where the food is prepared off-site and distributed to the schools daily. Ed says, "They are part of a catering operation called Fresh Start. The labor force is all ex-offenders. They developed a local produce distribution system way ahead of everybody else and they're cooking from scratch."

Seven other schools are in a pilot project being managed by the California-based social enterprise, Revolution Foods. The founders, a pair of U.C.–Berkeley business school grads named Kristin Richmond and Kirsten Tobey, have created a mission for the company to provide sustainably sourced foods, and to operate in a manner that is safe for the environment and ensures workers have fair wages and health benefits. The contract with Revolution Foods calls for them to operate within a break-even budget, a feat that had so far been impossible for Chartwells to pull off in the district.

Ed says that Parents United for Better D.C. School Food plans to have regular meetings with their food service director. The organization includes parents, chefs, the local Farm to School people, local food bank and food access advocates. At this point, the schools aren't cooking from raw meat products and they don't have a central kitchen. He says the "center of the plate" is still mostly a highly processed protein. His group plans to perform an evaluation to see what the possibilities are for building their own processing facility where raw products can be turned into healthier recipes. "What's the solution? That just keeps me up at night. It's easier to get the junk out than to make these other sweeping changes. We're still a tiny fraction of the population that cares deeply about all these food issues," Ed reminds me. "I'm still trying to sort it out and I'm as confused as everybody as to what the actual solution is. Schools have to at least not be part of the problem. Food service directors have to get the idea out of their head that we have to give kids what they want. We're selling them a lifetime of health problems. Every journey starts with a step."

Ed's story illustrates the power of the pen (or should I say keyboard?). From the superintendent, to the food service director, to the city council, his community responded. They got connected and the changes started to happen.

STEPS FOR VISITING THE SCHOOL CAFETERIA

- Make sure you are signed in at the front office. Bring a photo ID.
- Ask for ingredients lists. Read labels.
- Take pictures of the food and the food labels.
- Take note of food waste and other garbage.
- Report your findings to friends in a blog or news article.

TWO

GET CONNECTED

In order to make change you have to make change.

—Bruce Gluck, Food Service Director

A September 2010 study by Russell Research, a national research firm, found that while 45 percent of children buy lunch at school at least some days, 75 percent of parents think that the food offered at school is not very nutritious. Those numbers interest me for several reasons. Seventy-five percent demonstrates that there are a lot of parents who are aware of the need to improve school food. It also suggests that there are many parents who choose to have their children buy lunch even if they believe it's not healthy. And perhaps many more parents would send in lunch money (or these days put money on account) if they believed the food was nutritious. In marketing parlance, that's a lot of low-hanging fruit. What would it take to get those parents to become advocates for their kids? Maybe they just need to get connected.

Out of the Closet

Van Jones, author, activist, and former special adviser to the White House Council on Environmental Quality, told me, "Everybody has to come to that place in themselves where their own fear or shame about standing out is less important than the damage we're doing to our children. If you think about a mother lion, you know she's a pretty peaceful cat most of the time but when somebody is threatening the cubs, that's a different thing. And what's happening right now is if somebody ran into a school with a gun we would react very aggressively to try to figure out what we're going to do. The kind of food that we're giving our children is going to wind up killing more children than any gunman this year. We're setting our kids up for diabetes, for lifelong obesity; we're putting toxins in the food that goes into their bodies. That's an emergency. And in an emergency you have to respond."

One of the first and most important things you can do to get a local movement started is to speak out. I spent many years passively observing fast-food culture, without ever considering just getting out there and talking about it. When my kids were little, they'd have friends come over for playdates that often included a meal. Whether we were having stir-fried rice and veggies, or lamb chops with beans, I was often met with "No, thanks, I'm not hungry, do you have any soda?" I soon learned to keep chicken nuggets and bagels in the freezer, as these were the mainstays of my daughters' friends. Every now and then I would attempt to entice them with a carrot freshly pulled from my garden, but these kids were mostly set in their ways and the thanks I got from one dad was the title of "granolahead." By the time the kids were in middle school, the overheard carpool conversations often turned to a discussion of which medications each child was taking. "Oh, you're on Prozac too?!" is not a line of dialog from a cheeky Hollywood movie, it's an actual sound bite from the back seat of my minivan. So I began speaking up at home, preaching to my kids and their friends (eyes rolling) about the benefits of eating real food. By high school, both of my daughters had several friends who struggled with physical, emotional, and behavioral disorders that required hospitalization. Finally my younger daughter said to me, "So does this mean *we're* the normal ones?"

Could I have changed the outcomes of my kids' friends' health issues if I'd spoken up sooner? Probably not, but those kids helped me see my own struggles in a different light. Maybe if these kids had been exposed to a greater variety of fresh foods, maybe if they weren't offered junk food as often, maybe if there had been a bit more emphasis on developing their taste buds, maybe they would have been stronger and more resistant to the challenges of adolescence.

Our food ways had made my children feel different growing up, but my daughter's epiphany led to one of my own. Why should my family's healthy eating habits be considered marginal? Shouldn't our food be the mainstream "normal" cuisine, and junk food the weird stuff? In France, where my husband's family lives, mainstream culture revolves around real, whole food. As an American visiting there, I had been surprised by a culture in which the regular people, everyday middle-class families, shopped at farmers' markets, and prepared affordable meals from scratch. I thought it was quaint, and figured they would be thrilled when a giant Carrefour grocery store opened nearby. Although the village farmers' markets weren't necessarily cheaper than the new supermarket, the convenience foods and frozen dinners the big market offered were met with bemusement by a culture that lives by the joy of cooking. (With one notable exception—Granny, the ninety-plus-year-old matriarch of the family, adored the frozen pizza I sneaked in for my kids one afternoon.) In French schools and home kitchens, children learn about growing, preparing, and tasting real food. They eat the same food as their brothers, sisters, and parents. They spend time at the dinner table in conversation. This simple daily mealtime ritual covers all the bases of Popular Parenting 101—nurturing, sharing, quality time, focusing attention on the family. My daughter and my French family made me realize that if we could actually change our American culture and get real food back onto family dinner tables and into the mainstream, we could go a long way to reversing the crisis in children's health. I had to speak up!

Since I started speaking up, I've met many successful activists who have shared some great advice with me. Here's what Alan Khazei, founder of Be the Change, and former CEO of City Year, a program of AmeriCorps, has to say: "As a mom you are powerful. It's Mothers Against Drunk Driving that found solutions to the drunk driving problem and led a revolution. Recognize you are a powerful person. It's not rocking the boat when you're advocating for your children and other people's children. They can't advocate for themselves; they are too young. They're not eighteen, they can't change who is making the policy, so if you feel a little shy or a little intimidated, think about your kids and what they need, or think about other people's kids and what they need. Find another mom or two that you're friends with and say, 'Ya know, I've been concerned about the food in the lunchroom—What do you think?' They're concerned, too. You are needed. We can't afford for anybody to sit on the sidelines. If we don't rock the boat, then the boat's going to sink. Get out there and you will make a difference."

When you speak out, you find other people who share your passion. Maybe they've been afraid to speak up as well, or maybe you hadn't known they were out there talking about this. I found a community in my town that I had never known and they took on school food the way parents in the school district had taken on topics like school expansion, bullying, and ball fields.

Face Your Fear

Are you a skilled public speaker? I was not! Before taking on the mission of "angry moms," I was strictly a behind-the-scenes person. My knees would tremble and my palms would sweat when I attempted to ask a question at a school meeting. When my husband insisted that I step out in front of the camera as a way to demonstrate my commitment to this cause, my first thought was, They're not going to like me . . . it's going to be like the scene from *Carrie* at the prom. . . .

By speaking up, you are entering the fray and taking a side. When I finally did speak up, in some ways my worst fears came true. I started by writing an article about school food for a local magazine, which led to an invitation to speak at a PTO meeting. When I asked the PTO leaders for permission to film my presentation I subsequently received an un-invitation. I felt like a social pariah, having finally outed myself as a counterculture whole-food eater, and being rewarded with a smack-down. Then I was invited to speak at a district wellness committee meeting. I arrived with a basket of organically grown apples and pages of handouts. One of the items I shared was a list of ingredients for the Tater Tots served in the school cafeteria. I had Googled one of the unpronounceable ingredients and printed out the page

decorated with skull and crossbones that said "Danger—harmful if swal-
lowed." My audience did not appreciate that particular irony. Later I was
informed that I could attend subsequent meetings, but those not on the committee (me) were forbidden to speak at the meetings.

Fortunately, I had been warned to expect resistance to my presentation
at the wellness committee. The rebuff still stung. Since that time I have
received scores of letters from moms who have just seen *Two Angry Moms*,
and they usually read something like this: "I am soooooo excited to take on
this cause in my son's school!!! I am going to show your movie to our school
superintendent!!! I can't wait to get the ball rolling here in Kalamazoo!!! Do
you have any advice for me?"

Or this: "I am so upset. I sent my daughter off to kindergarten with a
lovely packed lunch and she came home with candy and Pop-Tart wrappers
in her backpack. I didn't expect the school would allow junk food in kindergarten. I really want to share my ideas about how we can clean up the school
food environment in my daughter's school here in Little Rock. I have never
done anything like this before and I don't want to make any enemies. I am
afraid that if the school administration doesn't like my suggestions they will
take it out on my child. How can I get started without offending anyone?"

I'm always encouraging in my response, but the encouragement is tinged
with a bit of caution. Like these moms, I thought if I just went to the school
administration, explained what a disservice we are doing to our kids, what a
missed opportunity school food is, and offered my vast knowledge of how to
make it right, they'd be so enlightened and eager to let me work my magic.
Since that time, I've spoken with many moms who thought the same thing.
So now, my first advice to everyone is to host a screening of *Two Angry Moms*,
or coordinate a film series, book club, or speaker series on the topic for your
local library. There are several new books and movies that also tackle the
subject of school food and each adds another angle to the conversation (see
the resources section in the back of this book). You can educate your community about the issue. Invite parents, students, school administrators, local
business leaders, farmers, and health practitioners to come to your event.
Once your neighbors have more information, they may want to join with

you to advocate for your cause. Hosting a screening is not as intimidating as it may sound, and we have gathered all the resources you need in our screening planner on the website (www.angrymoms.org). Usually a movie showing, especially if it's free, will draw a crowd. Advertise free healthy snacks or a light dinner—food is a great enticement. Get some local teens to offer free babysitting. Be sure to have a sign-in sheet at your event. Ask people for their e-mail addresses. This is the beginning of your local coalition.

Food Evangelism

There's no energy greater than that of a mom with a cause. As parents, we should all have high expectations when it comes to our children's well-being. The world is filled with thrills and dangers for our kids; what fills one parent with fear may seem warm and fuzzy to another. I let my daughters take the commuter train into New York City when they were fourteen. Several of their friends' parents were horrified, others were happy to send their kids along for the adventure. Food is even more personal. What I consider inedible may be the mainstay of my neighbor's pantry. We cling to our food fears and preferences the way we cling to religion. Most humans seem to be hardwired to form their food and religious beliefs early on and then stick with them unless or until they experience some kind of epiphany. Sometimes I do feel like a food evangelist, passionately trying to convince school systems to confess their sins, change their ways, and see the light, hallelujah! Being an advocate for better food in schools requires the passion, zeal, and tenacity of an evangelist but not necessarily the dogma. The sin and salvation metaphor rings true up to a point. Our kids are on track to being the least healthy generation of Americans, and a sustainable school food system could save them from that doom. Where I think we, as advocates, need to tread carefully is in imposing dogmatic food rules that smack of extremism or fundamentalism. Most important, when you speak out, seek common ground. Are you a vegan? Then by all means, focus all your efforts on getting more plant-based foods into the cafeteria. Lobby for a Meatless Monday menu. Got kids with food allergies? Surely your platform will include a call for disclosure of all the ingredients for meals, snacks, and vending items. Concerned about sugar and artificial sweeteners? You'll want to point out all the foods that these substances are hiding in. Maybe you simply want to see the junk food kicked out of school. You'll no doubt have to dialog with kids and parents who will argue that a range of choices should be available. Any of these angles can drive a wedge in your community, or be the basis for a policy that makes your school system a proud model of reform.

I asked Dean Cycon, community development advocate and founder of Dean's Beans, what lessons he's learned from his years of advocacy work. Dean's a passionate guy and he shared his wisdom with me.

"I find that as I've gotten older and really started to think deeply about my own behavior—the difficulty of knowing when to engage and when to let go—sometimes I wonder if you are a terrier and you don't let go, are you necessarily providing that much of a service to your cause? Or are you sometimes actually inhibiting it because you're alienating people by your own intense energy, your passion? And this is a good parenting skill, too. I think that in my advocacy over the last thirty years there have been times when I was over-engaged and I felt like I had to control everything, because it wasn't going my way or it didn't feel like it was going in the right direction. And there were other times where in reaction to that I said—you know I've got to let go and let people do this and let whatever's going to happen, happen, and then been disappointed because either it didn't end up the way I wanted or simply didn't reach its potential, and I actually could have had more of an impact if I had stayed involved. There is a wonderful Hindu expression out of the Bhagavad Gita that our role here is to add our light to the sum of lights. So it's not necessarily what are the actions we do but it's how we show up as a person. I really believe that reasonable people can be reasoned with and unreasonable people can't be reasoned with but they also can't be bludgeoned. So I think the struggle for me has always been how far engaged to be and how far to let go, both as a parent and as an advocate. It's a deeply personal balance that you have to find."

Dean's words really ring true for me and serve as a good reminder for me to practice listening and letting go as passionately as I practice sharing information.

A Legacy of Reform

There's a century of social and political history chronicling do-gooders' efforts to integrate immigrants into American society by weaning them off their native diets. We may now know the antibacterial benefits of garlic, and the cleansing powers of cabbage, but in the 1920s, well-meaning food reformers insisted that these odiferous ingredients had no place in a healthy American diet. In fact, our current state of dietary confusion dates back to the time when a scientific rather than cultural approach to human nutrition was first advocated. The field of dietetics was dominated by women from its inception at the turn of the twentieth century. According to Susan Levine, author of *School Lunch Politics*, "Women rarely found opportunities to pursue research in chemistry or biology. Instead, women drawn to these disciplines often ended up in home economics." Levine explains, "The women who ran school lunch programs worked hard to instill their domain with professional standards and the latest scientific methods. Indeed, by the mid-1920s professionals claimed control over the majority of the nation's lunchrooms." Nutrition sciences became one of the earliest careers in which women could excel. These scientists pointed out that America's farmers understood quite well which combinations of nutrients allowed their animals to grow and thrive; common sense dictated we should be able to do the same for humans.

Much of the current school food debate hinges upon this scientific argument. Between the two World Wars, home economists and dieticians developed human nutrient standards. Those dietary standards were applied to the original National School Lunch Program in 1946, and they are still in place today (see chapter four). Nowadays the dieticians' scientific approach has become conventional wisdom but their dietary standards haven't kept up with the proliferation of junk food, nor do they take into account the many additives that act as "anti-nutrients" when they accumulate in our children's diets. Despite the many new food studies and the need for systemic change they imply, many food service and health professionals cling to the old science, reluctant to consider that conventional wisdom may need an upgrade.

Can you identify with the well-intentioned food reformers of the 1920s and 1930s? I sure can. They saw malnutrition in as many as 25 percent of American children and believed they had the science-based knowledge to solve the problem. What they struggled with was the large gap between knowledge and practice. Changing behaviors became the real challenge for them, just as it is for school food reformers today. Understand that your school community may need education and a bit of seduction more than evangelism. One of the best bits of advice I ever received was "Meet them where they are." Don't be dismayed if people don't get you right away. What you are sharing with them is new and contradictory information for many people and it may actually freak them out. *So take your time, consider all the options, and don't do it alone.*

Communicate

There are many ways to connect with your community around school food. You don't have to become a superhero or make a movie. Think about the communication tools that you are familiar with. Does your town have a local paper or online news bulletin? If so, consider writing a letter to the editor. Grab some of the facts about children's health that are in this book, and use them to express your concern about your school's food environment. Your letter doesn't have to be long or scholarly, in fact it's better to just write plainly and share your passion. Our town gets a lively forum going in the op-ed pages, and I've bonded with many a local letter writer on a variety of topics. Does your school have a newspaper or PTO or PTA bulletin? Usually they are eager for content and might be willing to publish a short article or editorial about school food. Be sure to publish your contact information so readers can find you.

Be creative in your communication. Try to find a new twist on the school food story. A good way to get your message across is to make it personal. Rather than writing an article or a letter about childhood obesity, write about a specific child you know or have heard about. Here's an attention-grabbing introduction. "George Mungai may look like your typical high-schooler, but he has quite a story to tell. In the last year he's lost 125 pounds. 'People I hadn't been in contact with didn't even know who I was,' Mungai said." This article goes on to tell how the student credits his school's lunch staff with helping him by creating a special healthy meal option that became popular with lots of other students as well. Readers will respond to your own personal story—does your child have diabetes or a food allergy? You can use a personal story to create awareness of a larger issue. Add some statistics about childhood obesity and type 2 diabetes after you've shared something intimate. The statistics become more powerful and underscore how many children share the same challenges as the child you've just portrayed.

Communication is a two-way street, so expect to get responses. I used to take the negative communication personally, but have learned to remind myself that, just like the State Department says, "It's important to establish a dialogue." Any communication, even if it's critical, is a step toward raising awareness. When our local food committee began discussing some changes, the vice president of the high school student council was not pleased. An articulate honors student, he took us to task. What follows is an excerpt from his editorial in our local paper.

"A coalition of mothers has launched a successful coup d'état against the student-acclaimed food program. Their decision to supplant the current food program is intended to benefit us, whose grades and health they believe are compromised because of the toxins that enter our bodies via cafeteria food. We would like to warn these zealous mothers that they don't know what they're dealing with. For better or for worse, the WHS students have become accustomed to the chocolate chip cookies, Pop-Tarts, SunChips, and frozen yogurt. We know that white flour isn't the healthiest choice for our bodies. Most of us don't care. In a world where access to illicit drugs is practically at our fingertips, can you really hope to make a difference in the amount of high fructose corn syrup we consume? If we want junk food, we'll find a way to get it. We're prepared to fight for what we want. We are not going to capitulate to a bunch of mothers who banded together one afternoon because it was something to do and because being organic is in vogue."

This young man raises some important issues. What might work in elementary school might not go over so well in high school. Our high school has an open campus and students have the option of purchasing lunch at a nearby deli. His letter underscores the importance of getting students involved in food education from an early age, addressing the food environment of the entire school, and working with the whole community when considering changes to the meal program. It also reinforces something I heard over and over again in my travels.

Focus on the Positive

I've heard it said in many ways. In New Hampshire, food service director Tony Geraci said, "For somebody to go into a typical school district and get rid of everything all at once, and say this is how it's gonna be, you're going to get more resentment than you are cooperation." John Turenne of Sustainable Food Systems says, "Seduce them with taste." School board members around the country say, "Come to us with a proposal." Pointing out the problem and complaining is not a bad way to raise an issue, but to go from being an armchair critic to becoming an advocate, you need a platform and a program that can satisfy the needs of all the constituents in your school community. Better to volunteer to do recipe samplings in the cafeteria, smoothie days, themed dinners with students and parents, bring in speakers, connect with local farmers, and lead tours of model school food programs in nearby districts. Act like a politician and win over your constituents. You'll need to tailor a strategy specific to your district. Do you have a school principal who really cares about school food? He or she might be a great partner for a presentation to the superintendent. Maybe your school board will agree to try out some changes in one school as a test site.

Due Diligence

Find out if there's already a movement or group of concerned parents in your area. Do a bit of research on the Web. Call the school and ask if there's a wellness or nutrition committee that already exists. If so, talk to some of the people on the committee. This research really is important. You need to learn the history of school food in your school. Have there been other parents who have attempted to make changes and failed? Has there been some progress over the years that you can capitalize on? If so, who are the leaders? Are there people on the school board, in the administration, teachers, parents of older students, or students themselves whom you should reach out to? Very often I hear that there's a school nurse, or an athletic director, or some other staff person who would love to work with parents on this issue. Perhaps these people have been in the school system longer than you and they may be able to give you some perspective.

Find Your Tribe

Whether you live in a small town, big city, or somewhere in between, you will find that the issue of school food is competing with a lot of other burning local issues. In most towns, it's not even on the radar. Letter writing and research may lead you to a handful of allies, but you can also find your tribe in some of the places and groups you frequent for other purposes. Our local Unitarian Church has a very active social action committee and an environmental committee. Both of these committees have sponsored school food-related events that have drawn good crowds. Make a short announcement after a yoga class, cooking class, or book club. Put a little sign on the bulletin board at your place of worship, your pediatrician's office, your gym, local YWCA, Boys and Girls Club, grocery or health food store. Here, too, it helps to get creative. Start your notice off with a question—"Have you had lunch in the school cafeteria lately?" or "Do your kids bring a packed lunch to school?" Dr. Susan Rubin, founder of Better School Food (and the other "angry mom" of the movie's title) says even parents of kids who bring lunch "might be very surprised to learn how a brown-bagging student can be impacted by the school food environment." Chat with the parents at your child's ballet class, ball games, and piano lessons. Gather phone numbers or e-mail addresses from everyone who expresses interest in your cause. Send out short notes to your mailing list when you have a bit of news. If you later decide to become a more formal group, these people will remember those conversations and might want to support you.

Don't overlook the folks who are serving meals at the school. They may be feeling targeted as the bad guys, even as they struggle to serve something decent without badly needed funding, equipment, and training. Many of them are parents and grandparents themselves; they will have concerns about school food that outsiders would never be aware of. A mom who took a job in the school cafeteria when her husband lost his business wrote one of the most touching letters I've ever received. She says, "I am very conflicted right now. No one seems to care. I am sure if the parents of these children knew what the kids were eating, they would be very upset. It is scary. I don't want to get my boss in trouble, and don't want to lose my job. I am sick to my stomach working there." This mom is desperate for support and ready to join forces as an insider.

Reach out to your school's athletic director. Sports nutrition is a great way to win support for a school food overhaul. When we filmed in Peterborough, New Hampshire, we learned that before tackling the whole school, the food service director there had started with the sports teams. Tony Geraci, who was later hired to run the school food service for the city of Baltimore, began by putting his local hockey and baseball teams on a sports nutrition program. In just one season, both teams went from underdogs to state champions. After that, kids and parents were clamoring for the same meals that the teams were getting.

Take a step back and look at the big-picture issues that school food connects with. Perhaps you would find more allies if you go with a broader mission. Is there already a children's wellness initiative in town? Some of the strongest advocates for cleaning up school food are wellness, nutrition, and health care professionals. These professionals are important to have on your team, because they have expert credentials. School administrators may find it easy to brush off a group of moms, but more challenging when the moms' group includes a pediatric cardiologist, a developmental psychologist, a holistic health coach, and a naturopathic physician.

Some other groups that may have a children's health initiative are your local veteran's groups, Rotary, Kiwanis, Lion's Club, Junior League, or Young Women's Club. Nonprofits, whether specifically focused on school food, or those that include children's health and the environment in their mission, make great partners. Their 501(c)(3) not-for-profit fiscal status may allow them to act as an umbrella for your subgroup, enabling you to fundraise and run your accounting through their administration.

The Three R's

"Reduce, reuse, recycle" has long been the mantra of the environmental movement, but more and more the buzzword is becoming "sustainability." In order to sustain life on our planet and to sustain our local and global economies, one of the primary systems that must function is our food system. Conventional methods of food production and distribution require a tremendous amount of greenhouse gas–producing fossil fuel. Our nation is slowly waking up to the fact that oil consumption will soon outstrip production. Ten percent of the energy used annually in the United States is consumed by the food industry. Much of that energy is wasted; it takes an estimated seven to ten calories of input energy to produce one calorie of food in our current food system. The practices of industrial agriculture account for much of that wasted energy. Oil and other nonrenewable resources are used in fertilizers, pesticides, herbicides, and transportation of these inputs as well as refrigeration, processing, and long-distance transportation of the finished products.

The argument is often made that we need all these petroleum-based inputs to grow enough food for our own needs and to subsidize the world's food needs. However, there's plenty of good science that demonstrates that the human population of the world could feed itself on organically grown crops if there weren't the social problems of war, corruption, and hierarchical structures that create famines and prevent farming and trade. The Organic Center reports that pesticides actually reduce crop yields by one-third due to their disruption of chemical signaling between plants and soil microbes.

In her book *Diet for a Hot Planet*, Anna Lappé provides an in-depth exploration of the connection between America's system of food production and global climate change. Her closing argument for choosing a diet of locally produced, organic, non-GMO, mostly plant, made-from-scratch food is not about you or your kids' health. It's about the health of planet Earth. Sustainability is inextricably tied to our food system and many of the tenets of the larger sustainability movement, as exemplified by Anna Lappé's diet, are closely aligned with the principles of sustainable school food. The intersection of causes—sustainability for the planet and the fight for the health of our children—is the sweet spot for fixing school food. Fixing school food would have a profound impact on both of those problems.

Does your town have a green group or sustainability initiative? After the movie came out and I traveled with it for a year, I wanted to get more involved back home. I was introduced to a new organization called the Green Village Initiative (GVI). Founded and supported by a local philanthropist, Dan Levinson, these people *do* things. In the two years since its inception, the group, more than one hundred strong, has successfully renovated and launched a sustainable Town Farm, a CSA program (Community Supported Agriculture—shares of fresh produce and eggs from local farmers), edible organic gardens at over a dozen local schools and other public sites, created internship opportunities on the farm and at a shoreline nature preserve and banned the use of plastic bags at local stores. GVI was founded in Westport, Connecticut, the town made famous by Martha Stewart, but it now has a new claim to fame—the greenest town in Connecticut. It's a great success story of what can be done with a bit of expertise, a bit of money, and a lot of sweat equity. However, there's still a long way to go to make our own local schools' food system sustainable. To date we've hosted several well-attended workshops and the group is building school gardens wherever they're wanted, including some of the neediest schools in our county in neighboring Bridgeport. It's a low-cost, friendly way to get a foot in the door and begin educating students and school staff about real food in a hands-on way. The group has also sponsored film and lecture series on environmental topics, including several area screenings of *Two Angry Moms*. The initiative continues to grow, with Green Village Initiatives popping up in neighboring towns. The volunteers of GVI support one another's endeavors. They are a wonderful source of support and encouragement, and this group really gets the connection between school food and the local and global environment.

PTO/PTA

Parent–teacher organizations are notoriously conservative and avoidant of anything that smacks of controversy. Our local PTOs build new playgrounds, raise funds for new technologies, run bake sales, and bring in local experts to speak at meetings. Early on, these groups (each school in our town has its own) were fearful of bringing me in. Individually, though, many of the PTO leaders in my town and in other towns offered their support of my cause. They explained their fears to me, which essentially were about making waves with the school administration. After making me promise not to be too radical at meetings, I was eventually invited to speak and show the movie at PTO events in my town and in many other districts. It continues to baffle me how speaking out about how poorly we feed our kids is radical!

My local PTO leaders insisted that they were not part of a lobbying organization so they couldn't take a stand on the issue of school food. Although your PTO (parent–teacher organization) may be unaffiliated, the national Parent Teacher Association (PTA) website, PTA.org, actually *encourages* members to lobby on national issues. They have an action alert Web page that challenges state PTAs to take action on all kinds of educational issues:

All PTA members are being challenged to respond to action alerts by reaching out to their members of Congress. The state with the highest response rates to action alerts . . . will earn the title of National PTA Takes Action Challenge Champion. Encourage your friends and family to visit PTA.org/takesaction and join the PTA Takes Action Network!

From their website I also learned that the PTA was instrumental in fighting (yes, they use the word "fought") for the inclusion of a mandate for local school wellness policies in the Child Nutrition and WIC Reauthorization Act of 2004. According to their site, "These wellness policies give parents, students, school nutrition representatives, school board members, school administrators, and the general public the opportunity to formulate local policies that are tailored to the specific needs and capacity of their communities."

The PTA site has pages of recommendations for implementing, updating, and assessing the effectiveness of these policies. I'll discuss local wellness policies in greater detail in chapter three. If you're not a member of your school's PTO, PTA, or PTSA (Parent, Teacher, Student Association), consider joining. Share with them some of the information you've learned about how to make your school's food environment more sustainable. These organizations like a good project. Maybe they'd like to raise money for new kitchen equipment, staff training, an organic vegetable garden, a food budget subsidy, or for marketing new foods to students. Having the PTO on your side sanctions your efforts and will go a long way toward removing the perception that what you are doing is controversial. Now that my movie and its mission are more widely known, PTO and PTA groups all around the country are hosting screenings and tackling school food head-on.

To Committee or Not to Committee

Since 2006, every district that participates in the National School Lunch Program has been required to have a school wellness committee that must "engage students, parents, teachers, food service professionals, health professionals, and other interested community members in developing, implementing, monitoring, and reviewing district-wide nutrition and physical activity

policies." These committees can be really effective in setting a strong, meaningful, and sustainable school food policy. Unfortunately, most school food
policies are simply a boilerplate and sitting on these committees is often a
frustrating experience for parents who are truly engaged in the issue.

COMMITTED IN CONNECTICUT

Last year, personal chef and after-school cooking teacher Nicole Straight was
asked by her local PTA to serve on her district's wellness committee. The
invitation was extended with the assurance that she would only have to attend
four meetings over the course of the school year, and all she would have to do
at the meetings was take notes for the PTA bulletin. Having heard that the
meetings were boring and basically a rubber stamp of whatever policy was
already in place, Nicole graciously turned down the invitation.

As a whole-foods chef and parent of young kids, Nicole truly wanted to see
improvements in her school's food. With the idea that she could have a greater
impact outside the system, she hosted a screening of *Two Angry Moms* that
generated a mailing list of eighty interested parents. Nicole created a survey
that went out to her mailing list and received responses from each of them. All
but two (who were members of her district's wellness committee) responded
that they would like to see numerous improvements to the district's school
food environment. Armed with her surveys, Nicole attended a wellness committee meeting as a community member, but was not allowed to speak. "It
was there that I realized how much perceived power this group had. I felt it
was a David versus Goliath situation. I lost my steam."

Jennifer Boyd, a physician's assistant and ecological wellness practitioner,
had a son in kindergarten in Nicole's district. He came home from school
one day with a note about the 100th day of school celebration. The event
included a math exercise where the kids would count by tens to one hundred
using manipulatives—in this case, a variety of candies and sugary treats. She
called the teacher and asked if perhaps the math game could use some other

(continued)

objects—coins? Seashells? Marbles? The request stirred quite a brouhaha—the room mother resisted and, says Jennifer, "She even canceled a playdate because 'we were too far apart in our thinking.'" The teacher passed Jennifer's request on to the principal and Jennifer called the office to ask for a copy of the school's wellness policy. The policy contained a clause that prohibited the use of food rewards or incentives in the classroom. Although the policy actually called for in-service training on its guidelines, Jennifer notes that there seemed to be a lack of awareness about the policy. On the 100th day of school, the principal came to class and explained to the children that they could count the candy but were not allowed to eat any.

Feeling "ostracized and discouraged" but not ready to give up, Jennifer teamed up with Nicole, and the ad hoc group was revitalized. Since then, they've had their ups and downs. This year, Jennifer led the town's first-ever Green Halloween event—activity-filled, sugar-free. Raising awareness, she's garnered support from the parents of her son's classmates.

Meanwhile, Nicole was asked again by her school's PTA to be their representative on the district's wellness committee. This year, she decided to become an insider, as frustrating as that might be. "I'd be a hypocrite if I didn't do it," she says. Before the meeting, she e-mailed parents at the school to introduce herself as their new food committee rep. She received twenty-five comments from parents in response. At the first meeting, the food service director from Chartwells, the school's food service management company, proudly offered tastes of new pizza dough made from white whole-wheat flour. Apparently that was one of the larger changes since last year. When it was her turn to speak, she commented, "The wellness policy isn't being enforced. My son has homework counting Skittles. My daughter's third-grade teacher has never heard of the wellness policy." Another committee member calling herself the Cupcake Mom said the policy was purposely vague because the special education teachers can't motivate their students without candy. Nicole was incensed. "These are the kids whose diets we really need to be paying attention to! The people who get to make these decisions about what our school kids should eat know nothing about real food," she tells me. She kept her cool at the meeting, though, and by the end of the meeting, the assistant superintendent had agreed to inform teachers about the wellness policy. She also asked Nicole to collaborate with another chef on the committee to create some scratch recipes for consideration on the lunch menu. "We were given the guidelines and came up with a falafel meal, and a brown rice and black bean burger." Although her expectations were low, she recently heard back from the school's dietician, who expects to have one of the recipes on the menu by next month. Nicole says she's feeling good about being on the committee, working on the inside with the support of her group of parents on the outside. "We have each other's back. We don't have to feel like the only freaky food nut. And that is the most important thing."

It Takes a Village

Once you understand the nature and scope of the school food issue, you realize the enormity of the task. You need lots of help. How do you grow your numbers? Very often, parents will need to band together outside of the officially sanctioned wellness committee, and even outside of their local district.

After seven years of efforts, Dr. Susan Rubin wasn't making any progress in her district. Her tenacity motivated her to reach outside of her school district and form a countywide Better School Food coalition—the first of its kind. I met Susan shortly after the coalition formed. She had teamed up with moms from neighboring school districts. They held workshops and conferences for parents and school personnel. Their work began to have a ripple effect, drawing interest from beyond the county. By expanding her circle, Susan was able to affect a larger region, with tangible results. Better School Food now supports advocates all over the country. Community building around food is a cliché, but true. The sustainable food web is growing as a movement locally, regionally, and globally. Susan offers some very realistic advice: "Plan to spend a decade working on helping to build a better school food environment. As your kids get older, you'll look back on this as time well spent. I know ninth grade seems miles away to a mom of a kindergartener, but trust me, the years fly by."

Another national organization that supports local efforts is Slow Food USA. Through their Time for Lunch Campaign they have circulated petitions for policy change on the federal level. The Slow Food in Schools program focuses on local food education projects. Cooking classes, school gardens, and linking local farms with school cafeterias are some of the initiatives their membership has undertaken. Their website provides materials to help you get a project started, and resources for food-based curriculum, soil building, and gardening.

These organizations and others can be good umbrellas for your local group. For a small membership fee, your group can use their good name and be part of a nationally sanctioned movement. Some groups will allow you to use their nonprofit status and will administer any funds you may raise. The public perception of your group will be elevated.

Whether you've affiliated with a national group or created your own ad hoc committee, once you've taken the step of naming your group, you should issue a press release so that other members of the community begin to recognize your organization and your mission. Newspaper, radio, and television media are all looking for stories. Tie your launch story into a local issue, event, or personality and pitch it to all the media outlets in your area. Make the story simple, topical, personal, and just a bit sensational!

Friend Me

Susan Rubin taught me the incredible power of networking on the Internet through e-mail newsletters. These services (I use one called Constant Contact; there's another called MailChimp) are low cost and some are even free if your circulation is small. They offer preformatted templates for feature articles, events, sponsors, links, coupons, and photos. While there is a learning curve for the templates, you don't have to know HTML or any other technical stuff. The newsletter service will help you manage a mailing list; you can sort your lists, plan events with e-vites, and receive online RSVPs.

If you do a Web search for "school food," you will find pages of resources, and this is often the first point of entry for parents who feel isolated in their district. When I started making *Two Angry Moms*, I worked with a Web designer and programmer to create the first version of the angrymoms.org website. The original purpose of the site was just to let people know I was making the movie, and to solicit contributions to help with production costs. Over several years, and with the help of a generous grant, we've expanded the site to include resources and links. I am constantly amazed at the number of people who find their way to the site. Each month I receive a website traffic report; people from South Korea, Romania, Turkey, Brazil, South Africa, and Argentina are showing up and spending time there. If you're in a big school district, you might consider a simple website (there are lots of DIY templates) to help parents and others find out about local efforts.

I've been dragged kicking and screaming into the world of Facebook and Twitter. As a Facebook member, you can add a Cause page. Our cause has over 1,000 "likes." For those of you who aren't Facebook users (is anyone out there not on Facebook?), a "like" is when someone gives your page a thumbs-up, which is a recommendation to others in their network. You can create a local Cause page—check out the Westport Food Revolution page as an example. This is an effective and easy way to go viral. Twitter is even simpler to use than Facebook. You can open a Twitter account in a couple of minutes, and begin Tweeting your passion for better food in schools right away. You can link your Twitter account with your Facebook account and a post in one place will go to the other. The more you post, the more you increase interest in your Twitter feeds and Facebook Cause. I describe Twitter and Facebook as real-time communications applications because they are really like personal news feeds. If you don't follow these sites on a regular basis, the information gets buried, just like an old newspaper on the bottom of a stack you haven't read. You have to read the thread of notes and comments backward, which is awkward and usually reads like old news, so think of these services as more of a running conversation than as an information center or archive.

Groupsite

Although this chapter provides lots of suggestions, if you are a basically shy person, you might still be nervous about taking that first step. I often receive e-mail from moms wondering how to find other parents who are leading the way in their community. We started angrymoms.groupsite.com so that parents could have a social network dedicated to the topic of better food in schools. We've created a Discussion Forum called "Find Advocates in My Area." Once you've joined the network you can write a post on this forum with your zip code or school district name, and find other people who have posted in your area. You don't have to be the leader; in fact, every movement needs more supporters than leaders, and every supporter can be emboldened to become an advocate and eventually to take a leading role.

Write Now

Blogs are a great way to get your feet wet in the school food arena. Is there a community blog for your area? I just did a quick Web search for "Brooklyn Parents Blog" and found dozens of pages of results. One of the first, *Park Slope Parents*, had a post called "Let's (Re)Do School Lunch." By writing or commenting on posts in local blogs, your concerns will have an airing. Not a letter writer? "Take a picture and post it. I go into school and take pictures of the lunch. That is so powerful," advises Bettina Siegel, whose blog, *The Lunch Tray*, gets 12,000 page views each month. I would add just one caveat. Be sure you only photograph the food. As a filmmaker, I have had to be very cautious filming children in schools. I always have releases signed either from the school or the parents. There are children in protective custody whose whereabouts must not be revealed, and others whose parents are sensitive about their privacy. My own daughter declined to be filmed except fleetingly from the back as she got on her school bus!

THE LUNCH TRAY

Bettina Siegel, a Houston mom, writes a terrific blog called *The Lunch Tray*. Her kids didn't eat the school lunch and so she wasn't particularly interested in becoming a cafeteria crusader. She got started innocently enough by going to the school principal to discuss her concerns about treats in her children's classrooms. "I was appalled by the food environment of the school. They were given food rewards, candy, every day." As it turned out, the district was forming a food and nutrition advisory committee and Bettina was chosen to be on it. She wrote about the experience of her first meeting in an article for Slow Food USA. "HISD [the Houston school district] showed the parents the food it was serving for breakfast—Trix yogurt, high-sodium biscuit and sausage sandwiches, Uncrustable peanut butter and jelly sandwiches, and the like. Horrible stuff, but what really baffled me was that at every meal, kids were also required to take a packet of animal crackers. When I asked about the animal crackers, the HISD/Aramark [food service company] dietician explained that they were needed for the meal to meet USDA nutritional guidelines and thereby qualify for government reimbursement. That really stumped me. I started to realize I'd stumbled into an area totally outside my prior experience." Bettina's "prior experience" was as a lawyer, a skill that no doubt helped her unravel the system that required the vitamin-fortified animal crackers as part of a balanced breakfast. Her story is really an archetype of advocacy. She spoke up, and in so doing became a de facto volunteer on the nutrition committee. Bettina tells me she thinks parents who are concerned must take the time to educate themselves. She read Janet Poppendieck's book *Free For All*, a compelling exposé and sociological report on the National School Lunch Program. Bettina says, "I became an expert against my will." Bettina soon read the contract between her district and Coke. She is hesitant to tell me how much money (millions) is flowing to the district over the course of a few years (see chapter three). "I am very sympathetic to school districts and the pressures they are under. You are quickly marginalized if you are too passionate. You get known as an extremist. I try to be rational and calm," she tells

(continued)

me. But "when parents started finding out that I was on the PAC, it seemed like everyone had something to say to me. I was stopped in hallways to discuss everything from school food to Oreos at the 10 a.m. soccer game—people clearly wanted to have this conversation. And, armed with the new knowledge I'd gained through the PAC and my own research, I realized I had a lot to say, too. Hence, *The Lunch Tray.*" With the blog, Bettina quickly created not only a local, but also a national forum. She learned how hard it is to unite people around food issues. "There's something about food. Touring the school kitchen one mom said we shouldn't even be serving sweetened yogurt." While she's seen a few changes in her own school, she finds the slow progress disheartening. "People realize it's a thankless task and they thank me for serving on the committee." What has she learned from the experience so far? In her district, she feels, "I'm working at the wrong level. My sense is that if you're at the school level and you have a sympathetic principal you can do a lot. And Congress can do a lot. At the district level I'm not sure what I can get done here. I can't change USDA funding. I'm never going to shape that menu the way I wish to see it. I can only make little changes." As for the blog—her advice is to start your own. "I am so happy to have created the space for people to share with each other."

Get Political

Not all school boards are elected, but if yours is, consider running for election on a sustainable schools platform. Or support a candidate who promises to make the school food environment a priority. In my district, school board members serve a four-year term and a portion of the board is up for election every two years. Even if your campaign doesn't win, election time is a great moment to garner attention to the issue and move it up on the list of district priorities.

Attend local debates and ask some hard questions about school food contracts, sourcing, and quality of ingredients.

Involve Students

A discussion that comes up often when debating school food is the issue of choice. Should kids have lots of choices? Should they get to choose between good and bad foods in the school cafeteria and vending machines? Earlier in this chapter I quoted from a letter written by a high school student who argued that kids would find junk food even if it were forbidden. Many parents and educators will also argue that it's important for children to have choices. As a parent, I abdicate my authority to the administration when I send my child to school. Our schools have abdicated a lot of choices to our children, especially about food, without considering the consequences. Children need to be educated about making choices. While it's essential to involve students in school food, the kinds of choices they can be making are far more sophisticated than fries versus Tater Tots. Critical thinking, decision making, and leadership are educational goals for every school system. I've seen students learning these skills by involvement in model school food programs. As students learn about their food—where it comes from, how it was produced, its impact on their bodies and the environment, how it's being marketed to them—they begin to make choices, and they begin to demand food that is cleaner, safer, and greener.

The Robert Wood Johnson Foundation has a blog (http://community .rwjf.org/message/3285) that poses this question: "If you and your friends could change anything about the food served in your school cafeteria, what would it be? (Here's your chance, so be specific! What should your cafeteria NOT sell? Which foods do you wish were offered?)" Most of the kids write in asking for salad bars and more fresh foods. Some of the students ask for fast-food vendors to supply the meals because it's tastier and healthier than what their school currently serves. This blog, and others like it, are a great way to involve students and establish a dialog.

Teachers Are People, Too

An anonymous teacher, Mrs. Q, resolved to eat her school's lunch every day for a year, posting a daily lunch photo and writing about the lunch and everything else to do with school food. I promised not to blow her cover (though she may have revealed herself by the time you read this), but I can tell you that she's a mom of a young child and her blog grew out of her frustration with not being able to do more to change the system from the inside. As a teacher, she experiences the impact of poor nutrition on her students every day. Her suggestion is to be gentle and conversational with your child's teacher. "Be a sympathetic listener; teachers are people, too. 'You know, Ms. Jones, Joey came home with Dum-Dums in his pocket and I wondered, is that a special reward for performance?' Get an explanation for the reward. 'Would you mind giving him a sticker instead? It's too much sugar before dinner' (or whatever your reason is). 'You know, I know Rice Krispies and Cheetos are occasional snacks or treats, too. I can see how those kinds of foods are okay rarely, but I just worry that processed and sugary snacks aren't good on a regular basis. What's your thought on that?' Allow open dialogue. 'Maybe the parents can get together and brainstorm some healthier snacks like cheese and crackers, grapes, and carrot sticks that help them learn healthy habits and remain focused at school.'"

Having a teacher like Mrs. Q on your team is a real asset. Bear in mind that teachers have to protect their jobs, so they may be hesitant to confront school administrators, even when they feel strongly about an issue. I am looking forward to seeing what happens when Mrs. Q reveals her identity.

Mendy Heaps, a Colorado middle school teacher, wasn't as cautious as Mrs. Q. When her husband was diagnosed with cancer, diabetes, and high blood pressure, Mendy began selling fruit and other healthy snacks to her students. Her fruit cart was quite popular with the students, but her activism was rewarded with a "cease and desist" memo from the school principal. Apparently the school food service felt that her cart was competing with the lunch program.

In an interview with *The Slow Cook* blogger Ed Bruske, Mendy says, "I felt part of the reason I was so successful selling good food was because I had *only* good choices. I didn't have chips or cookies or ice cream. The kids could only buy healthy items. I wanted to show that kids *will* buy what's good for them if that's all that is offered. If they are hungry and have to choose between a Choco Taco and an apple they are probably going to choose the Choco Taco. *But* . . . if they are hungry and have to choose between an apple or a pear or a banana, then they'll choose something good. That's what I wanted to show people."

Mendy was obliged to sign the memo from the principal to avoid further disciplinary action. One comment to a blog post about Mendy suggests that hers is a case of "no good deed goes unpunished." The stories of both Mrs. Q and Mendy Heaps are cautionary tales. Enthusiasm and righteousness don't necessarily create change. When all the stars are in alignment, a school system can change very quickly—I've seen it happen—but you need to proceed with caution and create a strategy that is flexible enough to be modified when you hit an obstacle. Channel that enthusiasm into a thoughtful, simple plan that can be adapted depending upon the responses you receive. Take your time, go slowly, and try to avoid getting burned out. This business can really suck you in!

Two Steps Forward, One Step Back

Environmental activist Van Jones says, "You go through ups and downs because you're pushing yourself up against the limits of what you know how to do well and your comfort zones—those valleys are really important to go through because first of all they make the mountaintops a lot nicer but also you learn things from the valley that you need to get to the mountaintop. We all get discouraged . . . and it's so easy to stop, but the reality is often if you just go one more step, you find an ally, you go another step, and it turns out that somebody that you thought was your enemy just misunderstood something and it's amazing how quickly things can turn around. The challenge is not to give up hope. Change is hard but if you keep the hope, if you can nurture the hope, if you can stay in there, it's amazing how quickly things can turn around. And then you look back and you say, look at all these miracles that happened. They weren't miracles—they were just people determined not to give up when it looked really hard."

THE MARBLEHEAD MOMS

One of my school food heroes, Lolli Leeson, is a "pick up the phone and go for it" kind of gal. She's got a magnetic personality, and if Lolli asks you to help her with a cause, she'll make you feel like you want to be part of it. Lolli activated her network of friends, then she called me, and I was lured to Marblehead, Massachusetts, to both inspire and learn from them.

Marblehead is a picture-perfect New England town. A beautiful rocky Atlantic beach stretches along its eastern shore. Across from the beach is a patchwork of sidewalk-lined streets graced by comfortable suburban homes. A commercial lane replete with all the conveniences just inland from the residential area services the town's 22,000 inhabitants. Tucked in the northern corner of Marblehead is the historic eighteenth-century downtown—now a thriving, upscale shopping, restaurant, and café district. The entire town could be posing for a catalog of Norman Rockwell illustrations. Marblehead is reputed to have a top-notch public school system, with the average student scoring 30 percent above state average on standardized testing. Lolli Leeson wasn't lulled into complacency by the near-Stepford perfection of her town. She recalls:

"In the spring of 2007 I was having coffee with four moms. Some were friends and some were acquaintances. We started talking about the state of the school food and being very frustrated with it. All four of us have something unique to bring to the table. Mom #1, Laura Plunkett, had a son, Danny, who was diagnosed with diabetes in third grade. She had just spent the last four years dealing with his diabetes and had written a book on her ordeal and what she learned. Mom #2, Marybeth M., was a breast cancer survivor. Mom #3, Shannon L., had some serious health challenges and had been desperate

enough to spend a month at the Hippocrates Institute in Florida. Then there
was me.

"I had a food background and had graduated from the Cambridge School
of Culinary Arts. A few years later, as a volunteer for HealthLink, a grassroots organization on the North Shore that was pressuring the Salem power
plant to comply with modern air standards, as they are one of the 'Filthy Five'
in Massachusetts, I started to learn a lot about the depletion of our air and
water and how the soil is compromised from pesticides. I was learning oodles
about nutrition and becoming quite angry that I did not know this information about the supreme necessity of plant nutrition and how the nutrition in
food was not what it used to be. At the same time I started volunteering in
my son's third-grade elementary school as a lunch helper. We as moms took
turns helping out the one lunch aide for a total of eighty children. It was there
that I shook my head and said, 'This is outrageous,' and 'No wonder kids have
so many problems learning in school.' Parents have no idea what is going on
here. The whole environment was frenetic.

"We moms talked more and decided to approach the superintendent to
voice our concerns and to get his pulse to see if this was something that he was
supportive of us taking on. I think he saw the four of us coming and he couldn't
say, 'No, I am not willing or interested in taking up this cause.' He was thinking he was playing his cards right. Anyway, he agreed to start a task force
and we formed the wellness committee with the head nurse Paula Dubrow as
the chairman and Laura Plunkett as the co-chair. The superintendent figured
that the head nurse, who worked closely with him, would keep a lid on things
pretty well and things would go smoothly. Our committee was twenty strong
and we had the head of the farmers' market, the head of the YMCA, a local
pediatrician, a board of health member, a school nurse, teachers, and parents.
So, that is how it started."

The moms on the committee divided themselves into individual task forces.
Each mom had a mission. Laura researched local farmers who were willing
to supply the schools with fresh produce. Another focused on consciousness-
raising and technical skills training among the cafeteria staff. She cooked a

(continued)

breakfast for them, organized an appreciation day, walked them through some basic recipes, and helped get them some new tools. The school nurse worked on getting a school garden started. Lolli worked with the students. She got permission to teach a ten-week Food Appreciation course to a group of fifth-graders, which is now in its second year. They use Dr. David Katz's free *Nutrition Detectives* DVD that teaches kids how to read food labels and understand ingredients in their packaged food from the cafeteria and their lunch boxes. Lolli brings in her Vitamix and the kids get to make their own smoothies during the last ten minutes of class.

In the fall of 2008 the wellness committee brought me to Marblehead to speak after a screening of *Two Angry Moms*. They had a great turnout for the film and a lively discussion ensued. The group gained a lot of momentum over the course of the school year, and by the end of the year had convinced the superintendent that they needed a new food service director who could overhaul the cafeteria. The nearby Medford school system had recently hired chef Bridget Collins to create recipes and train the district's fifty-eight school food employees in nutrition and cooking techniques. Laura wrote and received a grant to get Chef Bridget to come up twelve times to teach the Marblehead lunch ladies scratch cooking. She brought in Melinda DeFeo, the woman who runs the Farm to School program on Martha's Vineyard, to do a full-day presentation on how to work school food into the curriculum. They were really on a roll.

It took until late August for the district to hire a new food service director. Lolli says, "She had just two weeks to get her kitchen in order. It was like someone jumping into the ocean and sinking. She wasn't able to swim back up. She started taking food away and got bad press about taking away cookies and ice cream. The superintendent and school board didn't support her when the parents complained. There were so many issues in the kitchen, from maintaining sanitation and food safety to how to use the equipment. We had a full day of in-service training but she never had a chance to get in there and do the job she was hired to do. She said the stress of the job was too much and she resigned before the school year ended."

At that point there were twenty-five people on the wellness committee. Lolli says the superintendent and the school board then put the kibosh on the wellness committee because they thought the committee had too much power and had moved too fast.

"We've had some failures," Lolli philosophizes. "It's two steps forward and one step back. The head nurse, Paula, who had been with the schools for fifteen years, quit her job because she was so disappointed by the fallout after putting so much of her effort and energy into this. We felt so dissed by the superintendent and school board. There has definitely been frustration with the political part but now there's a change in the wind. The good news is that we've built our coalition over time. We've kept up with letters to the editor, and there's a lot of talk now about school food in Marblehead. There's been a huge amount of education around this. We're not done yet; we're gearing up for round two. It will come full circle. In two weeks the newly rehired previous food service director will come to a meeting and our group will be there in force. The topic has not gone away; this has only fueled it from where we were a year ago."

I asked Lolli how she maintains her optimism and enthusiasm for this struggle. "I know what I know and I love what I do. I'm teaching and I'm educating and that is where I'm going to make the most change. Those kids just look at you with amazement and they want to learn more. And the kids are teaching their parents."

The Marblehead community was won over by Lolli's enthusiasm. She had a lot of popular support for her efforts and her coalition did a great job researching, educating the public, and persuading the administration to make some changes. Unfortunately, the administration didn't have a strategic plan in place. For the next round in Marblehead, Lolli's coalition will have to help implement steps toward building a sustainable food system in the school cafeteria (found in chapter six). Meanwhile, they're not discouraged.

Float Your Boat

President John F. Kennedy said, "A rising tide lifts all boats." He was referring to economic betterment, but the metaphor is apt for school food. Our small, scattered efforts are having an impact, even when we face setbacks like

Lolli's. "Find whatever floats your boat and get involved," says Susan Rubin. Susan left dentistry to become a nutrition counselor and school food advocate. Many of the school food leaders I've met left professional positions in order to raise their families. These women (and a few men) tend to be good at taking charge and managing others. Your coalition needs its leaders, but it also needs worker bees, so if you'd rather not be carrying the flag, think about what you're good at, and what you like to do. The reward you will get for taking part in this movement will mostly be the satisfaction of participation, so get involved on a level that feels comfortable. Do you have computer skills? Maybe you'll want to be in charge of publishing a newsletter. You can join forces with another mom who would love to write the content. Love to cook? Meetings and events tend to draw a good crowd when the invitation mentions food. Most schools will allow a parent to do a cooking and tasting demo in the cafeteria during lunch. If you're a good shopper, maybe you can help find resources for a school garden, or help find local sources for fresh produce and other healthy food products. Do you have good teaching or coaching skills? You might consider leading a workshop on shopping at the grocery store, healthy cooking, organic gardening, or whole foods for young athletes. Documenting your movement is an important way to tell your story, so reach out to someone who loves taking photographs. A contribution of business development, fund-raising, or bookkeeping skills is always appreciated. Most importantly, every volunteer effort needs lots of extra hands. The greatest skill you can bring to a local wellness effort is the ability to show up and do whatever needs to be done. Whether it's showing up in force at a public meeting, helping out in the cafeteria, bringing a healthy snack for a class, a game, or the theater group, or making phone calls and sending e-mails, you will be helping to build momentum and sustain a movement.

The Survey

A tool that many groups find helpful is a survey. Whether you are working with a district wellness committee, PTO group, or ad hoc community group, a school food survey will help you gauge community interest in the topic and also generate awareness. In Katonah-Lewisboro, New York, a district-wide school food survey drew more than a 50 percent response rate. If you're working within the school system, you should be able to use their e-mail list for your survey. Until recently, compiling results from a survey meant hours of data crunching. Now there are several free or low-cost online survey providers (search "free online survey creation"). We have used SurveyMonkey, a service that allows you to program your survey questions, send out a mass e-mail, and then tabulate the responses online. Most of these services offer free trials, and free service for small surveys. They may charge a minimal fee for a more detailed survey.

If you don't have access to your school district's e-mail list, you can publish an article about the survey in a school bulletin or local paper sending readers to your online link.

Surveys can be targeted for different populations like parents, students, staff, or you can create a broad survey for the whole school community. New York State's Board of Cooperative Educational Services created a sample school food survey for students with ten questions:

FOOD SERVICES STUDENT SURVEY

SELECT YOUR SCHOOL DISTRICT

DISTRICT: SCHOOL: GRADE:

1. Do you think that school lunch is a healthy meal?
   ☐ Yes   ☐ No   ☐ Somewhat   ☐ Not Sure

2. How often do you buy lunch at school?
   ☐ Never   ☐ 1 Time per Week   ☐ 2 times   ☐ 3 times   ☐ 4 times
   ☐ Every Day

3. If you selected "Never," why don't you buy lunch at school? Choose all that apply.
☐ Selection of Food   ☐ Nutritional Value   ☐ Quality   ☐ Cost
☐ Service   ☐ Portion Size   ☐ Other—Please specify:

4. How often do you buy breakfast at school?
☐ Never   ☐ 1 Time per Week   ☐ 2 times   ☐ 3 times   ☐ 4 times
☐ Every Day

5. If you selected "Never," why don't you buy breakfast at school?
Choose all that apply.
☐ Selection of Food   ☐ Nutritional Value   ☐ Quality   ☐ Cost
☐ Service   ☐ Eat Breakfast at Home

6. List your favorite school lunch entrees:

7. If you could add new menu items to the lunch menu, what would they be?

8. How would you rate the quality of the food served by the school food service program?
☐ Poor   ☐ Fair   ☐ Good   ☐ Excellent

9. Please list one or two things you think we could do to improve the quality of the food we serve.

10. How would you rate the quality of service from the cafeteria staff?
☐ Poor   ☐ Fair   ☐ Good   ☐ Excellent

http://www.gstboces.org/ms/foodservices/studentsurvey/

With input from a professional psychologist, chef Nicole Straight adapted a survey for parents published by the Better School Food coalition. Here's Nicole's version:

PARENT FOOD AND WELLNESS QUESTIONNAIRE

1. The food served in our cafeteria promotes a healthy diet.
   ☐ Strongly Disagree   ☐ Disagree   ☐ I Don't Know   ☐ Agree
   ☐ Strongly Agree   ☐ Elementary School   ☐ Middle School
   ☐ High School

2. Foods advertised on the menu are mostly available.
   ☐ Strongly Disagree   ☐ Disagree   ☐ I Don't Know   ☐ Agree
   ☐ Strongly Agree   ☐ Elementary School   ☐ Middle School
   ☐ High School

3. The foods, beverages, and snacks provided at school are healthy for my child.
   ☐ Strongly Disagree   ☐ Disagree   ☐ I Don't Know   ☐ Agree
   ☐ Strongly Agree   ☐ Elementary School   ☐ Middle School
   ☐ High School

4. Daily menus feature a sufficient variety of healthy choices.
   ☐ Strongly Disagree   ☐ Disagree   ☐ I Don't Know   ☐ Agree
   ☐ Strongly Agree   ☐ Elementary School   ☐ Middle School
   ☐ High School

5. My children are satisfied with the food served in the cafeteria.
   ☐ Strongly Disagree   ☐ Disagree   ☐ I Don't Know   ☐ Agree
   ☐ Strongly Agree   ☐ Elementary School   ☐ Middle School
   ☐ High School

6. The vending machines feature a sufficient variety of healthy choices.
   ☐ Strongly Disagree   ☐ Disagree   ☐ I Don't Know   ☐ Agree
   ☐ Strongly Agree   ☐ Elementary School   ☐ Middle School
   ☐ High School

7. My children are satisfied with the snacks and beverages available in the vending machines.
   ☐ Strongly Disagree   ☐ Disagree   ☐ I Don't Know   ☐ Agree
   ☐ Strongly Agree   ☐ Elementary School   ☐ Middle School
   ☐ High School

8. Cafeteria hours of operation should be extended to accommodate students with after-school activities at the middle school and the high school.
   ☐ Strongly Disagree   ☐ Disagree   ☐ I Don't Know   ☐ Agree
   ☐ Strongly Agree   ☐ Elementary School   ☐ Middle School
   ☐ High School

9. I would be willing to pay more for a daily school lunch that provides healthier and more nutritious foods for my children.
   ☐ Strongly Disagree   ☐ Disagree   ☐ I Don't Know   ☐ Agree
   ☐ Strongly Agree   ☐ Elementary School   ☐ Middle School
   ☐ High School

10. My impression is that the cafeteria is clean, pleasant, and appealing.
    ☐ Strongly Disagree   ☐ Disagree   ☐ I Don't Know   ☐ Agree
    ☐ Strongly Agree   ☐ Elementary School   ☐ Middle School
    ☐ High School

11. My children have enough time to eat lunch.
    ☐ Strongly Disagree   ☐ Disagree   ☐ I Don't Know   ☐ Agree
    ☐ Strongly Agree   ☐ Elementary School   ☐ Middle School
    ☐ High School

12. How many days per week do your children usually buy school lunch in the cafeteria?
    ☐ Never   ☐ One day   ☐ Two days   ☐ Three days   ☐ Four days
    ☐ Five days   ☐ Elementary School   ☐ Middle School   ☐ High School

13. My children attend: [List schools in the district]

14. Please make additional comments:

The types of questions on these two surveys get parents and students thinking about school food. Rather than complacency and complaints, survey takers will begin to see themselves as active participants in the school food conversation. Another question that could be added to both surveys: Would you be interested in joining our coalition to advocate for healthy and great tasting food in the cafeteria and throughout the school? Please add your e-mail here:_____.

Group Dynamics

Your group is growing. Whether you are the leader or a member of a community group or committee, you will inevitably run into issues of philosophical differences, personality conflicts, and members who just don't pull their weight. Annie Leonard, author and filmmaker of *The Story of Stuff* (storyofstuff.org), says one of the lessons she's learned from other organizers is, "If you like everyone in your coalition then your coalition isn't big enough." Group dynamics seem to be amplified among volunteers. When the group is working well it's a lovefest of pride and progress. When the going gets tough, though, you will see a lot of finger-pointing, stubbornness, and dropouts. It's important to nip those conflicts in the bud in order not to lose your momentum.

You may want to develop a short vision statement and some ground rules, including determining what the process will be for resolving conflicts before they happen. Make sure everyone has a voice at the table, all concerns are addressed, and everyone receives an active response. Decide upon a course of action for any concerns that do arise, and make sure there is follow-up. Some people will still part ways, but it's important not to burn your bridges. Don't let them go away grumpy! Those who leave the coalition may be interested in serving in an advisory capacity or on a per-project basis once some time has passed. Your group may be formal or informal, but you'll want to be sure you are all on the same page as you move forward with your agenda.

If you have a hard time growing your group, or if your group finds itself in conflict with factions in the community, the Massachusetts Public Health Community Action to Change School Food Policy toolkit suggests asking yourselves the following questions: "Are they poorly informed? Are they invested in keeping things as they are? Do they have a financial interest or need in keeping things as they are? Is this issue simply not relevant to them? Why not? Pay attention to cultures other than your own. Do you need materials in other languages? Are there cultural barriers that you have not considered?"

It's important to have diverse representation in your group, from all parts of the local community. With diversity comes a better understanding of the various interests at stake in the school food issue, and you'll have a better perspective as you develop an approach to working through the challenges.

Strategic Plan

You have a committed group of volunteers and you recognize that you're in it for the long haul. It's time to get very clear and set some short-term and long-term goals. Break them down into individual projects. Determine priorities for your projects and in what order they would best work. Make a chart of who will do what and when. Implement a decision-making process that allows for some discussion but also sets time limits so meetings don't drag on endlessly. Alan Khazei offers this advice: "Go for early wins. You don't have to change the whole world right from the beginning. It's good to set big dreams and goals but then take a step back and say, 'How can we get started?' For City Year [a year-long youth mentoring service program] our goal was and still is a million people in national service. We started with fifty young people for ten weeks so we figured, well, that's a doable thing." Alan quotes Sun Tzu from *The Art of War*, "Every battle is won or lost before it's fought." He says, "It's about the planning, it's about the preparations, it's about the training, it's about the strategy. Think where you want to be ultimately and then work backwards." You will need to determine not only where you want to be, but also how you want to start and what your point of entry as a movement should be. Can you approach your school administrators and form a partnership? Maybe now it's time to put out a press release, have a public meeting, and share your plans.

Press Release

I'm frequently asked for templates for various kinds of documents. I'll pop them into the pages of this book whenever the opportunity comes up. I had never done a press release until I made the movie, and we had to search a bit to find the right format. The one below is adapted from the Massachusetts Public Health Association:

The Health Advocacy Council of _____

Phone: XXX-XXX-XXXX
E-mail : XXX-XXX-XXXX
Contact Name and Title
Date: Month/Day/Year

PRESS RELEASEPRESS RELEASE***

FOR IMMEDIATE RELEASE

Strong title in bold, e.g.: COUNCIL RECOMMENDS THAT (Your Town/City) MAKES IMPROVING THE SCHOOL FOOD ENVIRONMENT A PRIORITY THIS YEAR

City/Town, State—The first paragraph should include the most important and powerful information and should answer the questions:

- **Who** founded the initiative?
- **What** will the initiative do?
- **When** will it be brought to the school committee?
- **Where** will it be instituted?

(continued)

Following paragraphs should answer **why** the initiative is important and discuss its relevance to your district.

- Be brief and to the point.
- The document should be double-spaced.
- Keep it to no more than two pages.
- Use quotes from parents, school officials, and students.

Finish with some information about your committee, for example: The (City) Health Advocacy Council was formed in (Year) to address the wellness needs of (City's) students by writing and recommending programs and policy. For more information, call_____.

At the bottom center of the last page of the release, type three pound signs (###)—this is standard journalistic practice.

Meet

Someone needs to play the role of facilitator at your meetings. You may have a lot of differing perspectives being expressed, and you want to make sure everyone gets heard, and that as a group you are working toward common goals. You may have to set time limits on individuals, or on specific discussion topics. The facilitator's job is to manage the process; she doesn't have to be an expert on school food. If there's someone in your group who has experience as a health coach or psychotherapist, he or she will have been trained in facilitation. If you don't have a trained facilitator, here are a few tips for running your meeting:

- E-mail a meeting invitation or meeting reminder. Send out a couple of reminders—one week ahead and one or two days ahead. Set an agenda ahead of time. Your agenda should list projects, tasks, discussions, and goals.

- Make it attractive. Ask for volunteers to supply coffee or tea, fruit, healthy treats, soup, or small sandwiches if the meeting falls close to mealtime.

- Open the meeting by introducing new members. If the group is a manageable size, ask each person to introduce him- or herself for thirty to sixty seconds whenever you have a new member join. Gently but firmly limit the time for introductions and any side conversations that may take off. Suggest that you can add an extra topic to the agenda if there's time later in the meeting, or suggest that people can remain after the meeting if they'd like to continue a specific conversation.

- In any group dynamic, listening is important, and as a facilitator, your role is to listen actively. You can repeat back the main idea of a comment, or paraphrase a question, then allow others to offer their answers and comments. Don't be intimidated by expressions of emotion; acknowledge feelings but don't allow passion to dominate the meeting. Remind people that you are there to create consensus and move forward on a project.

- Wrap up the meeting with a very brief summary of the discussion, action points, and individual tasks that people have agreed to follow up on. It's a good idea to schedule your next meeting at the close of each meeting, making sure the date works for the majority of attendees.

Educate

Film screenings and surveys are great tools for raising awareness but you'll want to follow up with more information. The next step is a concerted community effort to educate and involve more parents and school personnel, not only about the impact food has on our kids' health and development, but about the many cost-effective ways we can improve our local school food environments. Your group may want to host a larger event that brings in families and other diverse members of the community. Ask a high-profile neighbor—a doctor or chef, a published author or actor, a farmer or congressional representative to speak about school food or to participate in a panel discussion. You may want to target one group; invite school staff from around your region to a day of workshops on a variety of topics—school gardens, Farm to School, wellness policy, cooking demos, or curriculum development. I've seen these types of group immersion and constructive collaborations lead to big changes in attitudes, policies, and practices.

People Change

In my interview with Be the Change's Alan Khazei, he reminded me that the tipping point for change occurs because people change. He says, "There's always going to be skeptics, there's always going to be people who say it can't be done, it won't be done, it can't work." Alan taught his City Year members the Native American prayer: "Great Spirit, grant that I shall not criticize my brother or sister until I walk a mile in his or her moccasins." "Try to see it from their perspective," Alan explains. "What's making them skeptical? Maybe they've had a bad experience, maybe they've tried to do something that didn't work out, or maybe they've had other people around them that have said it can't be done. And then I try to present an argument or a case as to why in this situation it can be done. If I come up against . . . a roadblock, I go on to the next person or the next issue but I try to stay in touch so that if and when we are successful I can say, 'It actually did work out.' Try not to make enemies. There are people who are going to oppose you, there are people who won't believe it can be done but it's usually because of something that's happened to them in their life . . . understand that. You don't have to convince everyone, you just have to convince enough people who you need to support you or support your cause or support your efforts, so don't hit your head against the wall. We've also had people who at the beginning never thought it could be done, and we went and did it, and they became our biggest champions because we reached out to them early and they go, 'Oh wow, I couldn't believe that you could get that done!' So today's skeptic could be tomorrow's biggest supporter."

Alan's final words of advice to me were, "Remember the guardian angel axiom. If you're trying to be good for the world, if you are pursuing some kind of issue of justice, people will come out of the woodwork to help you. It's remarkable. There is a spirit of public service. There is an idealism that's out there, there is a desire within people to want to make a difference and once you put yourself out and people see that you're committed, they will be inspired by your commitment and people will come to help you. Not every day is easy and things get hard but you can count on that people will emerge to help you if you stick with it."

One pair of shoes you will need to walk a mile in are those of your school food service director. And for that, you will need an understanding of the morass of federal, state, and local policies that govern the school meals program.

STEPS FOR SCHOOL FOOD ADVOCATES

- Visit the cafeteria. Read labels, take photos, and share the results.
- Create partnerships with parents, community groups, school staff, and students. Reach beyond your district for resources.
- Survey your district and share the results.
- Show up, educate, and be creative.
- Hire a consultant in sustainable school food systems, and/or hire a chef.
- Audit the school food environment.
- Create or update your district wellness policy.
- Review and provide input for RFPs* and contracts.
- Stick with it—don't give up!

---

* RFP—A Request for Proposal is a document that school districts are required to write when they request bids from food service management companies. See chapter eight for complete details.

THREE

THE WONKY CHAPTER

No nation is any healthier than its children or more prosperous than its farmers.

—Harry Truman

You're now aware of the perils of the school food environment, and you're on your way to organizing a local movement. I've often heard school district business managers and food service directors brush off parent activism with comments like, "They don't understand how the system works. I have to follow USDA regulations. I can't make changes to the program." It helps if you can understand where these administrators are coming from and speak their language. So you need to know some history, understand a bit of policy, learn a handful of regulations, and then get your head around a whole lot of politics. The various federal guidelines, rules, and regulations governing school meals require periodic legislative assessment, review, and renewal by Congress. Essentially, federal policy is an attempt to provide minimum standards, just a floor, and barely enough (arguably, not nearly enough) funding for school districts to meet those minimums. Beyond that, federal policy leaves it up to the state and local school districts to raise the bar or sometimes skirt around it. The regulations are fairly straightforward and provide some measure of uniformity to the school meals program. An often-discussed issue is whether this uniformity is to the benefit of students' health. According to a recent USDA report, "One of the main goals of NSLP as identified by Congress is to promote the health and well-being of the nation's children. In recent years, questions have been raised about the program's ability to meet this goal, especially as the main nutrition problem has shifted from undernutrition to overweight and obesity. Public concern for the program has focused on whether it is contributing to the growing problem of childhood obesity and on the quality of foods available to schoolchildren . . . issues at the federal level include how to help school meal providers improve the nutritional quality of foods served . . ."

The same USDA that encourages us to join our children for lunch is hostage to the dairy and meat industry and agribusiness interests, which have heavily influenced federal regulations governing school meals. The above quote all but says, "Our hands are tied," and while recent federal child wellness initiatives sound promising, many of the current reforms lack adequate funding.

How Does It Work?

Despite its many flaws, the National School Lunch Program is one of the most successful public welfare programs in the United States. It's a federally mandated program that was signed into law in 1946 by President Harry S. Truman. According to the USDA, the program now operates in 99 percent of the public schools in the U.S. and it feeds 31.6 million children (about half of all schoolchildren) daily in over 101,000 public and nonprofit private schools. Sixty percent of those children receive their meals free or at a reduced price. The remaining children pay somewhere between $1.50 and $3.50 for a USDA-approved school lunch. Public or nonprofit private K–12 schools are eligible to participate, as are nonprofit nursery schools and day care programs. Schools are required to file monthly reports stating the number of eligible meals they are claiming for reimbursement. The federal reimbursement rates per meal as of November 2010 are $2.72 for a free lunch, $2.32 for a reduced price lunch, and 26 cents for a paid lunch. Recent federal legislation promises to raise those reimbursement rates by 6 cents per meal. Snacks are currently reimbursed at rates of 74 cents, 37 cents, and 6 cents, respectively. The school meals program costs taxpayers about $9.3 billion in school year 2010–2011.

The U.S. Department of Agriculture's Food and Nutrition Service (FNS) is the department that administers the school meals programs. In addition to the National School Lunch Program, the department also administers the School Breakfast Program (serving 11 million children), the Fresh Fruit and Vegetable Program, the Special Milk Program (for schools that don't participate in NSLP), and the Team Nutrition initiative (nutrition education and food service training), along with a number of other public assistance food programs such as the SNAP program (food stamps) and the WIC program (Women, Infants, and Children). The FNS also provides senior meal programs and summer feeding programs for children.

The Fresh Fruit and Vegetable Program is a collaboration between the USDA and the Department of Defense (DOD). These two agencies are the superpowers of institutional food—the DOD is the world's largest institutional meal provider, supplying food to the U.S. Armed Services, and the school meals program is the second largest. With access to DOD's purchasing power and distribution infrastructure, the Fresh Fruit and Vegetable Program provides a small but cost-effective stipend for the school meals program—$1.5 million in school year 2010–2011. It's meant to supplement districts with a high number of children eligible for free meals and is intended to result in an additional $50 to $75 per-student annual allocation for fresh food.

Free Lunch

Also known as Provision 2, a school district may be granted Universal Free Meal status and claim a 100 percent reimbursement rate in areas with a high eligibility rate for free meals. The provision is meant to reduce paperwork and administrative costs for the district. It also helps to reduce stigma for students and their families. Schools are only required to collect applications for free meals once every four years at most. Schools then are reimbursed at the federal rate for every meal provided. According to USDA regulations, any school that participates in the federal meal program may apply for Provision 2, although generally schools with 75 percent or more low-income students actually take advantage of the option. Schools that utilize Provision 2 are responsible for making up the shortfall between the reimbursement rate and the actual cost of the meals served. The School Nutrition Association estimates actual meal costs are 35 to 45 cents higher per meal than the reimbursement rate. Schools may receive additional funds from the state or local district.

TIM CIPRIANO, THE LOCAL FOOD DUDE

Prior to 2008, the New Haven, Connecticut, school meals program had been outsourced to Aramark, one of several food service management companies that vie for the school lunch market across the country. The troubled program had a deficit of close to three million dollars, and unrest between the unionized school food service workers and the management company was making local headlines. New Haven's active Food Policy Council decided to bring the lunch program back in-house under new leadership. By hiring a chef nicknamed the Local Food Dude, the council was sending a message that they were ready for some changes. Tim went back to basics. As a high-poverty district, New Haven was already serving Universal Free Meals to its students. Tim gets the standard federal reimbursement for every meal served, plus a stipend of 14.5 cents per meal from the state of Connecticut for complying with the state's healthy school meals requirements. In April of his first year, Tim stopped selling all competitive items except water. "We want our students to eat a nutritious reimbursable meal instead of snacks. The majority of our students qualify for free and reduced meals and by selling snacks we are basically taking food off of the dinner table at home so the kids can be cool like their friends. I don't want to be the guy taking food away from hungry families, so we removed all snacks."

(continued)

What I saw in Tim's lunchroom reminded me a lot of my school lunch from the 1960s. A simple pasta with meat sauce that looked and smelled good was accompanied by a side of decent-looking broccoli, a small apple, and a carton of white milk. The kids were eating the food. Almost all of it, including the apple and broccoli. Instead of the washable hard plastic trays of my childhood, each student had a recyclable/biodegradable sectioned cardboard tray. The lunchroom itself was sun-filled and clean with a noise level that enabled us to carry on a conversation.

The New Haven schools educate 20,000 students each year and Tim says he's feeding about 17,000 of them each day. Participation in the lunch program has gone up. He's now serving over 300,000 more meals per year than the district served with Aramark. As a result, revenue has gone up by $800,000 and expenses went down by the same amount. Tim has brought the deficit down by almost half and is working to find ways to save money and provide better-quality ingredients. "We were basically losing money to provide junk food to kids. Even with the snacks meeting the Connecticut Nutrition Standards the snacks were still junk. We want to feed our children healthy foods all the time but we also realize the importance of eating a good breakfast. Our menus aren't perfect and we struggle with breakfast and the fine line between feeding hungry children and feeding these children breakfast foods with less sugar. We are working with a local bakery to develop a whole-grain breakfast bread and we are meeting with food manufacturers to reduce the sugar in their popular cereals. Our sweet cereals are now required to be 9 grams or less of sugar per serving. We want to see that number drastically reduced and are challenging the industry to produce a great tasting, kid-friendly product with low sugar. Sugar is sugar, whether it's HFCS, brown rice syrup, dehydrated cane juice . . . it's not needed."

One way Tim is economizing is by preparing most of the district's meals in a large central kitchen. The facility is well equipped, although not all the staff is trained to use it. "When I started here two years ago I couldn't bring my team with me, so it's taking some time. It makes sense to spend money on training to get us going but we don't have the money to get started." New Haven is fortunate to have the Yale Sustainable Food Project nearby; as part of their community outreach they train six to twelve of Tim's cooks each year. "They are lined up wanting to do it, but I have two hundred workers, so it's gonna take a long time to cycle all those employees through the program." Tim is working all the angles to get the funding or in-kind services he needs for his district. One of his goals is for the district's schools to meet the HealthierUS Schools Challenge that mandates stricter nutrition requirements and comes with a financial incentive.

He's taking advantage of a five-year grant to bring in a nutritionist with culinary skills to help devise menus that will address the rigorous requirements as well as cater to children with food allergies and other special dietary needs. "And include more beans in the menu. This year we've already brought in 140,000 pounds of produce from Connecticut. Double that if you count fresh produce from the region. It amounts to about 15 percent of our produce." I asked Tim about the commodity program, if he'd rather have the cash instead. "Nothing would really change if the USDA gave us the money instead of the commodities. I would still want to support American farmers. No one is now overseeing who we order from. We can order vegetables from Chile if we want, but why should we be spending federal funds to support Chilean farmers?" Tim is also a realist. When he started as a food service director, he tried ordering whole, eight-cut chicken, what he referred to as "in the brown box" from the USDA. He soon learned that he didn't always get what he asked for when requesting whole commodity items. "If I order the processed products, they get allocated to me and I don't come up short. So what we get is a chicken patty—chopped and formed. I have no idea what's in them but we're always looking for a better product. We look for items that have the best yield [from before to after processing]—like 90 percent. Those beef crumbles have a yield like 150 percent, so you know there's something else in there. The USDA is working with us more and more to tackle these things."

One idea Tim has is to try to get quinoa, a high-protein grain, into the commodity program. He'd like to see it processed into flour to use in a pizza dough so they could put less cheese on the pizza.

During our conversation, a teacher recognized Chef Tim and complained about a boy who had brought his own lunch but wanted a carton of milk.

(continued)

In order to get the milk for free, the boy would have to take a whole meal. "He's just going to throw the food away. It's a waste!" That's USDA regulations at work. In this case though, nothing was wasted. As we watched, the boy handed off the tray of food to a friend who was still hungry. Chef Tim is working hard to end hunger in New Haven, and that challenge doesn't always mesh perfectly with his mission as the Local Food Dude. He's hoping that updated government regulations will make his job a bit easier. "What I'm doing now makes me the black sheep, the bad guy—'Oh he's trying to make our jobs more difficult.' But then Uncle Sam says, Well, this is what you need to do—then I have all these allies that come out of nowhere and they want to help, or they want me to help them, and we're all working as a team again. So I think its good that the feds are coming together to really take more control over the programs and it just helps us as the people who are doing it already."

School Food History

So do we need more regulations or fewer? That seems to be a constant political debate in America, especially these days. In order to understand both sides of this debate as it pertains to school food, you have to understand the structure of the National School Lunch Program, and for that, we need a little history lesson. There are histories of school food dating back to the eighteenth century in Europe. One of the most comprehensive early programs began in the city of Paris in 1877. Its inception is credited to the beloved author Victor Hugo, who had been previously exiled for his populist sentiments. The program provided a midday meal for all the schoolchildren of Paris. The city paid the tab for the needy majority; those who could pay did so. Hugo invented a system of lunch tickets, which were distributed to all children so that there would be no social stigma for the poor. This system worked well to encourage participation by all—something we could use as a lesson for today's American meal program.

In the early days of school in America (and even when I was a kid!), many students went home for lunch. (On a recent trip to Barcelona, Spain, I learned that kids in that city still return home at midday.) In rural areas school was too far from home, so usually children would bring a lunch pail to school. During the industrial revolution in America, immigrants arrived who couldn't feed their families as they had been accustomed, more students were concentrated in cities, and more families abandoned their farming backgrounds. As a result, dietary deficiencies among children became a focus of welfare organizations, social scientists, and the government. The Children's Aid Society of New York created the first free lunch program, in 1853, and that organization continues to feed New York City's needy children and teach them about food and nutrition today.

Social service organizations and schools teamed up to serve school meals in both cities and rural areas for the next hundred years. In the early 1900s, many schools, even those in cities, had vegetable gardens tended by students. An entertaining Library of Congress video shows the history of school gardens, which were considered an integral part of educating, nourishing, and providing fresh air, character building, nature study, and exercise for students. There are even tales of schools that kept cows for milk and chickens for eggs. In those days the gardens weren't considered quaint or avant-garde, they were merely a practical solution to raising food for malnourished students. Teachers reported rapid improvements in students' academic performance when they had access to school meals.

The following quote comes from a World War I treatise on the importance of healthy school food, but it could just as easily have been written today:

The expensive machinery of education is wasted when it operates on a mind listless from hunger or befogged by indigestible food. Whether the cause be poverty, ignorance, or carelessness, the child is the sufferer, and the painstaking work of the school lunch supervisors to secure wholesome and adequate noon meals for the schoolchildren at a minimum cost not only brings immediate benefit to the children, but exerts a widespread influence upon homes and parents, as the children carry to them reports of these concrete lessons in the science of proper selection, preparation, and hygiene of food.

Menu items included such staples as baked beans, vegetable soup, macaroni, creamed beef, milk or cocoa, and crackers or ice cream. Very often children were chosen to help serve the food to their peers in the lunch line. One early example from New York City describes a system where children had to first select a cup of soup before they could choose from the other items offered that day.

While child hunger was a chronic problem in America, the Great Depression caused an even greater increase in malnutrition among children and an increased demand for school feeding programs. In 1936, the government stepped in and began supplying excess farm commodities to schools. Yet as the Depression-era children came of military age during World War II, 150,000 young men were rejected due to nutrition-related health problems including rickets, pellagra, beriberi, and dental diseases. The poor constitution of the recruits that were enlisted accounts for 150,000 deaths that were ascribed to disease rather than battle.

During the war, the USDA paid farmers to grow crops to feed our hungry army. At the end of World War II, the government saw a win-win in the notion of feeding the nation's children while supporting farmers by continuing to boost the market for surplus agricultural commodities like wheat, corn, rice, eggs, milk, and meat. A 1946 Congressional Committee on Agriculture report stated:

> The need for a permanent legislative basis for a school lunch program, rather than operating it on a year-to-year basis, or one dependent solely on agricultural surpluses that for a child may be nutritionally unbalanced or nutritionally unattractive, has now become apparent. The national school lunch bill provides basic, comprehensive legislation for aid, in general, to the states in the operation of school lunch programs as permanent and integral parts of their school systems. . . . Such aid, heretofore extended by Congress through the Department of Agriculture has, for the past ten years, proven for exceptional benefit to the children, schools, and agriculture of the country as whole, but the necessity for now coordinating the work throughout the nation, and especially to encourage and increase the financial participation and active

control by the several states, makes it desirable that permanent enabling leg-islation take the place of the present temporary legislative structure. . . . The educational features of a properly chosen diet served at school should not be under-emphasized. Not only is the child taught what a good diet consists of, but his parents and family likewise are indirectly instructed.

In 1946, the ad hoc school meal programs were united under the compre-hensive National School Lunch Program with the declaration, "It is hereby declared to be the policy of Congress, as a measure of national security, to safeguard the health and well-being of the Nation's children and to encour-age domestic consumption of nutritious agricultural commodities and other food by assisting the states, through grants-in-aid and other means, in pro-viding an adequate supply of food and other facilities for the establishment, maintenance, operation, and expansion of nonprofit school lunch programs." In addition to surplus commodity items, the Child Nutrition Act provided funds for nonsurplus foods and required that meals be based on tested nutri-tional standards. Meals had to be offered to all children without discrimina-tion of any type and accountability, though record-keeping and reporting was required.

Since then, the act has been amended to add additional programs as men-tioned above, but the centerpiece of the legislation, and by far its largest com-ponent, is still the National School Lunch Program, which oversees more than 5.5 billion lunches a year.

Compliance

The federal guidelines for the lunch program (known as a Type A meal) have not changed much since the program was implemented. The 2010 Child Nutrition reauthorization takes the childhood obesity crisis into account by requiring both minimum and maximum calorie limits, as well as limits on sodium. Also new is the ruling that half of all grains must be from whole-grain sources and food labels must read 0 grams of trans fats per serving (less than .5 grams). However, upper limits on fat have gone from no more than 30 percent of the calories from fat to a new maximum of 35 percent, with less than 10 percent from saturated fat. Permitting more fat content is a response to complaints from food service directors that they were obliged to make up calories with sugary items in order to comply with the previous limits on fat. However, whole milk has been banned in favor of low-fat or fat-free milk, with sugary chocolate and strawberry flavors still allowed. In addition, meals must provide a proper balance of protein, vitamin A, vitamin C, iron, calcium, and calories.

Five key meal components must be served:

- 1 serving of meat or meat alternate
- 2 servings of fruits or vegetables
- 1 serving of grains
- 1 serving of fluid milk
- The actual foods served are the discretion of local school food authorities. In order to comply with these requirements, schools may choose one of three different methods to arrive at the proper proportions and serving sizes.

"Traditional Food-Based Menu Planning and Enhanced Food-Based Menu Planning" means that meals must be composed of specific quantities of meat or meat alternate, vegetable or fruit, grains or bread, and milk. The enhanced version requires each grade level to have slightly larger portions. The traditional option prescribes specified amounts for each food group but does not regulate different quantities per grade level. Only schools that have been participating in the lunch program prior to the 1994–1995 school year may use the traditional option.

"Nutrient Standard Menu Planning" requires the use of USDA-approved computer software that analyzes the nutrient content of each recipe in a week's worth of meals. Meals must meet the requirements when averaged over a week's time. This method seems more cumbersome, but actually allows for more flexibility—a meal light in one nutrient may be compensated for by a bit of excess in another day's menu.

Another term you may hear kicked about in school food service lingo is "offer versus serve." Many schools subscribe to this method of service because it cuts down on food waste. Offer versus serve means that a student purchasing or receiving a reimbursable meal must be offered all five components of the complete meal but may choose to refuse one or two of the items. As long as the student has at least three of the items on his or her tray, the lunch qualifies as a reimbursable meal.

Access

Children from families with incomes at or below 130 percent of the poverty level (for school year 2010–2011, 130 percent of the poverty level is $28,665 for a family of four) are entitled to free school meals. This is a tiered system whereby those with incomes between 130 percent and 185 percent of the poverty level are eligible for reduced-price meals (185 percent is $40,793), for which students can be charged no more than 40 cents. School breakfast and snack programs follow the same income guidelines, and in districts with more than 75 percent of children eligible for free meals, Universal Free Breakfast and Lunch may be provided. Each student on the free meal program brings a subsidy of more than $500 to the district per year.

Children receiving food stamps or other public assistance are eligible for direct certification, meaning they do not have to fill out an application for free lunch. As of 2010, roughly one-fifth of local education agencies had not yet implemented a system of direct certification as required by federal law.

All eligible children living in the United States, regardless of citizenship status, are entitled to take advantage of the National School Lunch Program.

It's incumbent on school districts to ensure that every eligible child applies for the meal program in order to receive the maximum funding for the school's meal program. In addition to school meals, the free and reduced-price qualification also leverages funding for academic assistance, library telecommunication services, summer and after-school snack and meal programs, and support from other public and private foundations.

Entitlement Foods

These are the USDA agricultural surplus foods that are doled out to schools on a per-child basis. For school year 2010–2011 a school received about 20 to 25 cents' worth of commodities for every meal served. Some schools I visited were able to request cash instead of commodity items. This isn't true for every school in the program; those that joined the program prior to the 1994–1995 school year are "grandfathered in," meaning they retain the choice while schools that joined more recently don't. Even so, many of the schools that have the option prefer the commodities because they claim to get better value from the commodity items. As discussed in chapter two, most of today's commodity items are sent to a processor before they reach the schools. Peanut butter arrives laden with hydrogenated oils, salt, and sugar added. Meat is generally very low grade and high in saturated fat. Most of the fruit is canned and contains added sugars, and most of the grains are not whole grains. The USDA is now making attempts to offer a greater variety of healthier commodity food items.

Not only do school food operators get value for the commodity products, they also get convenience. Many of the commodity items sent to food processors are delivered to schools in single-serve portions. These portioned products are stamped "CN (Child Nutrution)" compliant, meaning they meet the USDA nutritional guidelines for school food. The operator doesn't have to calculate their nutritional value—it's all on the label. The convenience foods reduce on-site labor needs, and permit the use of low-skilled cheaper workers instead of a skilled cooking staff.

Ketchup as a Vegetable

Several forces have conspired to degrade the National School Lunch Program and, along with it, the school food environment. Expansion, without commensurate funding increases, took place for decades. Beginning in the 1960s, President Lyndon Johnson, as part of his War on Poverty, added school breakfast to the program. America, the richest nation in the world, had a poverty rate of 19 percent at that time (in 2009 the poverty rate was 14.3 percent). The 1970s and 1980s saw day care and summer school food programs added to the package, while funding and other resources for what had once been a fully funded mandate eventually became stretched beyond limit. A Reagan administration directive that would have reclassified ketchup and relish as vegetables, allowing public schools to cut out a serving of cooked or fresh vegetables, epitomized these budget cuts. The Reagan White House estimated that the measure would result in an annual budgetary savings of $1 billion, but the proposal was loudly protested and never went into effect. School systems suffered budget cuts in educational resources as well, and most required their lunch programs to break even.

As costs for food items and lunch staff increased, district managers began looking for new models to fix their school meal finances, and many turned to selling unregulated competitive foods as a revenue stream. Students became customers, and the school cafeteria became a business. Rodney Taylor, a school food service director in Riverside, California, tells me, "Businessmen were brought in to use their creative thinking. Generate money, grow the business, be self-sufficient. So we brought in the McDonald's, the Taco Bells, the Pizza Huts. And we were innovative and we were successful. School district nutrition programs are a lot more healthy financially." The first half of the dual mission of the NSLP, "to safeguard the health and well-being of the nation's children," was conveniently ignored as we turned our children from students to consumers.

REALITY—JAMIE, THEN JOHN, IN WEST VIRGINIA

For those of you who don't watch TV, a quick recap on Jamie Oliver, aka the Naked Chef. Jamie's a British restaurateur who has had several successful television cooking shows and published numerous cookbooks. He's scruffily charismatic, like the doggy from the shelter that you just can't resist, and his U.S. TV series and campaign, *Jamie Oliver's Food Revolution*, has become a lightning rod for the school food movement. The Emmy-winning series created a lot of media buzz about school food in America, and Jamie's petition for better food in schools drew more than 600,000 signatures. The first season depicts what happens when a British chef with lofty ideas about feeding children real food attempts to transform a school cafeteria staffed by American lunch ladies who don't like to be bossed around. Along the way he works with a family addicted to junk food, converts the local radio DJ, and recruits a group of high schoolers to help market his healthy fare.

In addition to the ubiquitous lack of funds, Jamie's greatest obstacle for most of the series is the head lunch lady, Alice. The drama turns on winning over Alice, which after a predictable albeit satisfying head-to-head confrontation, he does. The district's food service director, Rhonda, proves to be an even tougher nut to crack. Though she seems somewhat supportive of Oliver's efforts, viewers may wonder whether she's responsible for restocking the cartons of chocolate milk that he's gone to great pains to remove from the lunch line. When he confronts Rhonda, she patiently explains that the milk is required by USDA regulations and that it's more likely kids will drink it if it's flavored—i.e., full of sugar. She also tells him that the chicken nuggets and other commodity junk foods are stockpiled and must be used up in order to stay within the district's budget. In the final moments of the final episode, Jamie turns to the camera for his revelation, and the cliff-hanger for season two: he realizes that he can't fix school food until he confronts the USDA!

In the aftermath of the cameras, chef John Turenne and his crew from Sustainable Food Systems continued to train the lunch ladies in the twenty-six schools of Cabell County, West Virginia. I asked John about the commodity food situation in that state. "West Virginia is tough," he reports. "We want to see whole-muscle chicken as opposed to nuggets or patties. Most food service directors don't usually ask for it, so it's not readily available. I had an opportunity to meet with the governor last year. I walked into the meeting with a plate that had a processed chicken patty and a whole chicken drumstick on it. I said, 'I need your help. We can't stop these [chicken patties] from coming in even though the USDA says we have those [chicken drumsticks].' The governor asked his people to help figure this out."

Apparently the governor had some influence and the whole chicken has now made its way into the cafeteria, for the most part. A year later, John went back to Huntington for a visit. He saw Alice and Rhonda and "all the girls at Central City." "They are executing a lot of recipes that we put in. However, Rhonda still had a lot of commodity food that she ordered last January. The day we went, we saw whole rotisserie chicken and real baked potato wedges, but the next day could be those commodity nuggets. We brought the lunch program from a very low grade to something much higher. Maybe they've gone down a notch or two, but they're way better than they were."

Back when I interviewed John for my movie, he had recently transformed a Yale dining hall and a private school cafeteria. In those environments, eager administrators and community members had encouraged him to go organic, and local, and cook from scratch and despite the challenges, his new programs had received accolades. John's Confucius-like response to my question "What advice do you have for parents?" at that time was simply, "If you want this, ask for it." After working in the public schools of West Virginia, he's amended his answer a bit. "Parents and community stakeholders need to take charge and not only ask for it, but help facilitate getting folks like me in the door to simply explain to school boards, superintendents, and school food administrators that improvement to the food can be done in a nurturing and responsible manner. Then, usually these stakeholders agree to allow our help. Then the parents sometimes have to fund-raise to cover our consultation services."

Subverted Subsidies

The second part of the lunch program's stated mission, "to encourage domestic consumption of nutritious agricultural commodities," was also diluted
over time by input from interests that were becoming more industrial than
agricultural. In the 1970s, Secretary of Agriculture Earl Butz proclaimed a
farming policy of "get big or get out." He told farmers to "adapt or die" and
family farms were quickly wiped off the map, replaced by giant agribusiness
conglomerates. The surviving farms were no longer diversified. Fields of
soybeans and corn were planted "fencerow to fencerow" and CAFOs (Concentrated Animal Feeding Operations) became the standard for chicken,
pork, and beef production. In 1940, 23 percent of Americans lived on farms;
today barely 1 percent of us are farmers. Those farm subsidies that were so
successful during and after World War II continue today, but the subsidies
that were once meant to help small farmers now support Big Food. The
USDA now props up the mass production of commodities like corn, soy,
and their derivatives—high fructose corn syrup, hydrogenated soybean oil,
grain-fed factory farmed beef, and so on. As a result, the surplus government
commodities supplied by the USDA are not in balance with their own stated
child nutrition guidelines.

Food policy professor Marion Nestle tells me, "The USDA could be doing
a much better job but the USDA was established to promote American agriculture. That's what its main mission has always been. When the pressure
started coming on the USDA to provide healthy meals, the USDA went into
a conflict of interest. It can't really be an agency that is meant to promote the
consumption of American sugars and American beef and be in a situation
where it's providing menus that cut down on high fat meats and cut down on
sugars. So it's stuck between a rock and a hard place. So this is politics. And
it's the ugliest kind of politics being fought over our kids' health."

For an active young man, the USDA's Federal Nutrition Recommendations (as of early 2011), known as the food pyramid, call for 10 ounces of grain
per day, 6.5 cups of fruits and vegetables, 3 cups of milk, and 7 ounces of animal

or vegetable protein daily with sugar, oil, and salt in sparing amounts. Yet from 1995 to 2005, our Farm Bill allotted 74 percent of government agricultural subsidies to meat and dairy outfits, 13 percent for grains, 10 percent for sugar, oil, starch, and alcohol production, 1.9 percent for nuts and legumes, and a mere .37 percent went to subsidize fruits and vegetables. This inverse subsidy pyramid explains why it's cheaper to buy a burger than a salad at most fast-food restaurants.

In 1946, the surplus commodities added much-needed calories, vitamins, and protein to an insufficient diet. Today, commodity and subsidized food products are a major contributing factor to the overfeeding and undernourishment of America's schoolchildren.

Food Costs

While it may sound simple enough to meet the USDA basic nutrition requirements, it gets more complicated with only $1 per meal for food costs, which is the national average left over once staff and other fixed costs have been paid. In St. Louis that amount was about 78 cents when I visited in 2008; some districts have a few cents more. Milk is a required item and not donated as a commodity, so roughly 25 cents of each dollar must be subtracted for milk costs. Fat is limited by the regulations, but meals must meet a minimum calorie count. Food service directors seeking cheap calories often end up adding an inexpensive sugary commodity item to the meal just to meet the calorie requirement.

I've met a lot of lunch ladies and they all tell me how hard it is to make a meal that meets the USDA standards. Those requirements seemed so minimal to me that I was skeptical—how difficult could it be? So I tried my own experiment. Using a free online nutrition calculator, I punched in some of our family's favorite simple dinner recipes. Proudly, I discovered that our meals were low in fat, high in nutrients. Next, I added up the cost for dinner for four, then calculated per person cost per meal. Our vegetarian quinoa pasta dinner came in at $1 per serving—right on target! Each of the other four dinners cost between $2.50 and $3 per person. I fiddled with the recipes, reducing the ground turkey and adding more beans to the tacos, swapping the fresh salmon for frozen cod, and got the food costs down to between $1.75 and $2 each. Not bad considering I'm paying retail prices, using mostly organic ingredients, and not using any free commodities. I was beginning to feel smug. Then I noticed there was virtually no vitamin D in any of our recipes. Recent studies show that nearly every American is deficient in vitamin D, and it's required by USDA standards, so fortified milk or some other supplement (we take cod liver oil all winter) really seems necessary. Next, I checked on the calories. Crestfallen, I realized that my meals provided a mere 350 to 500 calories each. The minimum calorie requirements for a teenager are 1,800 to 2,000 a day. We're not big milk drinkers, but for my experiment I added a cup of whole milk to the count. I was still okay with the fat, closer on the vitamin D, and much closer to the calorie target. The milk would add another 25 cents per meal to the budget, though. What could I do to get those last few calories? Fruit! I hadn't included a dessert in my meal, and a serving of fruit would get me where I wanted to be. In season, I could get a local apple for about 25 cents. Between the milk and the fruit, I just added another 50 cents to the price of my meal. Maybe I could sell some Pop-Tarts to help cover the extra costs? Okay, lunch ladies—you're right, it's impossible. And in fact, almost all the experts agree, a realistic number for food cost would be somewhere between $1.75 and $2 per meal, minus the value of subsidized commodity items.

The price of a school lunch may vary greatly from one district to another. In Watertown, Massachusetts, parents complained that they're paying $3 at the elementary school and $3.50 for lunch at the middle school and high school while other area schools charge less. This disparity may be caused by several factors. The reimbursement rate for a free or reduced price meal only covers about 82 percent of the meal, and schools have to find some way to make up the shortfall, sometimes by charging more to their paying customers. Watertown has a higher number of low-income families, so the school lunch service provides more free lunches. And while most administrators expect their lunch programs to be self-sufficient, their definitions may vary.

Equipment purchases and repairs may or may not be included in the lunch program's budget; some districts pay for food service employee benefits like health insurance while others don't, and some districts mandate better-quality food, which costs more. A study of three hundred school districts in Minnesota, published in the *Review of Agricultural Economics* in 2007, revealed that indirect costs paid by school nutrition programs to the districts negatively affect the quality of the meals. These indirect costs may vary from district to district. Some districts charge the lunch programs for electricity, custodial services, garbage removal, and so on, all of which adds to the cost of the program and takes money away from food quality and staffing.

The researchers also observed that the quality of meals is limited by equipment, training, and processes utilized to prepare the meals, not by student demand or per-meal costs. Therefore they recommended that more money be spent on capital investment for kitchens, equipment, and other resources that would streamline the preparation process.

At the State Level

At the state level, the state board of education usually administers the school meals program. A handful of states house child nutrition services in their departments of health and social services or state department of agriculture. Each state department of school nutrition services must administer the program and report meal counts to the USDA on a monthly basis. The state then distributes reimbursement funds back to the school districts. The states also select commodity foods from a list of foods purchased by the USDA and choose what food will be sent to a processor before being offered to local district school food authorities. States also receive periodic bonus foods from the USDA, which they in turn may distribute to local districts based upon available quantities. In addition to monitoring local school food authorities' performance and adherence to nutritional standards, state agencies are also in charge of providing technical assistance to schools in the form of training materials and templates.

States are also required to make a minimal contribution to the school meals program. In order to receive federal reimbursements, each state must cough up an amount equal to 30 percent of the funds they received in 1980. The funds are frozen at 1980 levels, so these contributions only amount to 5 percent or less of today's budgets. For states with a per capita income below the national average, the match is decreased by a corresponding percentage.

While it may seem as though states are just acting as a pass-through for the federal program, there's actually plenty of opportunity to advocate for better food in schools on the state level. According to the Health Policy Tracking Service, in 2005 there were nearly two hundred individual bills introduced to raise nutrition standards in forty states. About half the states had nutrition standards that were higher than the federal standards prior to the 2010 Child Nutrition Act reauthorization.

California and Texas prohibit or strictly limit fried foods and foods containing artificial trans fats. Other states have banned candy, soda, and sweetened beverages and other sugary snacks during the school day. In Mississippi, the 2007 Healthy Student Act limits choices and mandates serving a variety of fruits and vegetables on weekly menus. I notice a lot of states going in the direction of restricting certain ingredients (fat, sugar, etc.) more than they're mandating serving healthier whole foods. This type of "banning" reinforces the myth that food advocacy is a front for nutrition Nazis, and always invites a large helping of media backlash. It's easier to complain about taking away the fries than it is to complain about having to choose between orange quarters or a small apple instead of the Fruit Roll-Up. In March 2010, Massachusetts passed some of the strongest school nutrition legislation to date. The law requires standards for all food sold in schools, including competitive foods and vending machines. The bill bans deep-fried food and seeks to replace it with more fresh fruits and vegetables and require the purchase of local, farm-fresh produce wherever possible. School district administrators don't always welcome this type of state legislation because it doesn't usually come with all the necessary funding.

A number of states have lists of approved snack items that can be sold in vending machines. One such list is published by the John C. Stalker Institute of Food and Nutrition. Their "A-List of 'Acceptable' Vending Items" offers convenience to food service staff by listing items by product name and manufacturer. The list contains items that are lower in fat and sugar than most vending fare, and some items that are minimally processed, however, I found plenty of items on this list that have minimal nutritional value.

Some states have also passed bills aimed at assessing the BMI (body mass index) or physical fitness of students. These types of assessments can be stigmatizing for kids and I don't personally like the idea. Then again, my children have always had their vision tested at school and were screened for scoliosis, so some type of fitness assessment may become the new normal.

ALTERED STATE: BETH LOVERIDGE

When her daughter came home in tears after being called a nerd for bringing a healthy lunch to school, Beth Loveridge got angry. So angry, as well as weary of the concrete and traffic of Dallas, that she moved her family to the small peninsula town of Port Angeles, Washington. Here, Beth hoped that she and her family could be part of the community without having to make so many compromises. The move wasn't just about the Lunchables, but school food advocacy became a symbol of the possibilities of Beth's new life.

Beth found the school food environment in her children's new school district to be not much different from the one in Texas. Though her attempts to make change in Dallas had been thwarted, she dutifully started over in her new district. The meetings were slow and frustrating but Beth persevered. She knew she needed allies, so when she heard about *Two Angry Moms*, she quickly bought a bunch of DVDs and began hosting screenings at local libraries in her district and then all around the area. She tells me, "The *Two Angry Moms* movie was key for me because it was a tool to find out who else out there was interested in changing school food, because I knew I couldn't do it myself. Once I pushed the button to buy the movie, I knew I was committed. And then others started showing the movie. A gal out of Port Townsend recently showed it at the local movie theater. She invited school board members and

(continued)

got over a hundred people. So now we have a large e-mail list and I have this foundation of folks to keep me going."

At the movie screenings, Beth met up with some local VIPs. One of them, Kia from Nash's Organic Produce, invited her to a meeting where they were writing a nutrition policy. Kia wanted her fresh produce written into the policy, Beth explains. "This is a farming community. We see thousands of pounds of produce shipped off our peninsula and we get the Sysco truck. This promoted some interest from the press."

The Washington State Environmental Council got wind of Beth's efforts and tied the school food initiative to a bill supporting local farmers. "From there, the Local Farms–Healthy Kids legislation was proposed at the state level and Kia and I and a group of us went down to Olympia and lobbied our senators down there. We showed the whole state school board the movie and asked them to adopt a resolution in favor of this legislation. That meant adopting at the state level a Farm to School program."

The legislation was passed in March 2008. By mandating a preference for local food, the bill makes it possible for schools to obtain locally grown produce, even if the local producer's bid is not the lowest. It included funding for state department of agriculture staff to coordinate a Farm to School program with the state departments of public instruction and health. These staffers work with the farmers to help them market to the schools, and they work with the schools to provide curriculum on the nutritional and environmental benefits of consuming locally grown food. The Washington-Grown Fresh Fruit and Vegetable program was funded to provide snacks for low-income students. The legislation also authorizes schools to grow food for consumption in their meal programs, an issue that is sometimes in contention with local health regulations. Numerous publications credited the hard work of Beth Loveridge as the key to getting the bill passed.

"When I moved us up here it was a big change of life to get away from pollution and live in a community that's not based on fear of being run over or kidnapped. In Dallas I spoke to the school board about getting Cokes out of school. They were sitting on top of this dais and it was like speaking to the angels on high. You had to speak into a microphone in a hall equipped with

TV monitors. Here in Washington, the board were spitting distance away and smiled and nodded and asked us to be more specific and showed community support. They listened and put language into policy and they acted."

Enacting the state policy has been a challenge. A skewed distribution system makes the local produce more costly, even when produce from Washington State may be the least costly choice for a school in New York City! The law has spurred progress throughout Washington State, though. An Associated Press article from September 2010 reports:

Olympia spends 30 percent of its produce budget buying directly from local farms. La Conner students drink smoothies made from local strawberries and eat apples from the Skagit Valley. Food services manager Georgia Johnson said the district is hoping to buy its own cows next year, raise them on a Samish Island farm, and use them for meat.

The Auburn School District spent about $100,000 of its produce budget last year with Terra Organics, a Tacoma-area farm known for its home-delivered produce boxes. . . . The district got all of its potatoes from local farms, and served other produce. They also get produce fresh from their own school garden.

Too Fat to Fight

If there ever was a bipartisan issue, school food could be it. If liberals champion healthy food as a right for every child, conservatives argue the case from the national security angle. As was the case during World War I and World War II, America needs able-bodied soldiers. In September 2010, more than one hundred retired generals and admirals published an open letter to Congress elucidating the latest threat to American security and prosperity. Explains retired U.S. Army General Johnnie E. Wilson, "Child obesity has become so serious in this country that military leaders are viewing this epidemic as a potential threat to our national security. We need America's

service members to be in excellent physical condition because they have
such an important job to do. Rigorous service standards are critical if we
are to maintain the fighting readiness of our military." Only 25 percent of
today's young adults meet the physical fitness requirements for military service. The generals' report estimates that 9 million young adults, 27 percent
of all Americans age seventeen to twenty-four, are too overweight to join the
military. This, despite the fact that the military standard for body fat was
lowered in 2006 in order to encourage more recruits. The report declares,
"Improving nutrition in the nation's schools is a critical and necessary step to
combating obesity among young adults. We are calling on Congress to pass
new child nutrition legislation that would (a) get the junk food out of our
schools; (b) support increased funding to improve nutritional standards and
the quality of meals served in schools; and (c) provide more children access
to effective programs that cut obesity."

It was defense nutrition that founded the school nutrition program, and it
may well have been defense nutrition that motivated Congress to make the
recent changes to the reauthorization of the program.

The USDA Trilemma

According to the USDA's own analysis of the NSLP, the program faces a
"school meal trilemma involving the meal's nutrition, program cost, and
student participation in the program." The report states, "This trilemma
applies to competitive foods as well because revenues from these foods can
be important to the budgets of both the cafeteria and the school as a whole.
A change to one component of the trilemma can have unintentional effects
on either or both of the other components. . . . To defray costs, many schools,
and sometimes, the school food service itself, depend on revenues from
competitive foods, even though such foods have been found to contribute to
overconsumption of calories, increased plate waste of nutritionally balanced
NSLP lunches, and decreased intakes of nutrients by students. . . . Several
studies show that schools could reduce the fat content of foods offered and

increase consumption of underconsumed foods, such as milk and vegetables, while still maintaining revenue levels and NSLP participation levels. This can be done by exposing students to new foods, updating menus, changing the way food is presented, and providing nutrition education."

The trilemma always feeds back to lack of funding. To sum up—shortfalls in the NSLP cause school food authorities to sell competitive foods. Kids prefer the à la carte, unhealthy, fast food–style items. The kids who can afford it don't eat the school meal, so sales drop further. Food service directors try to make the reimbursable meal more like fast food, so they use processed commodity items. Kids eat the junkier foods and get fat and sick. The USDA's self-described trilemma is a self-fulfilling prophecy. As you'll see in chapters five and six, districts that are taking a sustainable approach to school food are finding creative ways to achieve a healthy bottom line and a healthy food environment.

The St. Paul, Minnesota, public schools serve more than 46,000 meals daily. The district is now an oft-cited model, as the percentage of kids eating school meals has increased since the district started eliminating junk food, offering more fruit and vegetables and healthier proteins. These increased sales have increased revenues, offsetting the higher cost of better-quality food.

Institute of Medicine

While making the movie, I filmed a public commentary session at the Institute of Medicine in Washington, D.C. The IOM is a quasi-government agency that conducts research at the behest of Congress and other federal agencies and independent organizations. At the time, in early 2006, the institute, in conjunction with the Centers for Disease Control (CDC), was holding public hearings around the United States for input on creating standards for competitive foods sold in schools. My mission was to film a statement by

Dr. Susan Rubin, and we figured we'd get to meet other parents advocating for better food in schools. Upon arrival, I queried a man waiting at the security desk—where did he hail from? Eyeing my camera equipment, he snapped, "You don't want to talk to us. We're the suits." I didn't understand his comment until later, in the auditorium where a stakeholder's panel was convened. The "suit" I had spoken with turned out to be Richard Black, a representative from Coca-Cola North America. Also on the panel were spokespeople from Kraft, PepsiCo, Schwan's, and ConAgra. We had mistakenly thought "stakeholders" referred to parents, school administrators, teachers, food service directors, and students. Nancy Green from Pepsi testified, "A lot of times the healthier products are the least profitable for us." Susan Waltman from ConAgra stated unconvincingly, "We are really wanting people to improve." A lot of the discussion focused on when and where children consume various food items at school, how they prefer the processed items, and why we should give them better, re-engineered versions of what they want. Hope Hale from Schwan's insisted, "The kids are pretty savvy. They have a real understanding of what they're consuming, what's bad and good." Although it was called a public hearing, "angry mom" Susan Rubin turned out to be the only unpaid citizen advocate in attendance.

Fast forward to April 2007. The IOM released their recommendations for regulating competitive foods in a report titled *Nutrition Standards for Foods in Schools: Leading the Way Toward Healthier Youth*. Apparently the committee heard from others outside of the processed food business, and no doubt they studied all the available literature. The report offered thirteen recommended standards. The first four standards proposed bringing competitive foods in line with the guidelines for a reimbursable school meal, for the first time since schools began selling à la carte and vended items. The next set of standards prohibited sale of caffeinated beverages, beverages containing nonnutritive sweeteners, and sports drinks during the school day. Standard 8 would require free and accessible drinking water during the school day. Standard 10 states, "Foods and beverages are not used as rewards or discipline for academic performance or behavior." The final three standards apply to high school vending machines, after-school activities, and on-campus

fund-raising. They create a lower threshold tier for elementary school competitive foods, requiring that these items have some nutritional value and
meet the existing reimbursable meal guidelines, while allowing Tier 2 snacks
(allowed only for high school students after school) a bit more latitude. The
report also suggests that the food industry must "Establish a user-friendly
identification system for Tier 1 and 2 snacks, foods, and beverages that meet
the standards per portion as packaged." Although they do suggest minimiz-
ing marketing and branding of Tier 2 items by locating logo-free vending
machines in low traffic areas, one compromise that was probably made to
win industry support is that the standards don't prohibit selling approved
à la carte items in the cafeteria in competition with the reimbursable meal.

In September 2009 the Institute of Medicine released another school food
report—this one proposed updates to the school meal programs' nutrition
standards. Those updates were subsequently largely adopted in the Child
Nutrition Act Reauthorization of 2010, and are scheduled to go into effect
by January 2012, although many schools are already working toward compliance. Based on the IOM report, Type A lunches now must not exceed 650
calories for K–5 students, 700 calories for middle schoolers, and 850 calories
for high school kids. Breakfast calorie limits are 500, 550, and 600, respectively. The report also recommended a ten-year incremental decrease in
sodium content. In addition to the emphasis on whole grains, the part I like
is the recommendation that schools should focus on food rather than nutrients. The new standards would increase the amount and variety of fruits and
vegetables offered and specify that dark green and bright orange vegetables
as well as legumes be served during the course of each week. It's expected
that the next federal nutritional guidelines for Americans (which we know
as the food pyramid) will be based on the IOM recommendations.

Child Nutrition Act

The original federal school lunch program is formally known as the Richard
B. Russell National School Lunch Act. Another acronym of the school food

world, the CNA (Child Nutrition Act of 1966), is the act governing all the national school feeding programs. Much attention gets paid to its reauthorization, which is due every five years, because of the opportunity it affords to update guidelines and lobby for funding increases. Although there's a misconception that they remain in limbo when the act is due for renewal, the School Breakfast Program and the National School Lunch Program are actually permanently authorized. The smaller programs—the Summer Food Service Program (SFSP), the Child and Adult Care Food Program (CACFP), State Administrative Expenses (SAE), the Special Nutrition Program for Women, Infants, and Children (WIC), and some other child nutrition programs have actual expiration dates. For thirty years prior to 2010, the only increases in funding for the program were adjustments for inflation. Advocates rallied nationwide to support the bill's renewal, proposing doubling or tripling the $1 allocated for food per meal. In November 2010, during a lame duck Congress session, the CNA was renewed with an additional $4.5 billion in funding over ten years ($.5 billion a year), and resulting in an additional allocation of 6 cents per school meal.

In addition to the token funding increase, the bill enacts most of the IOM guidelines for competitive foods, giving the USDA authority to set nutritional standards for all foods regularly sold in schools during the school day, including vending machines, the à la carte lunch lines, and school stores along with a restriction that all revenue from competitive foods must be turned back into the food service program. Although the specific standards aren't written into the bill, and don't entirely go into effect until 2012, it's expected that the IOM nutrition standards will be the basis of those regulations. The bill will increase the number of children who qualify for free or reduced lunches and simplify the qualifying process. This provision is expected to connect approximately 115,000 new students to the program. Schools will now be audited every three years to check on compliance with the act, and schools will also have to provide nutrition information to parents upon request. It establishes professional standards for food service workers and provides grants for additional training. The act ensures that more local foods will be used in the school setting with $40 million in grant aid for Farm to School and school garden projects. The bill expands access to drinking water in schools, particularly during mealtimes.

There's a provision for a better notification system for food recalls and a vague mandate to build on USDA work to improve nutritional quality of commodity foods. Without more varied and better commodities, or a signifi- cant funding increase, food service directors will have to be extremely cre- ative in finding shortcuts to meet the new standards. I fear more unintended consequences in the form of processed foods that may contain the required nutrients and food items but may not exemplify the spirit of the mandate.

The USDA released sample before-and-after menus to illustrate how the updated legislation would impact a typical school meal. A hot dog on a white bun with sides of canned pears, raw celery, carrots, and chocolate milk would be replaced by whole-wheat spaghetti with meat sauce, a whole-wheat roll, broccoli, cauliflower, kiwi halves, and low-fat white milk.

Let's Move!

With much fanfare in early 2010, First Lady Michelle Obama unveiled what will undoubtedly be historically hailed as the triumph of her tenure, the Let's Move! initiative. As a response to the childhood obesity crisis, the First Lady is campaigning for America to "raise a healthier generation of kids." Launched at about the same time as *Jamie Oliver's Food Revolution*, the syn- ergy of the two initiatives revitalized school food advocates. This popular groundswell is credited with sweeping the new legislation into existence. Perhaps the greater impact of the initiative is the tone of positive support it sets for the many community-based efforts currently underway.

The First Lady has demonstrated her personal commitment to healthy food by planting an organic vegetable garden on the White House lawn and inviting local schoolchildren to participate in the cycle of planting and har- vesting its crops.

White House Assistant Chef Sam Kass was anointed Senior Policy Adviser for Healthy Food Initiatives. He's the motivator behind one of Let's Move's volunteer efforts, Chefs Move to Schools. Administered by the USDA, the program calls upon skilled chefs to adopt a school and work with teachers, parents, school nutritionists, and administrators to help educate kids about food and nutrition. An interactive website (letsmove.gov/chefs) helps match up schools with chefs in their area.

Also under the Let's Move!/USDA umbrella is the HealthierUS Schools Challenge, which "establishes rigorous standards for schools' food quality, participation in meal programs, physical activity, and nutrition education—the key components that make for healthy and active kids—and provides recognition for schools that meet these standards." The Challenge uses the Institute of Medicine's guidelines as standards for the program. A tiered system of awards—bronze, silver, and gold—are given to schools that meet the standards and recognition comes with a one-time financial award as well.

Federal policy evolves slowly, and as advocates we must not only act locally, but also participate in a national dialog to constantly improve child nutrition and agricultural policy. While federal guidelines set minimum standards for school food, they also encourage districts to reach beyond those standards with programs like the HealthierUS Schools Challenge. In order to meet the standards promoted in the HealthierUS Schools Challenge, your school district needs to write and implement a local wellness policy that reflects those requirements. You and your group can have a huge impact locally by influencing the wellness policy in your district.

What You Can Do to Influence Federal Policy

COMMUNICATE WITH YOUR CONGRESSIONAL REPRESENTATIVES AND STATE SENATORS

Every citizen has one representative and two senators working for you in Washington, D.C. They need to hear from all of us when issues affecting our children's health come up in Congress.

SIGN UP FOR ACTION ALERTS FROM THESE ORGANIZATIONS

CSPI—Center for Science in the Public Interest
Center for Food Safety/The True Food Network
Organic Consumers Association
Slow Food in Schools/Time for Lunch
Two Angry Moms
ComFood
Community Food Security Coalition
Gmfreeschools.org

Action alerts make it easy to write or call your reps—when you click on a link for the action, you can usually link directly to the proper contact information just by typing in your zip code. They often provide a form letter you can customize, and a phone number if you'd prefer to call.

WATCH FOR THE REAUTHORIZATION OF IMPORTANT LEGISLATION

The Child Nutrition Act comes up for reauthorization every five years.

The Farm Bill is the big kahuna of legislation controlling the subsidies for commodity products. It, too, is renewed every five years. The next Farm Bill is up for renewal in 2012.

If your representative is on the Senate Agriculture Committee or the House Education and Labor Committee they can be particularly influential on these policies. These two committees oversee legislation about rules and funding pertaining to the USDA and the Food and Nutrition Service.

FOUR

LOCAL WELLNESS POLICIES

The job of the schools is to feed the brain. Not just what students eat but when and how.

—Dr. Stephen Cowan, M.D., FAAP

F ederal rules and regulations often seem to thwart any possibility of creating a sustainable school food environment. School business managers and food service directors will use the federal guidelines as an excuse for business as usual. However, local school districts actually retain a good deal of control over how they manage their school meals program. The USDA says, "Local school food authorities are responsible for serving meals, managing the administrative aspects of the program (i.e., enrolling students, processing applications, verifying student eligibility, negotiating food contracts), and maintaining data for reporting purposes." Beyond meeting those basic obligations, and meeting the minimum nutrition standards for a reimbursable meal, the federal government requires every school district in the NSLP to have a wellness policy in place. Wellness policies must address both the nutrition and physical education of students in the school district. These policies are the federal government's way of not offending the food business. The federal government, in essence, has dictated the quantities of food and nutrients, but has left decisions about the specific qualities of the food and the school's food culture up to each district to determine.

Five years ago, when I first began searching for school districts that were focusing on improving the school food environment, I had a tough time finding examples. Now, many districts are making improvements—some small, some grand—and in most cases those changes are based upon the creation of, or changes to, the school wellness policy. Beginning in September 2006, all schools participating in the NSLP were required to have a wellness policy in place. The mandate was created as part of the 2004 Child Nutrition Reauthorization. In the months preceding the 2006 deadline, school administrators were notified about the requirement and encouraged to form a wellness committee and start planning.

The USDA says, "The legislation places the responsibility of developing a wellness policy at the local level so the individual needs of each district can be addressed. At a minimum, the district school wellness policy must:

1. Include goals for nutrition education, physical activity, and other school-based activities designed to promote student wellness in a manner that the local educational agency determines appropriate;

2. Include nutrition guidelines for all foods available on the school campus during the school day, with the objectives of promoting student health and reducing childhood obesity;

3. Provide an assurance that guidelines for school meals are not less restrictive than those set by the U.S. Department of Agriculture;

4. Establish a plan for measuring implementation of the local wellness policy, including the designation of one or more persons within the local education agency or at each school, as appropriate, charged with ensuring that the school meets the local wellness policy; and

5. Involve parents, students, representatives of the school food authority, the school board, school administrators, and the public in development of the local wellness policy."

School Food Hierarchy

While the hierarchy of school food policy doesn't end at the wellness committee, this is where persistent parents and advocates can start to have some local clout. Here's a top-down schematic of authorities in charge of school food:

Congress (rules, funding)
  Senate Agriculture Committee
  House Education and Labor Committee
USDA (regulation, reimbursement, commodities, oversight)
  Food and Nutrition Services
  FNS Regional Offices (seven regions)
State Board of Education or State Health Department (regulation, commodity selection and distribution, monitoring compliance, program administration, funding match)
District Board of Education (funding, staff, contracts)
Wellness Committee (district wellness policy)
  Nutrition/Food Advisory Council (may be a subcommittee of wellness committee—mandated for districts subcontracted to food service management companies)
Local School Food Authority (compliance, budget, provisions, reporting)

Who's at the Table

According to language in the regulations, anyone can initiate a process to create a new policy or adopt an existing policy in a local school district. The law requires parents, students, representatives of the school food authority, the school board, school administrators, teachers, health care professionals, and the public to be involved in the process.

Beware

I had heard horror stories about wellness committees from a number of parents before I ever attended a meeting. My experience confirmed the stories.

At first, I was confused. I've sat on the boards of several nonprofit organizations and task forces, and those meetings were always purposeful and goal oriented. My district's wellness committee meeting was more like a hearing. Each member of the committee had a turn holding the floor, and each person was politely listened to. Parents and community members voiced their concerns over the quality of the food and some made suggestions on things we could do to improve it. One parent researched food brokers that could supply the district with organic produce, another commented on the fact that the food service was no longer serving whole roast chicken, although their marketing literature claimed they were. The board of ed members applauded the great job the food service staff was doing. One community member made an impassioned case for a thorough review and rewrite of an upcoming RFP (Request for Proposal) for renewal of the district's food service providers. As mandated, there were school administrators, teachers, health care providers, parents, students, and the food service director on the committee—a group of close to twenty people.

By the time we got around the whole table, the meeting was basically over. No new agenda was advanced, and very little discussion about follow-up ensued. Like Kafka's trial, the purpose of the proceeding was never quite revealed.

Unlike Kafka, though, I soon learned who the key players really were. The head of our wellness committee, as is often the case, is our district's business manager. At the meeting I attended, she opened the meeting, facilitated the discussion, and closed the meeting.

A school district business manager oversees all of the financial management of the school system. They also may manage human resources and health and safety policies, so the task of managing wellness policies falls to the business manager in many districts. The business manager must deal with building maintenance, waste management services, groundskeeping, heating and cooling services, school buses, and a myriad of other services and school staffing issues. School food is a line item in her budget, so unless your school business manager has a high food IQ, you can see why running the wellness committee isn't a priority on her to-do list.

What often happens is that the district school business manager will make closed-door decisions with the school board on important school food–related issues like contracts and RFPs. In order to follow regulations, the Kafkaesque wellness committee discussions take place, and for a brief moment the business manager may state that she is putting out an RFP, then changes the subject. In effect, the committee puts a rubber stamp on whatever decisions have been made by the board of education and the business manager.

This "what just happened?" phenomenon creates anger and frustration for the activists on the committee, and they often drop off after serving a single term, leaving the spot open for either another unsuspecting eager advocate, or for anyone willing to fill a PTO-appointed volunteer position.

Policy Requirements

The USDA and each state department of education publish wellness policy guidelines that are all quite similar. When the wellness policy requirement was first announced, my town published a set of goals and guidelines that looked like this:

I. Goals and Guidelines
The Board, following consultation with the Advisory Council, adopts the following goals and guidelines in order to promote student wellness:

A. NUTRITION EDUCATION AND PROMOTION
- Setting an average weekly minimum time for classroom nutrition education
- Providing a minimum number of hours per year of training to classroom teachers on how to integrate nutrition education into other basic subjects
- Setting rules for marketing and guidelines for promotion of nutritious foods and healthy habits outside the classroom

B. Physical Activity and Other School-Based Activities
  * Setting minimum physical education requirements including time, frequency, and intensity
  * Giving students and the community after-school access to school activity facilities
  * Creating after-school activity programs, a student health council, and community and family programs that encourage healthy habits
  * Providing school meals at appropriate times in appropriate settings
  * Working with food service providers to assure the marketing of healthy food in ways that increase its appeal
  * Removal from physical activity or recess should not be used as a consequence

C. Nutritional Guidelines for School Food
  * Addressing such issues as nutritional values and portion size
  * Regulating à la carte, vending machine, concession, and school store offerings
  * Regulating after-school activity, field trip, school events
  * Limiting the use of food as a reward
  * Encouraging the offering of healthy food as a fund-raiser
  * Training and certification of food preparation and food service staff
  * Evaluating food and drink contracts

At a minimum, all reimbursable school meals (i.e. free and reduced lunches) shall meet the program requirements and nutritional standards established by the USDA regulations applicable to school meals.

II. Measuring the Implementation of Wellness Policy

Pursuant to this policy, the Board shall designate at least one individual to be responsible for the oversight of the school district's wellness program. This individual will be responsible for ensuring that the goals and guidelines relating to nutrition education, physical activity, school-based wellness activities and nutritional value of school-provided food and beverages are met, that there is compliance with the wellness policy, and that all school policies and school-based activities are consistent with the wellness policy.

Having read the guidelines, a group of concerned parents (outside of the wellness committee) in my town wrote up a series of suggested specifications for the policy. We wanted the wellness policy to specify that the food offered in our schools contain better-quality ingredients. We wanted to see more real food, less processed food. We didn't want teachers handing out junk food as classroom rewards. We handed these suggestions to the board of education and a group of us of spoke at a board of education meeting in support of these and other specifications for the wellness policy. In another bizarre moment in school food history, rather than address the specific goals and guidelines set forth in the sample document, the board voted to adopt the sample guidelines themselves as the district's wellness policy. This vote established our district's wellness policy without any specifications for any of the areas the policy was required to address. After the vote, I pointed out that fact, and was met with the response from a member of the board, "Well, you wouldn't want us to be in breach of our own policy, would you?"

I soon learned that numerous other school districts had done the same! A 2009 report issued by Yale University's Rudd Center for Food Policy and Obesity found that one-third of the policies reviewed (from forty-nine states) did not address all of the mandated areas. The study also found that many policies are unenforceable because the language is so vague. Only half of the policies surveyed contained specific nutrition standards, and only a third of those required that the standards be met. In many states the researchers found that committees did not include representatives from all of the required categories, and that most policies did not address the issue of marketing items of low nutritional value in schools. The Rudd Center issued a report card for each school district's policy in the state of Connecticut. The categories they graded the policies on were nutrition education, school meals, other school foods and beverages, physical education, physical activity, communication and promotion, and evaluation. Out of a total possible score of 100, almost every district scored under 50 percent. Many districts reported lack of funding for implementation

as a barrier to creating a stronger policy, but interestingly, the only wellness policies in Connecticut that achieved a passing grade were from high-need, socio-
economically disadvantaged urban school districts. My district failed.

KATONAH-LEWISBORO, NEW YORK

Katonah-Lewisboro, New York, is the school district that I documented over
the course of a school year. I chose Katonah because they had a strong wellness committee, backed by a supportive superintendent and championed by
the then-regional Westchester Coalition for Better School Food. I had high
hopes that I could document the process of creating and implementing a wellness policy that had some substance. I got to know the moms on the committee who were really pushing for a nutrition policy that spelled out some
specifics—among them were an attorney, a nutritionist, and the board of education president. The district was in an enviable position because they had
some one-time funding that was earmarked for improvements to the school
food environment. After hiring consultant Kate Adamick of Food Systems
Solutions to survey the district and audit each school, the committee worked
with Kate to incorporate her findings into policy requirements that would
replace much of the toxic cafeteria food with less-processed alternatives. A
series of tense school board meetings ensued. Kate testified that her survey
revealed accusations from the students that the adults were being hypocritical
for teaching them one thing in class about nutrition and then providing them
with food that didn't meet those standards. A school board member worried
that the policy would prohibit hot dogs at the football games, and the business manager worried about the cost of the improvements. Assurances were
made by Kate and the committee, and by the end of the school year, the board
voted unanimously to adopt the policy, as written, along with a hike in the
price of lunch—the first in thirteen years. Over the summer, salad bars were
installed, sugary caffeinated beverages removed, a young chef was hired to
create recipes and train staff, and the committee went to work marketing the
changes through a newsletter and student leadership. When the new school

(continued)

year began, some students and parents were dismayed and confused, but the intrepid wellness committee members stood by their policy and spent time in the cafeteria helping to introduce the new items and explain why things had changed. After a shaky start, the kids got used to the new stuff, sales surpassed previous numbers, and the community proudly became a role model for others in the county.

Breakthrough

By now, almost every school district has a wellness policy in place, so ask to see yours. A well-thought-out policy can be a great asset. Every year your district is required to review their policy. If you have a strong group of advocates, you can work to strengthen your policy, or implement it more correctly. In districts with an impassioned administrator running the wellness committee, whether a business manager, assistant superintendent, school nurse, or principal, committee proceedings can go from rubber-stamp to active agenda. A pivotal piece of your advocacy work is bringing your committee chair, school board members, and other school personnel on board. With committed leadership on the part of any of these key players, and support from the community, your wellness policy can be a key tool in creating a vision for a sustainable school food environment.

PORT ANGELES, WASHINGTON— MICHELLE REID

Beth Loveridge (see chapter three) credits her assistant superintendent, Michelle Reid, with much of the success of her district's wellness committee. Michelle has been chair of the committee since its inception. Beth says, "She wasn't always on board, and definitely didn't have the support of her boss, the superintendent, initially."

I spoke with Michelle to get her perspective on what it's like to chair a committee that includes passionate parents like Beth. I learned that the committee was formed a year before Beth joined, and in that first year, had already made some changes, like eliminating caffeinated, sugary soda pop from the vending machines. Michelle has four kids, and two of them were still in district schools when the wellness policy changes took place.

In some districts the business manager heads the wellness committee. I asked Michelle how it was that she, as assistant superintendent, was chosen to chair the committee? Did she volunteer? Michelle explains, "No, I didn't volunteer, but I run several district curriculum committees and task forces. This was a committee about nutrition, health, and fitness so we were looking at physical education and the health curriculum as well as the food. I'm responsible for teaching and learning for K–12 in this district so anything we're doing with that I'm involved with. Our business manager's vision of what we could do was not as expansive as the committee's. The committee had a lot of energy, a lot of community people. My role was not to throw up roadblocks, but to see how we could support it financially and make it sustainable. We tried to assume that it would be successful. Originally I thought the topic was pretty benign and boring—something rivaling the safety committee."

The Port Angeles wellness committee was large and diverse. On it were teachers, a principal, a dietician from a local hospital, the school nurse, some high school students, and a coach. Michelle says, "We ended up making sweeping changes even in what goes in vending and the coaches had lots of input. We had local organic food activists and farmers, the local YMCA director, county health advisory board members, a school board member, and our local Sodexo food service director. It was important for him to be at the table or he was going to be on the menu. When the committee began to do something, people began to jump in. Beth was amazing; she kept pressing. Initially my boss [the superintendent] and the business manager thought I was nuts to keep pressing with them."

Michelle tells me that the wellness policy was well received by the board of education, because one of their members had sat on the committee. It's already

(continued)

been revised since its adoption in 2007. Michelle recounts, "We updated it to talk about purchasing more local food. We were already doing a lot of things that the new state legislation wanted. Our committee is expected to do an annual review of the policy and report to the board of education at the end of each school year."

I asked Michelle if she recalled how she was won over. She credits the enthusiasm and expertise of her committee members. "We had people who really knew what they were doing and could provide us a lot of factual information. You can't really shine on folks who know what they're doing, and we all had to learn a lot about the system. For example, the food service director explained to us how menu averaging is used. Not every meal has to meet the exact nutritional guidelines, as long as the weekly average of meals meets the guidelines."

With Michelle's support, the committee proposed a single elementary school trial project, which proved to be a learning experience for all involved. She says, "We learned we could get more unprocessed commodities if we asked for them—items with lower sodium, sugar, and added fats. The kids liked it. More kids started buying lunch. The food service director had an epiphany—maybe this could work! He became more excited as it became more obvious it was going to work. We didn't know we had done such a good job with our wellness policy until we got a $5,000 award from the state. So that was a tipping point."

When we spoke, Port Angeles was moving into the third of five elementary schools with changed menus and she was hopeful that the new program would be implemented district-wide by year's end. She tells me, "We have kids who had it [the new food] last year in elementary school and want it back for middle school."

For Michelle, another tipping point was "when I went up with other members of the committee and the regional director of Sodexo to observe the trial menus in the elementary school. We all saw that this is also good for business. So the food service RFP last spring was different from anything we'd ever written before. We didn't step forward as fast as Beth and the others would have liked, but we didn't step back."

The most important question I wanted to ask Michelle was for her advice to parents about working with school administrators on the wellness committee.

Her response reveals that she is clearly 100 percent on board. "The key is whoever is going to lead the committee, you want someone in the district who has the authority to make things happen. Find somebody in the system that has the authority to do something. Our job as school administrators is to provide excellent teaching and learning experiences for children. When you talk to administrators, emphasize that healthy kids have better attendance and do better academically. It's fair to say that in addition to the business manager on the committee we want someone from the instructional side of the house involved in that conversation. Wellness is part of the curriculum because it connects nutrition, health, and fitness." And, she adds, "Any time you initiate change, make sure it's the right change and far enough that you can't go back. Ask the question, 'Whose interests are you serving?' It can't be Sodexo's or the parents' interests. You have to find the balance and it has to be about the children."

Michelle writes an annual wellness committee report that includes data from surveys of students and staff. Their process is intentionally open and transparent, and really does reflect the input of the whole community.

Listen, Learn, Act

Engage key administrators and wellness committee members in a one-on-one dialogue. Make appointments to meet with your principal, assistant superintendent, superintendent, wellness chair, and others. Ask them what their priorities are and how wellness fits into their beliefs about student success. Rather than trying to sell them on your agenda, ask them what you can do to help fit wellness into their agenda. Get their input as to how you can make adoption of a top-grade wellness policy more appealing for them. If their main concern is improving test scores, bring them studies that show the positive impact of real food on academic achievement (see resources) as well as attendance and behavior. Let them know who else in the community supports school wellness reform. Suggest a pilot program in one school or other alternatives if they are hesitant to adopt a broad-based program right away. Be willing to negotiate; set a strategy for working through the goals over a period of time, or focus on an area that has more consensus to start off.

If your wellness committee is mired in bureaucracy, don't be afraid to take matters into your own hands. Set up a working group or policy council or work with an existing organization to draft a sample policy that you think would work for your community. Inform your school board and seek input from all of your community's constituents, including local businesses that also might be willing to donate funds and in-kind products and services that would help offset the cost of proposed improvements. Local hospitals, insurance agencies, caterers, grocery stores, restaurants, and health clubs are some prospective contributors. Publicize the proposed policy and solicit signatures on a petition to pass the policy. Your school board and school wellness committee will listen and respond when the public pressure builds.

Specifications

Your wellness policy should be specific. Studies of policies around the country find lack of specificity to be one of the main reasons for low evaluations. How does your school district define wellness? This is a helpful place to start as it can set the stage for a policy that embraces an integrative approach to wellness. Model wellness policies often begin with a vision statement and some basic assumptions about children's health, their right to a healthy school environment, the right to a healthy meal or meals, and the role of food literacy in a school system that seeks to educate the whole child. Define the school's responsibilities, mission, and goals in creating the policy. These goals will make it easier to then specify the programs and strategies that can be implemented to meet those goals.

Here's some sample opening language adapted from the British food and farming group Sustain:

The Board of Education recognizes the positive benefits of a healthy diet and physical activity upon a student's ability to learn effectively and perform well at school. The Board also recognizes the role a school can play, as part of the larger community, to promote family health, and sustainable food and farming practices. The Board of Education recognizes that sharing food is a fundamental experience for all people; a primary way to nurture and celebrate our cultural diversity; and an excellent bridge for building friendships and intergenerational bonds.

The educational mission of the Board of Education is to improve the health of the entire community by teaching students and families ways to establish and maintain lifelong healthy and environmentally sustainable eating habits. The mission shall be accomplished through food education and skills (such as cooking and growing food), the food served in schools, and core academic content in the classroom.

The three aspects that the wellness policy governs—nutrition education, physical activity, and school food—should each be addressed clearly by the policy. These three areas may go hand in hand, as suggested by the mission above and also by a model wellness policy from California's Center for Ecoliteracy, which requires the following:

- Each school in the district shall establish an instructional garden (tilled ground, raised bed, container, nearby park, community garden, farm, or lot) of sufficient size to provide students with experiences in planting, harvesting, preparation, serving, and tasting foods, including ceremonies and celebrations that observe food traditions, integrated with nutrition education and core curriculum, and articulated with state standards.
- Staff shall integrate hands-on experiences in gardens and kitchen classrooms, and enriched activities such as farm field studies, farmers' market tours, and visits to community gardens, with core curriculum so that students begin to understand how food reaches the table and the implications that has for their health and future.

- Sampling and tasting in school gardens and kitchen classrooms shall be encouraged as part of nutrition education.

- Staff members are encouraged to utilize food from school gardens and local farms in kitchen classrooms and cafeterias based upon availability and acceptability.

- Schools shall use food as an integrator and central focus of education about human events, history, and celebrations, and shall encourage classes to use food and cooking as part of a learning experience that sheds light on the customs, history, traditions, and cuisine of various countries and cultures.

- Eating experiences, gardens, cooking classes, and nutrition education shall be integrated into the core academic curriculum at all grade levels.

GOAL #1—NUTRITION EDUCATION AND PROMOTION

When you discuss nutrition education, consider making the focus on culture more than on calories. Policies that require a lot of measuring and data crunching are difficult to implement and monitor, and there are already a lot of federal regulations that do just that. You shouldn't need a nutrition degree to read, write, or understand a local wellness policy. Use language that moves away from nutrition (food guru Michael Pollan calls this "nutritionism") and toward food. Is food education a dietetics unit in Health class, or is it integrated into all subjects and grade levels? The following language for nutrition education was adapted from the National Alliance for Nutrition and Activity (NANA). Try reading it and substituting "food" everywhere you see "nutrition":

SCHOOLS SHOULD PROVIDE NUTRITION EDUCATION AND ENGAGE IN NUTRITION PROMOTION THAT:

- is offered at each grade level as part of a sequential, comprehensive, standards-based program designed to provide students with the knowledge and skills necessary to promote and protect their health;

- is part of not only health education classes, but also classroom instruction in subjects such as math, science, language arts, social sciences, and elective subjects;
- includes enjoyable, developmentally appropriate, culturally relevant, participatory activities, such as contests, promotions, taste testing, farm visits, and school gardens;
- promotes fruits, vegetables, whole-grain products, ethically raised animal products, healthy food preparation methods, and health-enhancing nutrition practices;
- emphasizes caloric balance between food intake and energy expenditure (physical activity/exercise);
- links with school meal programs, other school foods, and nutrition-related community services;
- teaches media literacy with an emphasis on food marketing; and includes training for teachers and other staff.

Note the inclusion of media literacy and training for teachers and other staff. Even the best-written policy cannot be implemented without understanding from your school staff. This may necessitate a training session or development day, and if so, that should be written into the policy as an annual or ongoing program.

Regarding food service staff, a growing and generally successful trend is the wellness policy requiring a trained chef, specifically a culinary school graduate, to run the food service or supervise the kitchen. Traditional food service directors come from management or dietetics backgrounds, and often do not have formal culinary training. If your policy specifies scratch cooking, make sure it specifies a trained chef.

The nutrition promotion policy should also be specific about the source of nutrition information and promotion. A good policy will address the use of food company logos and brand names on/in vending machines, books or curricula, textbook covers, school supplies, scoreboards, school structures, and sports equipment.

GOAL #2—PHYSICAL ACTIVITY AND OTHER SCHOOL-BASED ACTIVITIES

Kids need to move. Not just to develop strong muscles, but to wire their brains correctly, to promote proper breathing and circulation, and to facilitate digestion and elimination. Wellness policy should address how much time each day children should have for physical activity. Experts suggest that sixty minutes during the school day is optimum. Not only the amount of time, but also the types of physical activities offered by the school should be specified.

The Center for Ecoliteracy suggests, "The district's physical education program shall include a variety of kinesthetic activities, including team, individual, and cooperative sports and physical activities, as well as aesthetic movement forms, such as dance, yoga, or the martial arts. Students shall be given opportunities for physical activity through a range of before- and/or after-school programs, including, but not limited to, intramurals, interscholastic athletics, and physical activity clubs."

My daughters both tried team sports and found they didn't enjoy competitive physical activities. Our district really emphasizes team sports and didn't offer many opportunities for individual or group athletic activities that were noncompetitive. We were fortunate to be able to take advantage of community-based programs outside of the school system, but the wellness policy is an opportunity to discuss this issue in your district and consider devising an athletic program that is more inclusive.

Your policy should also insist that staff not withhold opportunities for physical activity such as PE or recess as a punishment, unless absolutely necessary.

Some school districts are using the wellness policy to assess safety issues around students' ability to walk or bike to school. NANA suggests the following language: "When appropriate, the district will work together with local public works, public safety, and/or police departments in those efforts. The school district will explore the availability of federal 'safe routes to school' funds, administered by the state department of transportation, to finance such improvements. The school district will encourage students to use public transportation when available and appropriate for travel to school, and will work with the local transit agency to provide transit passes for students."

The NANA guidelines also suggest including a clause about access to school grounds for activities outside of the school day, such as, "School spaces and facilities should be available to students, staff, and community members before, during, and after the school day, on weekends, and during school vacations. These spaces and facilities also should be available to community agencies and organizations offering physical activity and nutrition programs. School policies concerning safety will apply at all times."

FUELING UP!

Children become more organized and "recharge" when they play in random and purposeful ways. As muscle fibers activate and joints get stimulated through movement, the corresponding nerves send messages to parts of the brain that reenergize, helping to reboot neurological areas responsible for attention and focus. Movement also helps build connecting pathways, important for flexible, integrated thinking. Professional athletes will attest; you need fuel to move! When children have foods with the necessary complement of proteins, fats, and complex carbohydrates, they can extend their motor play, build endurance, and move more effectively. Sugar-filled foods give one big burst of energy and then the child is left depleted, with no reserve left for extended play. No wonder so many children prefer to plop in front of a television or electronic device!

(CONTRIBUTED BY JILL HOWLETT MAYS, AUTHOR OF *YOUR CHILD'S MOTOR DEVELOPMENT STORY*)

Recess Research—Recess First!

A study of kids who walked to school, then ate breakfast, went to class, then went to recess, then had lunch, showed a significant increase in IQ scores. Other studies demonstrate reduced plate waste when students go to recess before lunch, and teachers report that students settle back into class faster when they come in from lunch rather than recess. In Las Cruces, New Mexico, the director of Nutrition Services studied plate waste at two different elementary schools by rifling through the garbage. She found that at the school with recess before lunch, children consumed 30 percent more fruit, vegetables, and milk than students who followed the traditional schedule. Kids say they prefer recess before lunch because they have time to digest their food without running around, which made some feel nauseous, although they also report feeling sleepy after lunch, which has as much to do with *what* they're eating as *when* they eat. Recess comes after lunch in 73 percent of schools, and that's something your wellness policy can change.

The Dining Experience

A wellness policy from the regional school district of Oneida, Herkimer, and Madison, New York, interprets the "Other School-Based Activities" goal as a mandate for standards in the dining experience of its students. Here's an excerpt from the policy:

1. Dining Environment
   a) Provides clean, safe and enjoyable meal environment for students;
   b) Provides enough space and serving areas to ensure all students have access to school meals with minimum wait time;
   c) Drinking fountains and hydration resources are encouraged and available in schools, so that students can get water at meals and throughout the day;
   d) Encourage all students to participate in the school meals program and protect the identity of students who eat free and reduced-price meals.
2. Dining Time
   a) Adequate dining time for students to enjoy healthy foods.
   b) Schedule lunchtime as near the middle of the school day as possible.

Time for Lunch

Scheduling lunch gets complicated in overcrowded school districts. If your child winds up having a lunch period at 10 a.m. or 2 p.m., there may be no negotiating, but with some creativity, your wellness committee may be able to work with the food service director to find a work-around. The policy should also address high school students whose schedules don't allow any time at all for a lunch period. Some policies allow overscheduled students to bring their lunch to class.

Another policy from New York State—this one from Mount Kisco—also addresses the dining experience quite elegantly:

Meal Times and Scheduling

SCHOOLS

- will provide students with at least ten minutes to eat after sitting down for breakfast and fifteen minutes after sitting down for lunch;
- should schedule meal periods at appropriate and reasonable times;
- should not schedule tutoring, club, or organizational meetings or activities during mealtimes, unless students may eat during such activities;
- will schedule lunch periods to follow recess periods (in elementary schools) whenever possible for all students; if not possible, a rotational schedule to achieve this goal should be implemented;
- will provide students access to hand washing or hand sanitizing before they eat meals or snacks; and
- should take reasonable steps to accommodate the tooth-brushing regimens of students with special oral health needs (e.g., orthodontia or high tooth-decay risk).

Free and Reduced-Priced Meals. Schools will make every effort to eliminate any social stigma attached to, and prevent the overt identification of, students who are eligible for free and reduced-price school meals. Toward this end, schools may utilize electronic identification and payment systems; provide meals at no charge to all children, regardless of income; promote the availability of school meals to all students; and/ or use nontraditional methods for serving school meals, such as "grab-and-go" or classroom breakfast.

And while Mount Kisco's policy discourages food sharing, the Center for Ecoliteracy's policy *stresses* the cultural importance of sharing food:

Students will be encouraged to share food, as food sharing is a fundamental experience for all peoples. Despite concerns about allergies and other restrictions on some children's diets that can cause schools to discourage students from trading foods or beverages with classmates, sharing can be encouraged through service styles in the cafeteria, such as "family style," that provide students with the opportunity to serve themselves from a common platter and to pass platters of food to tablemates.

I would add to that, "The special needs of students with severe food allergies will be addressed and every effort made to accommodate them in the least restrictive manner possible." In nearly every culture, the tradition of regularly sharing a communal meal runs deep. Traditional cultures teach that ingesting the same nourishment induces harmony among a group—you are what you eat—a good reason to encourage the family-style meal. Family-style service and limited options in the lunch line can also save time and money and enable your food service to put out a better product.

GOAL #3—NUTRITIONAL GUIDELINES FOR SCHOOL FOOD

As much as possible, the food policy should be as specific as the audit categories in chapter one. By all means, include what you don't want, but also be really specific about what you do want. Food quality must be mandated. Address sourcing, wholeness, freshness, seasonality, and nutrient balance and density. A Web search will find you numerous model food policies in addition to the ones sampled here. Some of them may seem like pie in the sky—requiring scratch cooking when your district doesn't even have a kitchen, or organic food when the food budget is less than $1 per meal. Don't let the present reality get in the way of your goals, first in the minds and words of those who conceived of them, and then in their execution. Wellness policy can articulate and dictate your process. A policy can call for a gradual transition, or can state that a fund-raising initiative will be implemented to cover capital expenses or food costs in low-income districts. I've culled from several policies, particularly that of Katonah-Lewisboro, to create this menu of sample food guidelines:

NUTRITIONAL QUALITY OF FOODS AND BEVERAGES SOLD AND SERVED ON CAMPUS

Food served through the National School Lunch and Breakfast Programs and all other foods on campus will:

- be appealing, attractive and colorful to children, with an emphasis on displaying the healthful choices at key locations and in the front of the line for immediate student access.
- be served in clean and pleasant settings, with attempts to provide a calming atmosphere conducive to quieter, relaxing eating environments (i.e. live plants, piped-in soft music, etc.).
- meet, or exceed, nutrition requirements established by local, state, and federal statutes and regulations.
- not contain partially hydrogenated oils or similar trans fats; high fructose corn syrup or other artificial sweeteners; genetically engineered ingredients; preservatives, colorings, or flavorings (natural and artificial).
- be prepared locally or regionally from scratch.

- offer a variety of fresh fruits and vegetables:
  - To the extent possible, schools will offer at least two non-fried vegetables and two fruit options each day and will offer five different fruits and five different vegetables over the course of a week.
  - Fresh fruit and appropriate vegetables are to be washed thoroughly using a product to eliminate residues and pesticides.
  - The district is encouraged to source fresh fruits and vegetables from local farmers when practicable.
  - When fresh is not available or practicable, frozen may be used.
  - Canned vegetables may periodically be served.
  - Canned or jarred fruit (in its own fruit juice) may be used seasonally as necessary.
  - Select organic only for the "dirty dozen" fruits and vegetables that have the highest measured pesticide residues: apples, bell peppers, celery, cherries, imported grapes, nectarines, peaches, pears, potatoes, red raspberries, spinach, and strawberries.
- serve a variety of non-rBGH white milk (preferably organic, grass-fed) including whole, 2 percent, and skim and nutritionally equivalent non-dairy alternatives (to be defined by USDA).
  - All other beverage products, including those used as part of a daily meal item and those sold à la carte, shall meet the standards as set forth in this policy under "Beverages sold or served at school."
- ensure that half of the served grains are whole grain and that more types of whole grains and beans are served regularly.
- offer vegetarian options on a daily basis.
- discontinue use of oils that do not tolerate high heat, particularly in uses where they are repeatedly reheated (try rice bran oil).
- decrease refined carbohydrate foods (refined sugars) in snacks, and
- increase availability of more nutrient-dense snacks.

Schools should engage students and parents, through taste-tests of new entrées and surveys, in selecting foods sold through the school meal programs in order to identify new, healthful, and appealing food choices.

Breakfast. To ensure that all children have breakfast, either at home or at school, in order to meet their nutritional needs and enhance their ability to learn:

- Schools will, to the extent possible, operate the School Breakfast Program.
- Schools will, to the extent possible, arrange bus schedules and utilize methods to serve school breakfasts that encourage participation, including serving breakfast in the classroom, "grab-and-go" breakfast, or breakfast during morning break or recess.
- Schools that serve breakfast to students will notify parents and students of the availability of the School Breakfast Program.
- Schools will encourage parents to provide a healthy breakfast for their children through newsletter articles, take-home materials, or other means.

Water. All school eating areas shall contain free, safe drinking water sources and facilities for washing hands.

Food Allergies

Food allergies can be life-threatening, and a first-time reaction may occur during school. Your policy should call for staff training to recognize and react to symptoms of food allergy and anaphylaxis. Children with food allergies are often teased and bullied, so an atmosphere of tolerance and understanding should be fostered. The Educational Solutions Global Network advises schools to have written emergency protocols and to implement practices that minimize exposure to allergens. Most students with severe food allergies will have a Section 504 Plan (for students with disabilities) in place. This plan is separate from the wellness policy but will overlap in many areas. The ubiquity of food throughout the school premises may be addressed, as well as the student's right to be placed in the least restrictive environment rather than being segregated because of a food allergy.

Lunch Lessons

Your wellness policy can also determine whether lunch is viewed as an inter-ruption of the school day, or as part of the curriculum. In most schools I've visited, it's fifteen or twenty minutes of pandemonium. Staff dreads cafeteria duty and kids know they're able to get away with behavior that wouldn't fly in a classroom.

On the other hand, I've been to many schools, including elementary schools, where the food environment has been carefully considered and the students' behavior at lunch reflects that tone. Even in cafeterias with less than desirable acoustics, I've been able to have normal decibel conversations with both students and adults. Lunchtime can be an opportunity to reinforce positive messages about food and integrate lessons learned in the classroom into the lunchroom.

A positive attitude, combined with decent food, makes all the difference.

Positive Policy!

As I write this, potatoes are the new scourge in the school food world. Based upon Institute of Medicine recommendations, the poor spud is being banned from the school lunch and from food stamp programs, at least temporar-ily. "Less Banning, More Planning" might be a better motto. Our policies need to provide, not deprive. Rather than vilify a vitamin-rich, albeit starchy vegetable that has sustained entire populations for generations, we need to focus on the quality of the product that's going on the plate. In the form of a Tater Tot or a greasy fry, they're not a healthy food option, but roasted or baked, especially in combination with other root vegetables, potatoes can be as nutritious as they are delicious. As you ponder your policy, beware of unintended consequences. Have a "what if" discussion about every tenet in the policy.

Sustainability

You can address planetary health as well as children's health when you specify your strategies. Is your school's wellness policy part of an overall school district/town/city sustainability policy? Many town governments have, or are working on, such policies. Since schools play a large role in the business of a town or city, a study of how schools manage their energy consumption and waste can offer significant savings. There's a wealth of opportunity to utilize wellness policy to institute money-saving and planet-saving policies that will teach our kids to create a future that produces less waste and less pollution. Nearly 80 percent of the food waste generated at schools could be composted or recycled according to a recent study out of Hennepin County, Minnesota. The study recommends some easy, low-cost options schools can take to boost recycling. Properly placing and labeling composting and recycling containers, and forming a green team to track and improve performance are two suggestions that can be written into a wellness policy.

An audit of elementary school waste reveals that up to 30 percent of a school's trash is food waste and 24 percent is food-packaging waste. Your school district is paying for both the food and the waste disposal. You can be a school food hero by writing policy that saves cash and saves trash. Make sure the students on your wellness committee consider the environmental and social impact of their food options. You can have a table where students put uneaten whole fruit or packaged snacks for donations to local shelters or food banks. Teaching children what foods go into compost and which ones don't is a valuable biology lesson and one that can be practiced daily in the cafeteria. Students who bring lunch to school can be encouraged to use washable, reusable containers in their lunch boxes. Styrofoam and disposable plastic lunch trays and containers are still quite common in schools, but more and more I'm seeing compostable, post-consumer recycled cardboard lunch trays. Some schools have dishwashing equipment; those that do can switch back to the old-fashioned washable trays.

Although it's technically against USDA regulations, the Berkeley, California, school meals program serves milk from a large dispenser. Students take the amount they will drink (not always the required eight ounces), so less milk gets wasted, there's no milk carton trash, and the cups get washed in the dishwasher.

The Green Team at the Edna Louise Spear Elementary School in Port Jefferson, New York, reduced the garbage in their cafeteria by 25 percent during the school's No Waste Week. They set up recycling bins for plastics, aluminum, paper, and drink pouches alongside the garbage pails. Parents volunteered to show students how the recycling worked during the first two weeks of the program, and now the student government has taken on the task of monitoring the kids to make sure they are sorting the waste properly.

Wellness Policy in the Classroom

In addition to the lunchroom, wellness policy must address the food environment of the classroom—celebrations, snacks, food rewards, and curriculum. *Cupcake Wars* is now the title of a popular competition series on the Food Network, but the original cupcake wars began with the battle over school food policy. In her 2005 documentary film, *Let Them Eat Cake*, Lisa Kaselak chronicles the saga of the Texas Cupcake Controversy. When the state legislature, presiding over a population of children declared the most obese and least healthy in the nation, implemented a policy banning junk food in schools, the cupcake became the semaphore waved by opponents. The legislation was criticized as one more power grab by the "nanny state," while proponents argued that the $1 billion-plus cost of obesity in Texas was being borne by all the citizens of our largest state. A compromise was eventually reached in which the Texas state wellness policy remained in effect alongside a provision for a Safe Cupcake Amendment.

BREAKFAST IN THE CLASSROOM

Study after study shows that eating a good breakfast is one of the single most influential nutritional factors affecting student performance. As many as 48 percent of girls and 32 percent of boys skip breakfast on a regular basis. To counteract this trend, whole-grain muffins, breakfast burritos, a bowl of oatmeal, cups of yogurt with fresh or dried fruit, a hard-boiled egg, or even good-quality dry cereal with milk are some of the items that schools are sending into classrooms or offering in brown bags when students arrive at school. Despite concerns about potential for distraction from the lessons and the challenge of messy waste disposal, breakfast in the classroom is on the upswing, particularly in low-income school districts. I'd like to see this catch on everywhere. Eating a healthy breakfast is also key to setting a child's metabolism for the day, aiding in a balanced intake of calories and reducing blood sugar peaks and valleys and their corresponding mood swings.

SNACKS

Some policies refer to an approved list of classroom snacks, especially for the younger grades, but even the idea of snacking in class is controversial. If breakfast and lunch are scheduled at appropriate intervals, some parents and nutritionists wonder why children need to be given an additional opportunity to eat every couple of hours, preferring them to eat a complete meal at proper mealtimes.

If you're going to allow some snacks, you'll want to create a list that includes lots of healthy options that are simple to prepare and easy to serve. Here's a list you can pull from or add to:

Fresh fruit: small apples, bananas (cut in half), blueberries, sliced cantaloupe, cherries, peeled grapefruit sections, grapes, cubed honeydew, halved kiwis, mandarin oranges or clementines, nectarines, quartered oranges, peaches, pineapple rings, plums, raspberries, strawberries, tangerines, watermelon chunks.

Also unsweetened applesauce, dried fruit, mixed fruit salad, whole fruit smoothies with or without yogurt, and coconut-rolled pitted dates.

Veggies: Any kind of cut-up vegetables with dip—bell peppers, broccoli, carrots sticks or baby carrots, cauliflower, cherry tomatoes, cucumber, snap peas, snow peas, string beans, sprouts, summer squash.

Great veggie dips include bean dips, guacamole, hummus, nut butters or sunflower seed butter (depending upon allergies), pesto, salsa, tahini, and all kinds of homemade or good-quality salad dressings. You can jazz up the veggies by making ants on a log (celery spread with nut butter and topped with raisins), a mini salad bar, or stuffed pita pockets with dressing.

Whole grains: Non-GMO popcorn, puffed rice, or kamut cakes with nut or sunflower butters or fruit spreads, granola or muesli, whole-grain muffins or cereal-based cookies.

Protein: Trail mix with peanuts, cashews, almonds, sunflower seeds, pumpkin seeds, and dried fruits like raisins, apricots, apples, pineapple, or cranberries. (A few chocolate chips in the trail mix go a long way.) Deviled eggs or egg salad spread on pita.

Snack policy should specify no unpronounceable or artificial ingredients, colors, or flavors with a preference to whole foods rather than packaged bars, chips, or cookies.

Water: Water should always be available to students during snack time. Your policy should also dictate how and when students can have access to drinking water at other times of day. Are water bottles allowed in class? If not, do students need permission to get a drink from a drinking fountain?

CELEBRATE!

It's kind of ironic that teachers sometimes complain about breakfast in the classroom, yet we also hear teachers complain when wellness policies prohibit food rewards and cupcakes at classroom celebrations. A clear, well-reasoned policy, with lots of input from both teachers and parents, can help settle the cupcake wars in your district. Kids and most teachers love to celebrate birthdays and holidays and wellness policy shouldn't get in the way of having some fun. A good policy will provide guidelines for food and fun, and refer to documents that offer ideas for classroom celebrations that don't undermine wellness. A good celebration compromise I've seen allows for a shared monthly birthday celebration in the classroom, and specifies that the goodies can only be served after lunch, and a healthy alternative such as fresh fruit must be offered along with the cupcakes.

Stopping in at Dunkin' Donuts and picking up a box of Munchkins is easy and pretty much ensures your party will be a success. It takes a bit more effort to put on a fun-filled food-free celebration. A dance-a-thon, party games, or school building scavenger hunt can be fun party themes. The Massachusetts Public Health Association offers these suggestions:

- Celebrate with physical activity—allow them an extra recess or gym class.
- Have the children design, build, and run an obstacle course.
- Celebrate with art and music—have an art party. Divide the classroom into four stations and at each station have a craft activity. Play music in the background.
- Single out the birthday child with a "V.I.P." button/badge or crown.
- Have the birthday child be the first to do each classroom activity and/or be the line leader for the day.
- Book donation—A great way to build up the classroom library and recognize the child. Have the child's family donate a book and inside label it: "This book was donated to Mrs. Smith's classroom in honor of John Jones's 8th birthday."
- Sing the birthday song!

Holiday celebrations traditionally involve food as well. If your policy allows snacks, involve the students in planning and preparing a healthy holiday-themed meal or treat.

FOOD REWARDS

When my older daughter was in elementary school, she would often come home very sad from school on Fridays. She'd sigh and tell me that she took too long to do her work and didn't get the Friday treat, a reward her teacher gave to kids who finished their work early. Usually it was candy and extra recess time. It still makes me sad to think about my little girl struggling to complete her ditto sheet so she wouldn't be left out of the fun. Classroom rewards can turn into punishment for a child who needs extra time or extra help. In my daughter's case, the punishment was a one-size-fits-all policy that never rewarded her effort. I eventually spoke to the teacher and she agreed that the policy wasn't fair and made accommodations. At the time, I was worried less about the weekly candy than about my child's frustration and self-esteem.

What the teacher and I might have also discussed was the subtle yet firm reinforcement she was making to the belief system: "I did well, so I deserve candy (or substitute your favorite confection here)." Using food as a reward sends the wrong message. The reward comes with the promise of feeling good for a job well done, and then conditions us to believe we need the sugary treat to feel good. It's tempting to excuse a little weekly candy reward, but when Friday treat gets added to Saturday at the birthday party, Sunday with Grandma, Monday at the ball game, etc. . . . all those treats and rewards create patterns and habits that are very hard to break. The treats encourage children to eat between meals, eat for comfort, eat when they're not hungry, eat empty calories, seek immediate gratification—all the behaviors that any health counselor or diet guru will counsel you to correct if you're trying to lose weight, conquer type 2 diabetes, or heal a digestive disorder.

Teachers use rewards to encourage good behavior, and children often respond to a system of rewards with a desire to perform correctly. Psychology 101 refers to this as "operant conditioning." We used a similar system of positive reinforcement to train our puppies. First, the reward is given every time the pup exhibits the desired behavior; eventually you only need to give an occasional reward to reinforce the habit. The goal of operant conditioning is for the subject to internalize the behavior so they will no longer need a reward. The system works well for dogs, not so well for humans who are able to replicate the rewards by treating themselves as they get older.

Alternative Rewards

The Center for Science in the Public Interest has a comprehensive list of alternative classroom rewards and incentives that they recommend for inclusion in local wellness policy (adapted from CSPI).

Social Rewards

These involve attention, praise, or thanks, and are often more highly valued by children than a toy or food. Simple gestures like pats on the shoulder, verbal praise (including in front of others), nods, or smiles can mean a lot. These types of social rewards affirm a child's worth as a person.

Recognition

- Trophy, plaque, ribbon, or certificate in recognition of achievement or a sticker with an affirming message (e.g., "Great job")
- Recognizing a child's achievement on the school-wide morning announcements and/or the school's website
- A photo recognition board in a prominent location in the school
- A phone call, e-mail, or letter sent home to parents or guardians commending a child's accomplishment
- A note from the teacher to the student commending his or her achievement

Privileges

- Going first
- Choosing a class activity
- Helping the teacher
- Having an extra few minutes of recess with a friend
- Sitting by friends or in a special seat next to or at the teacher's desk
- "No homework" pass

- Teaching the class
- Playing an educational computer or other game
- Reading to a younger class
- Making deliveries to the office
- Reading the school-wide morning announcements
- Helping in another classroom
- Eating lunch with a teacher or principal
- Listening with a headset to a book on tape or CD
- Going to the library to select a book to read
- Working at the school store
- Taking a walk with the principal or teacher
- Designing a class or hall bulletin board
- Writing or drawing on the blackboard/whiteboard
- Taking care of the class animal for a day
- Being allowed to choose an extra recess activity for the class as a birthday treat

Rewards for a Class
- Extra recess
- Eating lunch, holding class or reading outdoors
- Going to the lunchroom first
- Extra art, music, PE, or reading time
- Listening to music while working
- Dancing to music
- Playing a game or doing a puzzle together
- "Free choice" time at the end of the day
- A song, dance, or performance by the teacher or students
- A book read aloud to the class by the teacher
- A field trip
- School supplies
- Sports equipment and athletic gear
- Toys/trinkets

- Gift certificate to the school store
- A plant, or seeds and pot for growing a plant
- Books
- Magazine subscription
- Board game
- A token or point system, whereby children earn points that accumulate toward a bigger prize. Possible prizes include those listed above and:
  - Gift certificate to a bookstore or sporting goods store
  - Movie pass or rental gift certificate
  - Ticket to sporting event

Children can be given fake money, tokens or stars, or a chart can be used to keep track of the points they have earned. Points can be exchanged for privileges or prizes when enough are accumulated.

A point system also may be used for an entire class to earn a reward. Whenever individual children have done well, points can be added to the entire class's "account." When the class has earned a target number of points, then they receive a group reward.

CURRICULUM

The how-to of integrating food into the curriculum is the subject of chapter seven. Your wellness policy should discuss why it's important to have consistent messages about food throughout the school environment, and should include a mandate for staff and teacher development. Teachers need to know how junk food is marketed to kids, how to read ingredient labels, and what subtle and not-so-subtle junk food messages may be promoted in their textbooks and other classroom materials. Teachers need to learn how to incorporate positive food lessons into every subject area in every grade. They need to be comfortable and familiar with some aspects of growing, shopping, preparing, cooking, and tasting whole foods so they can share these experiences with their students.

Food Policy Around the School

The school food environment extends beyond the cafeteria and classroom. Wellness policy should include school fund-raising activities, fairs, field trips, athletic practices, and games.

FUND-RAISING

Your PTO/PTA/PTSA relies on fund-raising to enrich the educational resources of your school system. Funds raised by these organizations are used to pay for computers, library books, SMART boards, video equipment, playgrounds, and even curriculum and teachers in these school-budget-strapped days. Many of the traditional fund-raising venues—cookie and candy drives, bake sales and fairs, label, coupon and receipt redemptions and rewards—are mostly targeted at selling food to kids, and most members of the school community hold these activities sacred. With that in mind, even some of the strictest wellness policies exempt bake sales and other fund-raising activities—the cupcake clause.

When you examine some of the ready-made fund-raisers more closely, though, they begin to resemble the vending machine conundrum. Lots of corporate marketing dollars are poured into glossy order forms with easy-to-follow instructions, but what's really going on is that the school is given a cut of sales for the work that our kids are doing as unpaid salespeople for the marketing firms. As our children are being pressed into service in this fashion, it's worth a look at the products they're selling and the ethics behind them. Recently, a number of companies have begun offering fund-raising programs based on fair trade items that pay a fair wage to the growers and producers in faraway lands. Equal Exchange offers high-quality snack foods: fair trade nuts, dried fruits, coffee, tea, and chocolate. Fundraise Naturally sells artisan-made soaps and candles; Global Sistergoods supports women artisans in developing countries.

While it might seem like a challenge to raise money without selling junk food, the Center for Science in the Public Interest reports that nonfood and healthy food fund-raisers generate profits for schools "equal to or greater than profits from fund-raisers selling low-nutrition foods." A great resource for nonfood fund-raising is *Nojunkfood.org*, a blog started by fed-up Los Angeles teacher Jacqueline Domac. Her list of alternative fund-raising ideas includes things kids can do and things they can sell. Here are a few sample suggestions:

Things You Can Do
- Auction
- Bike-a-thon
- Bowling night
- Car wash
- Carnival
- Dance
- Fair/festival
- Flea market
- Walk-a-thon
- Jump-rope-a-thon
- Magic show
- Raffle
- Read-a-thon
- Recycle cans/paper/ink cartridges
- Skate night
- Spelling bee
- Talent show
- Scavenger hunt

Things to Sell
- Books and calendars
- Buttons, pins, and stickers
- Candles
- Cookbooks

- Coupon books
- Emergency kits for cars
- First aid kits
- Flowers, plants, and bulbs
- Football game shout-outs
- Football seats
- Fruit and vegetable baskets
- Fruit smoothies and slushies
- Gift baskets
- Gift wrap
- Greeting cards
- Healthy snack items
- Holiday ornaments
- House decorations
- Jewelry
- License plate frames with school logo
- Magazine subscriptions
- Mugs
- Personalized stationery and pens
- Scarves
- School spirit gear and accessories, including Frisbees
- Stadium pillows
- Stuffed animals
- T-shirts and sweatshirts
- Temporary/henna tattoos
- Tupperware

ATHLETICS

There's not been a great deal of discussion about school food policy in regard to athletics, and most wellness policies specifically exempt league athletics and after-school programs from adhering to the food guidelines, but your committee might want to consider setting some guidelines for any program that takes place on the school grounds. Student athletes are often seen as role models and leaders in the school community. In my film, there's a scene in which Susan Rubin speaks with a group of high school athletes about Gatorade. When Susan suggests fruit and water might do just as well for hydration and electrolyte balance, the boys tell her that their coach says they need the Gatorade. One boy points to the label, insisting, "Look, Gatorade's better than water. There's a little chart on the back." Student athletes can have a really positive influence on the culture of school food when their training includes an active sports nutrition component. Consider inviting your school's athletic director or a coach to be part of the wellness council and working with the athletic department and league coaches to include a food component to team training.

Local boosters clubs often raise money for uniforms and sports equipment by supplying the team and spectators with a variety of burgers, hot dogs, and chips through a concession stand on game days. Your food advisory group might offer to supply some healthy alternatives such as a homemade soup or salad.

IN THE FIELD

My experience chaperoning the junk-food fueled kids on that field trip to Washington, D.C., exemplifies the need for a food policy specific to field trips. The teachers were desperate for some control over the kids' behavior and they recognized that the candy, chips, and soda were not helping matters. Meals on the field trip were prepaid in the fees that families had paid. Most of the meals once we got to D.C. were quite good, but little consideration had been made for the bus rides. A food policy governing field trips could specify that all meals should at least meet the USDA minimum guidelines and that three meals a day must be offered to students on the trip. School food service could provide a bus breakfast, or a local deli could provide muffins, egg sandwiches, fruit, and so on.

STAFF WELLNESS

Wellness policy may affect your staff and some districts have a staff wellness subcommittee to address issues and concerns regarding staff wellness. As school staff will be tasked with implementing and upholding your policy, they need to be committed to the process. Make sure staff are well represented on the committee and give input about how policy will affect them, and what policies could support their own wellness. Be sensitive to their concerns without creating a double standard; adults have the right to indulge in things that wellness policy may deem inappropriate for kids—even on school grounds. Policies may insist that they set a good example for students, but staff shouldn't be made to feel policed or harassed for their personal habits and choices.

Finance

Good food does cost more and the method your district uses to pay for it will depend upon the number of children eligible for free or reduced meals. Whether you have many low-income students or few, your wellness policy must call for marketing the meal program. Successful implementation depends upon student acceptance and increased participation. One of the many myths I hear about school food is that the district will lose money if it improves food quality. Just as with the vending machines, in nearly every case, what happens is that sales initially drop off, then rebound and surpass previous numbers in a matter of weeks.

The Berkeley, California, wellness policy took a responsible approach to financing its famously successful food policy:

> The Board of Education shall do a comprehensive cost/benefit analysis and business plan. The plan shall include an examination of different development models of increased fresh food preparation at the central and satellite kitchens.

And in Katonah-Lewisboro the policy commits the district to "maintaining the financial stability of its food service program and ensuring that an affordable, reasonably priced lunch is available for all students," and "re-evaluating the cost effectiveness of the National School Lunch Program after the nutritional guidelines set forth in the wellness policy have been implemented."

Administration

The vague policy my district voted on in 2006 has not changed in five years because there was never a provision for updating it. Your policy needs a plan for implementation, monitoring, evaluation, and renewal. Institutional oversight is critical; I've seen great programs fall apart when parent volunteers had children who aged out of the school system. Many school districts have created part-time positions for a school wellness coordinator to see that the policy is implemented and monitored throughout the school district. The wellness coordinator sits on the wellness committee and often acts as a liaison between the food service, the district, and the community at large. He or she has an active role in promoting wellness and food education in local media, via food events, tastings, school gardens, Farm to School programs, and classroom instruction. These jobs are being filled by trained chefs, experienced parents, and also by AmeriCorps/FoodCorps volunteers.

Presenting the Policy

Any proposed changes to your wellness policy will be subject to approval by your district's board of education. Your superintendent's office can tell you what the exact process is in your district. Most likely you will have to request a public hearing prior to getting the policy placed on the agenda for a board of ed meeting. Make sure your key supporters show up at the public hearing and again at the vote. Be prepared to hand out fact sheets and copies of your proposed policy. Expect to hear what Janet Poppendieck calls "disabling myths" and come prepared with preemptive solutions to the roadblocks that will be thrown in your way.

DISABLING MYTHS

I've been collecting this list of myths since I began my quest to learn what could be done to improve school food. They've been chanted to me like mantras, repeated by force of habit. Henry Ford famously stated, "If you think you can do a thing or can't do a thing, you're right." It's all about attitude. Here are some of the myths, and some ideas for addressing them to help change attitudes about wellness in your school community.

- The kids won't eat it; the kids won't like it.
  - Most kids are more flexible than we give them credit for. If new foods are introduced properly (tasting, learning about what the food is and where it comes from), children learn to like them readily. Not all kids like every food, but in every example I've found, more students preferred the new food, with some exceptions like nuggets and fries— these were tough to wean from and were phased out over time.
- Kids need choices so they can learn to make good choices.
  - Offering children unhealthy foods and drinks at school contradicts what they are taught about good nutrition and sends a mixed message. Why shouldn't all the choices be good choices? We don't ask kids if they'd rather have recess or math! Limiting choices, especially in the younger grades, helps kids develop a taste for good food, and good eating habits. When kids choose soda, candy, and junk food instead of eating a meal, they don't get the nourishment they need to learn properly.
- We don't have many obese kids in our school, so the food is not a problem.
  - Obesity is only part of the problem. Most of the nutrition messages we hear are focused on obesity, but America's children are developing chronic diseases at earlier ages and emotional, behavioral, and

learning disorders are epidemic. These behaviors have demonstrably improved in schools that have eliminated junk food.

- There's no such thing as bad food; you're contributing to eating disorders by making kids anxious about food.
  - This is a myth perpetuated by the food industry. Junk food addiction is its own eating disorder and causes disease. Our children are being exploited by the food industry and that shouldn't be allowed in school. Teaching children a healthy skepticism about processed food and exposing them to a wide array of real food choices will enable them to make decisions based on knowledge rather than fear.
- It's calories in, calories out. Kids just need to get more exercise.
  - A common myth is that protein is protein, regardless of its source, and that feeding children manufactured, standardized, industrialized food products fortified with vitamins is a healthy diet. This myth blames the kids for being fat and lazy but doesn't take into account that their lack of energy may be due to the lack of life force in the calories they are consuming.
- It's only one meal a day.
  - 180 days a year x 12 years = 2,160 meals—double that if there's a breakfast program. That's a lot of food. For many kids, especially low-income kids, school food makes up two-thirds or more of their diet.
- It's the parents' fault kids don't eat well.
  - America is now raising its third generation of fast-food babies. Many of today's parents did not grow up in households where food was freshly prepared. As a culture, we are losing our food knowledge. We also have become a society of single parents or two working parents who have little time to prepare meals. Schools therefore need to help teach children what their parents often cannot.
- This is a matter of personal choice; parents should decide what their kids should eat, not the schools.
  - That's basically what Sarah Palin is saying. Unfortunately for her argument, educators make decisions on behalf of their students every day. From curriculum content, to where they should go on field trips,

to whether the district must cut the music and arts budget or the athletics budget, parents can give input but must ultimately rely on school administrators to act on our behalf.

- Who needs it—let's just drop the meal program and let them bring lunch.
  - I heard this argument in Darien, Connecticut, one of the wealthiest school districts in the country. I've also seen it in conservative op-ed pieces. According to USDA regulations, as long as one child in the district qualifies for a free meal, the school must sponsor the meal program. It exists for the kids who need it; those who don't can bring their own.
- Sales will drop.
  - Districts that have improved food quality report that sales may go down initially, but recover and surpass previous numbers within about six weeks. Out of sixteen schools surveyed in California, thirteen reported that sales of à la carte items dropped, but more children bought school meals, which increased overall revenue. Maine, Minnesota, and Pennsylvania school districts have also reported positive results.
- It costs too much.
  - This is the pay now or pay later paradox. We can spend money on good food for children now, or spend far more on their health care down the road. Annual costs for treating diet-related diseases in America have increased by 400 percent over the past thirty years.
- It's too much work.
  - It *is* more work but it's not too much work. A return to real food in schools means increasing job skills and part-time local employment opportunities. Even staff members who are initially resistant to change will come around when they receive proper training.
- We don't have trained staff.
  - There is technical assistance and skills training available from the government as well as local volunteer efforts. You may find that your staff morale increases as they gain skill, confidence, and positive feedback in the cafeteria.
- We don't have a kitchen.

- Smaller districts in some regions are banding together to share a central kitchen. Others may contract with a local caterer to provide food that meets their specifications.
- We don't have the right equipment.
  - Ask your PTA, apply for a government grant, find out if your district has a fund or a bond for improvements. Kitchen equipment manufacturers and local appliance stores are also good places to seek donations.
- We can't do this in every school.
  - How about beginning in one school and growing from there?
- We can't get better food from our approved vendors.
  - Food service management companies (FSMC) may make this excuse and if they do, then fire them. Your district has hired the FSMC to deliver a meal plan that meets your food policy guidelines, which should be specified in their contract. If they signed a contract that specifies local or organic ingredients, then that is what they must deliver. They need to find better vendors.
- We can't purchase fresh food.
  - Even a district that relies heavily on commodity food has some flexibility in the food budget. If the food service director (FSD) can't or won't find sources for fresh food, parent volunteers can take on this task. Once the initial arrangements have been made, the FSD may find it simpler to manage than anticipated.
- We can't store or process fresh food.
  - In that case, your district may need to team up with another by pooling resources and developing a campaign to build a kitchen that has the capacity to store and process enough food to supply several schools. This model is proving efficient and economical even in some rural areas where the schools are spread out.
- If we made fresh food, how could we ensure it's safe?
  - Every school cafeteria is required to have a HACCP plan and a ServSafe-trained employee. Nearly every one of the food-borne illnesses that have made headlines in recent years have come from the

industrial food sector, not from local farms or small producers. Proper food handling procedures are not difficult to learn.

- The school food movement is elitist.
  - Some of the best examples I have seen of model school food programs are in districts where more than half of the students qualify for free meals. New Haven, Connecticut, and Berkeley, California, are just two examples. In fact, research shows that children from low-income families take up the new foods more readily than those in more affluent districts.
- We have too many other academic priorities—school food isn't an educational issue, so it's not my job.
  - A school superintendent told me this one. The USDA requires nutrition education and a school food policy, so clearly the government feels that it is an educational issue.
- We're already doing a great job. Our food is healthy; we meet all the USDA requirements.
  - Yes, you are. The families in our district want to support you and help you go beyond the USDA standards. We want to work with you and help figure out what resources you need to meet the standards of our new food policy.

DANA'S DECADE

Across the bay from the famous Edible Schoolyard in Berkeley, California, San Francisco mom Dana Woldow sank her teeth into the school food challenge and hasn't let go for ten years.

Dana, like most of us, says she fell into this by accident. "My children didn't eat school food. My oldest son was too impatient to wait in line but when he was in middle school I heard from kids in our car pool that they were selling all this stuff at school. When my next son got to middle school, he was interested but I didn't give him money. By the time my third son got to middle school I was friendly with the principal, who had two kids who were going to middle school the next year. She told me she was horrified." The principal had approached the food service director to stop selling the junk. The food service director refused and made it very clear that she did not want to be told what to do. Dana vividly recalls the astounded principal asking her if the food service program was getting some sort of incentive from Pepsi. Dana replied, "I don't know. Would you like me to look into it for you?" and then she was off and running with it.

Dana discovered that her kid's friend's parents didn't know that the kids were buying giant Pepsi's, enormous bags of Cheetos, or six huge cookies as their lunch. She says, "The reimbursable meal was horrible, too. I knew we could do better than this. I went to the superintendent to go over the head of the food service director." Dana proposed a six-month pilot program in the middle school. They would make some changes and track the revenue. "Because people always say if we stop selling junk we would lose money. I asked her to let us do this pilot for six months. And if it breaks even and makes money we can extend it. That was in October of 2002." She formed a nutrition committee with other parents, the principal, and Ed Wilkins, the supervisor who worked just under the food service director.

Although Ed was expected to represent the food service director, he appoached Dana after a first meeting and arranged to meet her for lunch the next day. "He said he wanted to help," Dana recalls, and the two began meeting clandestinely to craft a plan. "We got rid of the soda the first week of January of that year. The second week we got rid of the chips, the third week snack cakes and ice cream. We surveyed the students to see what healthy options they would be willing to eat. Once they realized that we didn't want to hear hot dogs, etc., they gave us reasonable suggestions, like subway-style sandwiches, salads, yogurt, and soup. These were all things that we could do. For drinks we served only bottled water, milk, and 100 percent juice—no more Gatorade, Snapple, juice drinks, no more enormous pizza, chicken wings, and hot links. Now we have a cookie made with pureed prunes instead of fat. We stuck with cookies because we had taken away every other thing the kids love, so we kept cookies and they bake them fresh."

(continued)

That first week, sales plummeted because sodas were the single biggest seller. By March, though, the cafeteria, which had been operating in the red, had gone into the black. Dana's was one of only two schools that showed a profit that year.

The San Francisco Board of Education passed a resolution in January 2003. Dana proudly proclaims, "We created a district-wide wellness committee three years before the federal requirement. The committee decided to get junk food out of the district by the start of 2003–2004 and it was up to the committee to figure out how to do that. We had an enormous committee—forty-five people—representatives from the public health department, the whole community. We had only a six-week timeline but we plowed on through, turned the policy in and then we waited."

After all the work, the board of education sent the policy back to the food service director. "It came back incomprehensible and was in no way what we had recommended. I went to a friend who was close with the superintendent. The superintendent called all of us into a meeting in her conference room. She said, 'This is not the policy written by the committee.'"

The superintendent proceeded to remove the administrators who had been co-chairs of the committee and appointed Dana as the chair. She's filled that role ever since. "We got the soda out of the vending machines. One principal said she used to walk through the halls and feel the caffeine buzz. We compared suspensions for the same time period the previous year and it had dropped by 50 percent. She attributed it to better counseling but also to the removal of the caffeine."

The momentum began to build. Dana recounts, "The second year we tackled the sorry-looking hot lunch. We were a completely self-run operation. We would divert our commodities to two or three different processors. The hamburgers, chicken nuggets, and hot dogs. It would go to a dirty middle school kitchen with workers assembling meals by hand." Much to Dana's relief, the food service director took early retirement, and her ally, Ed Wilkins, took on the job. Unfortunately, San Francisco did not have school kitchens equipped to cook from scratch, so instead they went looking for a local caterer that could supply them with better-quality food.

"We started working with an outfit called Preferred Meal Systems," says Dana. "They are not a food service management company. They don't come in and take over. They provide you with the meals. They have different levels of quality. We started with the lowest quality because at that time our concern was just about food safety. Over that year we looked at what they were serving and said the corn dog had to go. Then we started going through the menu and making tweaks. Potatoes were served as the vegetable four or five days a week. First of all, we said no more fried potatoes; they had to be mashed, boiled, or roasted. Now we serve potatoes only a few times a month. We looked at what vegetables were being served and what they were being served with. We changed the disgusting chicken nuggets to whole-breast-meat nuggets. We added whole grains. Over the last five years we have gradually improved. There's no more canned fruit, only fresh fruit, and the grains are entirely whole grain. No trans fats, no high fructose corn syrup. They produce a menu for us that is unlike the menu they do anywhere else."

When the district-wide changes began, the school food program faced a deficit of $1.5 million. Dana says it decreased to $140,000 after several years but then went up again with food, fuel, and labor increases in 2008. "We made a concerted effort to get more applications returned for free and reduced meals because we had thousands of kids who never filled out an application. We promoted the idea that every family needed to return the form—those who could afford to buy lunch could write 'not interested.' Kids didn't want to turn in the free meal form. By sixth grade the stigma is really pronounced, particularly for African-American and Latino students. The numbers drop off in middle school and high school because of the stigma. This year 60 percent of kids qualified and 92 percent of kids have already turned in forms. San Francisco is a sanctuary city; we have a lot of undocumented immigrants here who won't fill out forms. We spend probably a million dollars a year on kids who are uncollectable, but that's the cost of doing business in a big city. You have to spend the money. We can't afford to not feed them."

Dana continued advocating for the welfare of those kids. "We needed POS [Point of Sale—electronic] technology. We agitated for it for years. We tried

(continued)

to get grants. Our new superintendent in 2007 said he would find the way, and . . . last year it was installed. The kids all swipe cards and no one has to bring cash." And they did away with à la carte items entirely. The students now have three to five choices every day—the main meal or a sandwich, rice bowl, pizza, or hamburger. Dana explains, "Every choice comes as a complete meal. You can't just go get a bagel. The bagel comes with raw vegetables, fruit, and milk. At one school the participation has gone up 49 percent this year. So not only are kids eating a full meal, we get the 26 cents for the fully paid meals, and in two years we'll get an additional 20 cents' commodity allotment for those extra meals."

Over these many years, Dana has developed a deep understanding of the system. One of the big issues with making changes, she says, is that "it takes years because the school food service won't close the books until December of the following year. Commodity allotments get done in January of the calendar year, so the most recent figures will be from the year before. You submit your reimbursements but are lucky to see them many months later."

When I first met Dana she was irate that San Francisco wasn't getting the attention that Berkeley was getting, because they didn't have a celebrity chef or any outside financing or resources. What they did have was Dana, and her persistence is paying off. This year, she hopes the city will finance a central kitchen and they will be able to establish whole new job categories with job descriptions requiring culinary skills. Many of the current food service employees are unskilled and at or above retirement age, unable or unwilling to take on new tasks. With the new kitchen, Dana says she can bring in people who can actually cook—maybe even a budding celebrity chef?

I'm exhausted just from hearing about Dana's saga. I asked her what advice she has for parents who face similar challenges advocating in their districts. "After people get educated they have to get connected. You need to make friends and once you've got your core group of ten or fifteen people you can count on, then you have to look at your school board. Get to know who is on your school board—there's always one who cares about this. Your school board can then influence your superintendent. That one person can help you find out who else on your school board could be influenced."

Then, she says, "Once they've gotten educated and connected, they need to get going. You can get on the grant list from the federal government. Whenever there's a state or federal grant they'll send you an e-mail. My son's high school got a $70,000 grant for two years to go and buy vegetables. The kids were looking for a project. It made such a huge difference. In elementary schools now, once you're on [the fresh fruit and vegetable program] you can be on it forever."

And like many advocates working on the district level, Dana's philosophy is, "You can't sit around waiting for Congress to act, although ultimately that's the only fair and equitable way to fix school food."

Implementation

Implementation can occur all at once or may be phased in over time. Experts recommend a marketing and tasting phase first, and then gradual implementation when it comes to changes in the meal program. This allows for a feedback interval and time to make adjustments to the process as you go.

A large aspect of the food education piece of the policy at this point will be integrating the new food with positive food messages, stories, and hands-on experiences. In the most successful programs I've seen, those messages and experiences are consistently woven into the culture of the school in the cafeteria, the classroom, and throughout the entire curriculum.

Half a Sandwich

You may not succeed with your policy your first or second time around. Don't be discouraged—you are paving a path. Five years ago, a school nurse, Amanda Stone from Marion, Massachusetts, told me that her one accomplishment after years on the wellness committee was obtaining an agreement to serve a slice of whole-grain bread on one side of the peanut butter and jelly sandwiches. I wish I could say that was ancient history, but sadly another mom from elsewhere just told me the same story recently. I'm going to say it again—Don't give up! There are many things you can do outside of the school meals program to improve your school's food environment. As a guest food teacher in the classroom or a volunteer in the school garden, you can have a great impact on the students in your school.

And if your policy isn't adopted, get your group together for a debriefing. Discuss what aspects of your campaign did work, and what steps you'll need to take to get back in the fray. Maybe you need to grow your caucus, publicize the issue more widely, and tie it to other concerns in your community. Make sure your media contacts know that the policy wasn't approved. Were there members of the board of education who voted for the proposal or were there members who sympathized but didn't vote for it? These people are your allies and you need to firm up their support. Find out what they think happened and ask them to help you strategize for your next round. The Massachusetts Public Health Association counsels, "Don't give up! You may not have gotten your policy passed, but you *succeeded* in forming a committee and raising public awareness of the issue. After you have evaluated your process, try again. For the health of our children . . . don't take no for an answer!"

And if your policy does fly, *congratulations*! The following chapters illustrate wellness policy in action, along with some examples of what can be accomplished even without a strong policy.

STEPS FOR WELLNESS POLICY

- Research existing policy, contact key school administrators, request a meeting, share your agenda, listen and learn from them, and then request a policy review.
- Build a team, either on the district wellness committee or an outside wellness, sustainability, or food advisory council.
- Meet regularly, create goals and tasks, and report to school administrators and community.

- Assess the school's existing environment in terms of food education, opportunities for physical activity, and the food environment in the cafeteria and beyond.
- Write a detailed policy proposal for your district, promote it, and adopt it at a school board meeting.
- Have team members lead task forces to implement the policy throughout the district.
- Evaluate and update the policy regularly.

FIVE

TIPPING SCALES TO TIPPING POINTS

Be who you are and say what you feel, because those who mind don't
matter and those who matter don't mind.

—Dr. Seuss

ixing school food is a matter of degrees and clearly there's no single solution. Wellness policy can set the stage for changes large
and small, but beyond that, it's the people and the community that
make it happen. People, not policy, drive the movement for better food in
schools. My mission as a chronicler of the movement has been to learn and
share lessons from its leaders. Some of the dedicated leaders I've met are
pragmatists—they put one foot in front of the other, are willing to move forward in increments, baby steps—and over time, they can look back and see
some great progress. Others are visionaries with enough charisma to attract
the resources to implement their vision. I've seen success (and failure, too)
from both types of leadership. In every case, these leaders have articulated
an approach, and a sequence of actions that built momentum and led to a
series of tipping points at which the school food culture shifted, changed,
or in some cases was completely reinvented. Leadership and community
engagement are essential components of these tipping points, but also coming strongly into play are elements of luck, timing, and some good publicity
and PR.

Ultimately, it's the mission and clarity of the end goal that defines the process. School districts that define success as reduced BMI scores for students, or stronger nutrition regulations, may be able to achieve those goals without questioning or debating the entire culture and educational philosophy of the system. However, I've been truly inspired by the people and places that are willing to host that debate. These conversations can lead to deep and lasting reforms, and the schools that have taken a holistic approach to food policy and wellness are at the vanguard of the school food revolution.

One of the most celebrated of school food revolutionaries is chef and cookbook author Alice Waters. She coined the phrase "Delicious Revolution" for a social movement that invites Americans to discover the sensual pleasures of dining with family and friends on simple, fresh, locally grown foods in their season. It's a movement that embraces family farmers and small businesses, retains local dollars for the local economy, and fosters sustainable practices that cause the least harm to the local and global environment. This movement is now more than the latest foodie trend; it's one of the few bright spots in our sagging economy and its impact can be measured by the speed at which all things green and local are being promoted and mimicked by the food industry it shuns. The local food movement cuts across political, religious, and socioeconomic divides. The nutritional benefits of eating fresh food are almost secondary to the mission of building community through the shared experience of connecting with food at its source. Programs like double value for food stamps at farmers' markets, Community Supported Agriculture, and a resurgence of college grads choosing organic farming as a career are all validations of the success of the delicious revolution.

Alice and many other delicious revolutionaries are literally reinventing school food. They have taken the opportunity afforded by the mandate for local wellness policies to put everything on the table, beginning with the values, goals, and philosophy of a given school district. They see school food as a fundamental component of the local food movement, and they see building community as intrinsic to the program as building strong bodies. Against all odds, these delicious revolutionaries are creating school food systems that play by the rules (mostly) but step way out of the box, and they're making it work.

When I interviewed Alice Waters in the Edible Schoolyard in Berkeley, she explained, "This isn't a matter of just an upgrade of food that we're talking about. We're not talking about giving them a lot of choices. We're engaging them in the process of cooking and serving that food. And that's what gives them the investment. And that's what begins to change their eating habits. They love setting the table. They love washing the dishes. They like being part of this kind of feeling of family."

How do you tell the difference between an upgrade and a paradigm shift? Thomas Kuhn used the term "paradigm shift" to define a revolutionary change in basic scientific assumptions, with the resulting change invariably causing old assumptions to be discarded in favor of the new, which is proven to be better or more correct. Even in the world of science it takes some time for a paradigm shift to take root, but once that "aha!" moment occurs, there's no going back. I experienced that moment in Berkeley, and in several other schools around the country. You know it when you see it—food that looks and smells good, children engaged in learning, adults engaged with the children, and a general aura of calm and focus. It's not something that can be simulated; it's palpable, and once experienced, it's hard to deny.

The current school food revolution has its roots in decades of food politics, but its manifestation is little more than a dozen years old. One of the earliest models of the school food revolution was initiated by a group of parents in 1999 at the progressive Calhoun School on Manhattan's Upper West Side. Dissatisfied with the content and message of the highly processed meals provided by the school's food service management company, they performed a thorough assessment of the school's food environment. After exploring all their options, they hired the now-beloved Chef Bobo, a Culinary Institute–trained chef, to run their school food service. At the time, it was truly a radical idea to hire a chef to run a school food program. Chef Bobo soon became famous for his daily made-from-scratch soups, like roasted cauliflower, Indian tomato, and kabocha squash and adzuki bean soup. He's published a cookbook of his students' favorite recipes and now plays a vital role in teaching students the culinary arts in the school's rooftop vegetable garden as well as in the classrooms and cafeteria.

City kids in America are disproportionately overweight and obese, and it's in our city schools where we arguably need to make the greatest changes in the school food environment. The challenges of reimagining school food in an urban environment are compounded by lack of access to safe parks and playgrounds, overcrowded cafeterias, and fast-food joints on every corner. The city parents I meet always express the most urgency and desperation for change, and they're often cynical when I share examples from smaller districts. While some of the most comprehensively holistic school food programs I've seen are in private schools like Calhoun, or in small, self-operated suburban school districts, the school food revolution really is alive and well in our cities, although it just can't spread fast enough for most of us. Many of the models that the current crop of school food revolutionaries are rolling out and adapting to our big cities were first developed in those small-scale environments. What follows are a few examples.

Though she's become famous for her tenure as food service director in Berkeley, I first met Ann Cooper at the Ross School, a private day school on the eastern end of Long Island, New York. The school's founder, Courtney Ross, widow of Steven J. Ross, former chairman and CEO of Time Warner, had lured Ann away from a "white tablecloth" restaurant in Vermont. Perhaps inspired by Chef Bobo at Calhoun, she put Chef Ann in charge of the school's wellness and food program with high expectations. Ann delivered— she hired a handful of her fellow culinarians to help run the program and set to work integrating the progressive culture of the school into the food program, and integrating the food and wellness program into the school's curriculum. The day I visited the Ross School, I observed a tai chi class, a student meditating by a rippling koi pond, and a group of kids in the "café" dressed in head-to-toe Renaissance-era velvet costumes. The café, with its picture windows overlooking a wooded lot, and its high ceilings and natural wood beams, resembled an Aspen ski lodge. The open-hearth wood-fired pizza oven was running full tilt; the rest of the menu offered mu shu with cabbage and vegetables, braised duck ragout over pasta, mashed butternut squash and roasted turnips with chard. I had a fleeting fantasy of uprooting my family just so my daughter could attend this idyllic institution, but soon rationalized that she was better off learning how to cope in the real world of public school. Nevertheless, I came away inspired, wondering if the model Ann had created there could possibly be replicated, even in part, in public schools.

One of the first and best large-scale model programs is the school district of Berkeley, California. Since the 1960s, Berkeley has made a name for itself as a hotbed of activism, so it's not surprising that the school food revolution in the United States has Berkeley as its ground zero. My visit to Berkeley was the capstone for *Two Angry Moms*, and the district is still the gold standard for a healthy and delicious school food environment. It all began when Alice Waters started the Edible Schoolyard in 1995, inspired by an overgrown vacant lot on the property of a middle school she drove by every day on her way to work. That was the year she created her private foundation, the Chez Panisse Foundation, with the mission of using food to nurture, educate, and empower young people. The Edible Schoolyard has been growing fruit, vegetables, chickens, and children at the Martin Luther King Middle School for fifteen years, and today every school in the city of Berkeley has an edible school garden.

Alice's vision extended well beyond the garden. With her encouragement, the city of Berkeley adopted one of the most comprehensive wellness policies in the country, but they had a long way to go to implement many of their goals.

Next, the Chez Panisse Foundation built a kitchen classroom adjacent to the Edible Schoolyard, where students at the middle school could learn how to prepare the food they'd grown. I spoke with Annie Leonard, author of *The Story of Stuff*, whose daughter is a student at the Martin Luther King Middle School. She is thrilled about the food education her daughter receives there. She comments, "That school is absolutely incredible. They have a program that all the kids participate in that's called 'What's on Your Plate.' They learn basic things about food, about nutritional information, about serving size, about where it comes from, about how to compost. It's such a basic, fundamental part of being human that we've lost touch with. So my sixth-grader went in there not eating vegetables and she comes home now not only wanting to eat vegetables but she cooks them herself! She's doing more composting at home, she's aware of food, she's actually gained like five pounds since she started there, which she desperately needed so I am a huge fan of that. The food is mostly local; it's mostly organic, and best of all I don't have to pack lunches every day anymore. So I'm a big fan of their fabulous food program."

For years, the school had no cafeteria, and the kids were buying junk food from a snack shack in the schoolyard. News of Ann Cooper's work at the Ross School had made headlines, and Alice Waters brought Ann, aka The Renegade Lunch Lady, to California to transform the school food for the Berkeley Unified School District.

Ann Cooper's brash personality and notoriously curse-peppered words were a bit of a jolt for the laid-back Berkeley crowd, but they soon learned to respect her leadership and boundless energy. During her four-year turnaround tenure, she located local, often organic sources for all of her noncommodity food items, trained her staff in food safety, knife skills, and the rigors of scratch cooking some 5,000 meals a day. She refused to serve the worst of the processed commodities, and over time was able to order more whole foods through the program. She coordinated deliveries of breakfast and lunch from the district's central kitchen to the sixteen schools in the district, including the King Middle School, and she left the system with increased participation in the program, and a budget that is still running in the black.

There's been much debate about the extra funding that sustains the Berkeley model. Chez Panisse funded Ann's salary and some other startup costs, and Ann discovered entitlement funding from a California program called Meals for Needy Pupils that subsidizes the cost of breakfast and lunch. And the price for a school lunch is high—$3.25 for elementary lunch, $3.75 for middle school, and $4.25 for high school. Socioeconomically, Berkeley is a very diverse district; about 40 percent of the students in the district are eligible for subsidized meals. Yet Berkeley is home to a wealth of resources—in addition to the Chez Panisse Foundation, the Center for Ecoliteracy sponsors environmental education in its classrooms and the University of California at Berkeley has conducted longitudinal studies of the impact all of these programs has on Berkeley students. Advocates in many larger cities envy Berkeley's resources and activist population, and many wonder if the program is replicable. Ann Cooper insists that it is.

In fact, she's busy proving that claim in Boulder, Colorado, a much larger school district in a well-heeled community with only 20 percent of its students eligible for free or reduced-price meals. A wealthy school district presents a different set of challenges, because improving the lunch program depends on revenue from paying students as well as subsidized meals. Parents who can afford the time and cost of sending a healthy packed lunch to school may be reluctant to allow their kids to buy lunch. The goal in Boulder is to increase participation, and to do that, Ann and her crew will have to change not only the reality, but also the perception of the school meal program.

Ann claims she won't take on another district after Boulder, but if she could be persuaded to turn around a city like Detroit, Houston, or even Oakland, California, her detractors would surely be mollified.

By any standards, New York City is one of the most challenging school districts in America. In some of the boroughs, rates of childhood obesity are close to 25 percent. The district meal program, SchoolFood, led by chef Jorge Collazo, serves more than 860,000 school meals a day. The city has made a lot of progress in ridding the food of some of the worst ingredients, like trans fats, high fructose corn syrup, artificial flavors, colors, sweeteners, palm oil (usually hydrogenated), BHA, BHT, and MSG. There's still lots of processed food on the menu, though, and Chef Jorge welcomes collaboration in finding and implementing alternatives. A handful of parent advocacy groups have sprung up around the city, like NYC Green Schools and the Safe and Healthy Schools Coalition. I spent a day touring some city schools with the leaders of Wellness in the Schools, a nonprofit that is stirring up a food revolution in some of the city's school cafeterias and classrooms.

COOK FOR KIDS

As Dorothy Brayley of Kids First in Rhode Island says, "There are plenty of local organizations like us out there filling in the gaps in the school food system, but you're not going to find them in a Google search right off the bat. Most of them fly under the radar because they're not big, national, self-promoting dot-orgs. But there are people out there taking this on, building partnerships in their community."

One such organization is New York City's Wellness in the Schools. Founded in 2005 by a mom who's a former school principal, Nancy Easton, the organization's three-pronged mission is to improve the environment, nutrition, and fitness of New York City's public school kids. In a few short years, they've accomplished a great deal, albeit in a small slice of the city's 1,600 schools. Much of what they've done is based on soliciting and providing resources that the school system doesn't have. On the physical education front, Coach for Kids provides trained coaches to mentor the least active kids at recess. Green for Kids ensures that schools use bio-based, effective cleaning products that are healthy for children and the environment.

Cook for Kids partners with the city's Office of School Food, sending culinary-school graduates into school kitchens to prepare fresh meals from scratch and to educate food service staff, kids, and families about the importance of eating whole, unprocessed food. Despite her background as an educator, Nancy claims she was terribly naïve about advocacy when she started the program. "We started in one classroom four years ago. I had a series of volunteer chefs who would quit when they found a real job. I had two young kids and was pregnant with my third. The following year we did three schools. And then at the end of 2008 we met Bill."

Chef Bill Telepan, a NYC restaurant owner, is the driving force behind Cook for Kids. He's an unassuming guy with some strong convictions about taking better care of New York City's kids. His first year working with Nancy, they piloted the program in eight schools. The staff was still all volunteers, taking turns, each working a day a week for five weeks. The daily rotation was complicated and confusing, but Nancy says they learned a lot.

(continued)

"We learned from this pilot that we needed more consistency. We tried to model ourselves on the Teach for America model. And now, we are in nineteen schools and have nineteen of the most passionate, dedicated change agents. The other piece that was missing was the classroom-teaching piece. Now our chefs go into classrooms and do seasonal tastings. We make applesauce in the fall, grains in winter—oatmeal, then carrots and potatoes in the spring."

At P.S. 84, a bilingual elementary school on Manhattan's Upper West Side, Bill introduced me to Holly, a petite, articulate, no-nonsense chef who was busy filling the steel pans of a low-rise salad bar. Sliced cucumbers, baby carrots, chopped lettuce, and pesto pasta salad are some of the bar's offerings. Bill explains to me that the salad bar comes as an option with every meal, regardless of what else the students have on their tray. Strategically placed past the hot lunch line in the doorway before the checkout, students filing by are more likely to add some veggies to their plates. Holly has bonded with the school cafeteria's staff. They take pride in telling us about the success of yesterday's zucchini, bean, and basil stew. One of the staff offers a recipe for her homemade mac and cheese, the other item on yesterday's menu. She tells us that some of the kids mixed the stew in with the mac and cheese and while not every kid loved it, most tried it, and that's encouraging.

The Cook for Kids menus use a template for each day of the week: Meatless Mondays might be a chili, or a burrito, Trayless Tuesdays are sandwiches, rollups, and other finger foods, Wednesday is pasta day with a variety of sauces prepared from scratch, Thursday is chicken day, and they've kept Friday as pizza day, but the pizza is now homemade. The chefs work closely with the food service managers to bring in better quality and varieties of items. They've been able to procure olive oil, organic couscous, beans, quinoa, and even grass-fed beef.

The kids at the other elementary school we visited were having their favorite meal—the homemade pizza on Italian bread. Accompanying the pizza was a nice selection of vegetables—peas, corn, carrots—and every child had a perfect kid-size apple. For the most part, it looked like the kids were eating everything. The kitchen vibe at the second school was tense, though. Bill explained that the staff wasn't taking kindly to the young chef and there was resentment about the added workload. Bill had brought in a second chef for reinforcement, and they were optimistic that the school staff would come around. "We don't go where we're not wanted," he said, and they had actually pulled out of one school where the atmosphere was untenable for the new chef. Bill feels they're making good progress in most of the schools, introducing new items this year like the grass-fed beef, organic grains, and dried beans that come from a supplemental list subsidized by the PTA. WITS (Wellness in the Schools) is paying for the chefs, and the food costs are keeping at or close to the allocated amounts for the school system—about $1.10 per lunch.

The nineteen schools are distributed around the five boroughs of the city, and some of the schools are in the toughest neighborhoods. Nancy says the school principals are key to the success of the programs. "Before we go into a school the principal must sign a memorandum of understanding about the program. The district requires a monthly wellness partnership meeting with the school committee. They never really did it till we came along. We require that the school has a wellness committee and writes a policy and we ask that they put a green sustainability element in the policy. We enforce the meeting—it's our partnership meeting," and it keeps the school community involved.

Cook for Kids is also taking over science classes for a week in each of their schools, integrating food lessons with the chefs into a hands-on science lab.

Next year, they're hoping to expand the program from twenty to fifty schools, which would still reach just about 4 percent of New York's 1.1 million schoolchildren. Bill's not going to stop at that. "If we can get the kids eating unprocessed food for that 30 percent or 50 percent or 80 percent of their day [New York City has a breakfast and dinner program as well as lunch and snack], then they can leave school and eat whatever. The job here in New York City is much bigger than food service management. We all need to be out there lobbying, raising funds. The fight continues. These kids deserve better."

BROCCOLI BITES

Washington, D.C., has seen a number of recent tipping points (see chapter one) that resulted in some citywide improvements and several smaller pilot programs. Valerie Strauss, a *Washington Post* writer, visited the Elsie Whitlow Stokes Community Freedom Public Charter School and was awed by what she saw. In her report, titled "Yes, You Can Teach Kids To Eat Broccoli," she writes, "I wouldn't have believed it if I hadn't seen it, but chef Lisa Dobbs runs a food program that has young students relishing broccoli, tilapia encrusted with panko, *boureks* with beef or vegetables, and other foods not commonly embraced by kids." The meals are part of an overall wellness program that is intrinsic to the charter school's philosophy of caring for the whole child. Strauss expresses initial skepticism but admits that the program proves that even the pre-K kids "will eat healthy food—if the food is good, and they are given a chance to adjust to the fare." The article relates that most of the kids at Stokes are from low-income families, and the school provides a number of them with three meals a day.

The whole-foods program gets help from grocer Whole Foods Market, "which donated equipment and food (180 pounds of fresh tilapia a month), establishing a successful public-private partnership." It's part of the national No Kid Hungry Campaign championed by actor and activist Jeff Bridges and the nonprofit Share Our Strength. The goal of the campaign is to create such partnerships to help hungry families get the food they need.

Strauss reports, "The kids at Stokes didn't quite know what to make of the nutritious foods they were introduced to when Dobbs started the program early this year. They threw food around, crawled up under the sneeze guards on the salad bar, and piled up their plates with food that they ended up throwing out." By the time Strauss visited in November, the children were helping themselves to just what they could eat and they were following the rules.

The article concludes that a version of this program could and should be put in place at every school, and Strauss is convinced that it is possible. In fact, she writes, "Anybody who says it can't be done should talk to Lisa Dobbs."

The Debate

A couple of interrelated debates have arisen among school food advocates over fairness in the school food movement, and over whether a Berkeley-style school food revolution can be applied to every district. Can the local, organic food movement and its attendant community-building agenda fix school food universally? Policy makers continue to support economies of scale and the relative merits of reheating mass-produced frozen meals versus the potential staffing, financial, sourcing, and food-safety liabilities that come with meals cooked from scratch in the district. Fear fuels the debate, and every district needs to find its own comfort level, but the working models exist. Whether it's a single chef cooking vegetarian fare in a charter school, a large urban district working with a local caterer, or a regional consortium sharing a central kitchen, what each of the delicious revolutionary stories has in common is strong leadership, an integrative, community-focused approach to school food, and a dependence upon that community to come up with the necessary funding to implement a sustainable wellness program. Like any revolution, it begins in places that are most ripe and ready, and in those places that are willing to go the distance and create fundamental changes.

Those arguing for fairness insist that the federal government has to come up with greater compensation for the neediest communities in order to cover the inherent volatility in food pricing, and other escalating costs such as health care for kitchen staff, who, by the way, are generally paid less than school custodial workers. Dana Woldow in San Francisco argues that in the current recession, economically devastated communities don't have the extra dollars to pay for staff training, PR, facilities upgrades, utilities, waste management, repairs, and deliveries. She says the current reimbursement rate can only be expected to cover food and labor. It's the gap between covered expenses and additional costs that lies at the heart of the fairness debate. Dana rightly points out that some schools and school districts have the capacity to fund-raise enough to fill in that gap, and many others do not. Bettina Siegel adds, "If we rely on local communities to raise funds to improve food, we'll soon have a patchwork of either wealthier or more committed districts with good food, and poorer districts (where, I would note, more children are reliant on school food) with less healthful offerings."

"I'm not saying this to be boastful, but when Jamie Oliver visited there, he and his crew said that they'd never seen anything like it anywhere else in the U.S. *or* in the U.K.," says Kate Adamick, a former attorney and chef who now makes her living as one of the leaders in the school food revolution, consulting with districts that are serious about making changes. She's talking about Santa Barbara County, California. What makes Santa Barbara County special is that it's home to the Orfalea Fund, a resource that exists to help create sustainable collaborative and systemic change in the county, with a focus on educating children and families. One of the foundation's key initiatives is s'Cool Food, a program that provides training and resources for scratch cooking in all the schools in the county.

Kate Adamick has traveled from her home base in New York to her work consulting on the s'Cool Food initiative on a monthly basis over the course of several years. She spent the 2007–2008 school year conducting a comprehensive needs-assessment and educational campaign, focusing on the connection between school food and the health of the community. She tells me, "One of the reasons it's successful is because we took on the whole county at once on the theory that the school districts within the county would start to put pressure on each other. Both in terms of peer pressure and the more positive aspect of sharing best practices and building confidence in each other—for one school district to try one thing, like limiting chocolate milk and realize, oh, their participation didn't drop, and their milk consumption didn't drop, so then the others nearby were willing to do the same." Part of Kate's role was to communicate these experiments and discoveries from one district to the other within the county.

"They wouldn't have done it without us being there. In another district taking on the task of cooking raw poultry, overcoming that fear and then realizing, in their words, 'It's no big deal,' and then calling the other districts and telling them, 'It's nothing and we're saving a ton of money.'"

Kate says it takes a couple of years to implement such a comprehensive program. Her work in Santa Barbara entailed not only connecting meal programs with resources, but also some intensive staff training, which she does in weeklong boot camps that transform lunch ladies into lunch teachers. "Why I started this was all about being worried about all the kids. Where I saw the biggest change on a personal level was with the lunch teachers and how they are truly transformed from—you can really feel that they're treated like the bottom rung of the totem pole in a school district—to people who are suddenly empowered to be the solution rather than the problem. We had two seventy-eight-year-olds in camp who hadn't been students for sixty years. My first job in boot camp is to teach them that they still know how to learn. That's their biggest fear and once they overcome that, you just see them go from terrified to confident to angry. They're angry because all of a sudden they get it and it completely changes their lives. The first day they're there, some of them are resentful. By Wednesday they're telling us this is the greatest experience of their lives!"

As schools are experiencing major budget cuts across the board, it might seem futile to take on the task of improving the food quality. Not so, insists Kate. In fact, she claims, "The big secret in school food reform is that there really is enough money in the existing system to serve scratch-cooked meals. The poorer the district, the more that's true." Kate says, "Almost all of my public speaking at this point is addressing school lunch money—serving healthy school food in a sick economy and it's all about where the money is in the system. So for administrators the big key is demonstrating to them that the money is there in their system. And for the rank and file, it's convincing them that there's the time. And often those two things are one and the same. There's a tremendous amount of labor hours being spent—wasted—in ways that also cost money. The incessant packaging, prewrapping, portioning in plastic cups that are three cents apiece requires hours and hours a day of labor. For fruits and vegetables, just put it on a salad bar. Takes almost no time to prepare a salad bar. And there's no need to serve both hot and cold vegetables. If you have a salad bar, that's enough, which means your serving line goes faster. If you don't have a salad bar, then you just portion as the kids come, right onto

(continued)

their plate, because otherwise what happens is the same person who just spent three hours portioning into cups is then putting the cups on kids' trays."

Kate has now branded her lunch teacher training and expanded into instructor training as well. Her Cook for America boot camps are being rolled out statewide in Colorado. She's found her new niche, proudly recalling, "To see these chefs from twenty-two to sixty-two so excited about having meaning in their lives. One of them said, 'It's one thing to make somebody's evening better with a great meal, but this is a chance to change people's whole lives.'"

Kate's personal mission is to find a way to offer access to her services and programs on a broader basis. "My next project is to look for a local place to house the instructor training for Cook for America, so that chefs who want to be trained to teach the boot camps would come here for their training and the funding stream would be at the national level instead of the local level. I get calls from people every day who want the training, so a lot of people and places that would like the benefit aren't getting it." She is certain that districts would begin to realize a return on such an investment immediately.

"I get calls from lots of people in outsourced districts, not just parents. I tell them that they need to take the food service back. I tell them that children learn every waking moment of their lives, and just because the school has abdicated its responsibility to teach students during the lunch hour, it doesn't mean that the students aren't still learning. Consequently, what the students are learning are all the wrong messages. They're learning to eat quickly, to throw their food away, that something that is not food is food."

"When a publicly traded company is managing the food service do you think they're more concerned about your child's well-being or about their bottom line? In the twenty-first century, concerned parents have to be constantly vigilant that industry is not profiting at the expense of their children. That is the bottom line."

At this point in the game, it still takes extraordinary effort to realize fundamental change in the school food system and it's true that the school food revolution is in some way responsible for creating greater disparity among our public schools. The American system, with all its cruelties and inequalities, has its way of rewarding the hardest workers and most innovative thinkers, and that phenomenon applies to school food. The government is stingy but there is public money for grants and other programs available for the neediest districts that the wealthier are excluded from. Many private foundations also favor the most needy in their mission statements, and some programs, like s'Cool Food in Santa Barbara, offer resources to a large community that encompasses districts of varying means.

Nearly every business manager and food service director I spoke with, in wealthy and poor districts, in districts with awesome programs, and those struggling just to keep the nuggets on the table, were running meal programs at a deficit of some sort. There seems to be a universal acknowledgment that school food costs more than its budget, but not a universal acceptance of that fact. Those districts that do accept this as fact, and then endeavor to create the best quality program, are the ones that see the deficit as an educational expense. The others are stuck in the rhetoric of closing the deficit spending by finding ways to make the school meal program economically sustainable without fully taking into account its impact on the well-being of the students. I found this to be the crux of the matter and much more of a factor than whether the district was wealthy or poor. In willing communities, the ability to fund-raise certainly helps accelerate the process but with creative leadership some of the poorest districts are creating excellent models using resources within the community.

CAFETERIA MAN TONY GERACI

Tony's friends told him to "put up or shut up" when his kids' school district in rural New Hampshire was searching for a new food service director. A restaurateur and a food broker, he'd long been a critic of the local school food. The ConVal school administration was looking for someone who could design and implement a program that would integrate food education with healthier food throughout the district's schools. They were impressed with Tony's unconventional credentials and his can-do approach.

(continued)

Figuring he'd need to enlist popular support for his mission, Tony kicked off his district-wide overhaul with a sports nutrition program. Working with the coaches, he provided balanced meals for the school's athletes, and within the first year of the program, the district's hockey and baseball teams went from underdogs to state champions. He instituted school breakfast (real food, not doughnuts!) and had the students design menus for lunch that met all the federal guidelines without using processed foods. The meals, including salad bars and breads baked from scratch, became so popular that staff purchases became an additional revenue stream for the meal program. Tony understood the importance of involving the whole community in his mission. He invited all municipal employees to dine for free in the local schools, so the students could get to know their local police officers and firefighters. Parents and younger siblings eagerly participated in monthly ethnic-themed dinner parties in the school cafeterias.

Tony raised money for a greenhouse so that students could learn gardening year-round. A beekeeping class is the highlight of fifth grade, and an annual culinary scholarship has been established for one lucky graduate. Special education students help stock the district's vending machines with water, and they are some of the district's most fanatical gardeners. Tony's work in the Con-Val school district became the final five-minute segment of *Two Angry Moms*, proving that within the confines of a public school systems, an entrepreneur with a wide-ranging skill set and vision could re-create a better school food environment and even source food locally in the Northeast.

When I met Tony, he weighed close to three hundred pounds and was on daily medication for diabetes. During our first interview, he said, "I get the irony of the fat guy talking about nutrition." His personal struggle with diabetes and obesity is at the heart of his passion for doing right by America's children. "It's unrealistic to expect educators to teach a kid that's hungry or jacked up on sugar. My job is to serve education a meal at a time." After three years as food service director in his New Hampshire district, Tony accepted the job of food service director for the city of Baltimore, a city with a 75 percent school dropout rate and one of the highest poverty rates in America.

In 2008, I visited Tony at his new post in Baltimore. He'd lost one hundred

pounds and had been off his diabetes medicine for a year. This personal transformation seemed to be symbolic of the ambition he had for Baltimore. He
wasn't about to let anything get in his way, not even the politics of big-city
bureaucracy.

A revolutionary, but far from a radical, Tony believes school food can be
fixed by applying basic principles of American capitalism.

Over the course of two and half years, Tony instituted a breakfast in the
classroom program, creating his own colorful cardboard packaging to compete with the familiar branded products the students had come to expect.
"The cereal boxes aren't the end-all, be-all. We started with cereals and said
now we're going to substitute the juice box with an actual piece of fruit—
bananas, apples, and peaches. Part of the way you make the change is getting
them in the habit of eating the meal every day, and then you can start to raise
the bar. A lot of schools would like to serve hot oatmeal or grits, but the reality
is there's no place to cook it, no way to transport it. A lot of districts don't want
to reinvest in their own infrastructure. We went to hot cereal once a week,
then twice a week. We figured out we had about twenty cooking kitchens
around the city. In the other schools we used thermoses with hot water so we
could do the instant hot cereals. Not my best choice, but it was better than
what we had. The other thing we found that started working was we actually had parents volunteering, even if it's lugging the stuff up the stairs. I used
the ConVal model where the kids were breakfast monitors. They would take
turns bringing it up to the classrooms and then getting rid of the trash. We
gave them community service hours for the work. It's the simplest approaches
that work the best."

One of the first things Tony did in Baltimore was take over an abandoned
thirty-three-acre city-owned property and turn it into the Great Kids Farm.
In just over two years, the farm has hosted over 4,000 field trips and provided
more than one hundred interns with summer jobs learning to plant and grow
vegetables, fruits, and herbs, tending chickens, goats, and honeybees and then
selling the farm products at farmers' markets, restaurants, and a Community Supported Agriculture program. He also established numerous school

(continued)

gardens where the students could take back lessons learned on the farm and apply them on a regular basis in their own schoolyards.

Tony says his meatless Monday program is more about introducing new foods to kids, rather than on denying them the usual meaty fare. All the district's produce is now sourced in Maryland. That's $2.3 million of income for Maryland's fruit and vegetable farmers, and an opportunity for students to learn the taste of fresh food. I asked Tony how he made that happen. He says that since he's been in Baltimore, his focus has shifted more toward providing access to healthy food for all his students, especially those who live in communities where fresh food isn't available, and those who suffer from poverty and chronic hunger. "I found some obvious stepping stones where people hadn't really connected the dots. The state department of agriculture turned out to be my best partner. I connected with the secretary of agriculture for the state of Maryland. All that food grown in the state was shooting out of here on the highway and I told him I wanted to build some off-ramps from the highway to get to the food. Just the public school system alone spends $800 million a year on food. And that's not counting parochial schools and colleges. Why would you want to ship your money away? The secretary said, 'You're right.' We started doing cold calls with farmers. I said I use x amount of metric tons of fruit and vegetables. What do you grow besides GMOs and corn and soy? We started generating business models to show farmers that they could make more money doing this than growing GMO corn for Monsanto. They're not doing it exclusively for schools and they're making better money. We've made great partnerships with the local farmers."

Tony tells me that other states are starting to do this, too. Georgia, Louisiana, and North Carolina have tobacco money. He says, "Instead of paying farmers not to grow tobacco, we take the same money and start paying farmers to grow food for the school system. It's just a real simple sort of shift in thinking. Not having to create anything new. People forget that these farmers are also parents and grandparents and have siblings with kids. 'Let's go to the government and say let's figure out a way to keep our money here' is a conversation that's not falling on deaf ears. And we've started identifying processors that have freezers, so we go to farmers and say, Grow carrots, corn, lima beans, green beans, and spinach. And we freeze it and package it under Maryland's Best brand and sell it to hospitals and schools. The farmers and processors make money and we eliminate the middle guys. Now the food service director in Chicago did this for the Chicago public schools and it's working. So we're taking a model that works and replicating it. We can stop re-creating the wheel."

Tony now has an architect and a feasibility team starting plans for a central kitchen in Baltimore. "That's been our biggest hurdle, fighting the bureaucracy and building a place where you can actually cook," he tells me. "I fundraised over the last year and now have $18 million to build this thing."

He's hired a new operations director in Baltimore and cut back his hours so that he can fulfill the many requests he receives to put his business models in place in other urban districts. When I spoke with him he'd just helped get breakfast in the classroom for twenty-five schools in New Orleans, Universal Free Breakfast in Memphis, and was on his way to Atlanta. He's working with Chartwells, one of the global school food service corporations, who, Tony says, "finally figured it out that building school gardens and teaching kids about food makes business sense." Tony has helped initiate school garden projects for the company, and now he's working as a consultant creating how-to manuals for their many programs. Tony consults with other food industry giants to help them reformulate their cereals and other products to be healthier, cleaner, and less processed. "They've figured out that the pendulum is swinging."

Tony has created a marketing campaign for Breakfast in the Classroom by getting national sports teams involved in the promotion. "The colorful breakfast boxes—the sports organizations are getting on board with that. We're tying their philanthropic outreach into that. As a result we're now feeding 110,000 kids in Memphis. And Memphis has this enormous central kitchen that they aren't utilizing. They have a new business manager and a new food service director that called me up and said we have all this stuff and we want to make our food program better. They're one of the few districts that's actually in the black and wants to make improvements."

(continued)

He's also working with the White House on Chefs Move to Schools. "Once you get involved in this stuff it's hard to head in another direction, the work is so compelling and so important. What I'm finding more and more is that the trash on the ground is what people are eating in that community. We are building a bridge from that trash to whole food. Doing this work I've had a revelation. Putting food on the tray is the byproduct. Putting healthy kids in front of teachers is really the product."

Like I ask everyone, I asked Tony for his advice to parents. His response echoes the words I've heard from many others, but Tony adds an element of gospel to the task.

"Be an ingredient in the recipe for change. Come to it with a sense of 'How can I help?' Start looking at and identifying other champions in your community. There are pockets of people on the same page. Pull those pages together to make a book. Start doing resource assessment. Start identifying the pieces. Start working with the superintendent and the food service director and ask what are the hurdles in your way. Hold the hand of that person in the process. Do it in a nonconfrontational way that appeals to the needs of the community. We keep forgetting that the only reason school systems exist are for children. Not for [administrators'] careers. We have to keep reminding them of that."

Every revolution needs its leaders and this one happens to be led by an unlikely collection of parents and chefs instead of politicians and soldiers. These revolutionaries are doing what revolutionaries do—they are breaking ground and creating a template for others. There are talented chefs and managers willing to transform school districts in every part of the country, and the reality is that the school food revolution will look different in every district. The school food environment in Berkeley is different from those in Baltimore, Boise, Biloxi, or Boston. And that's the idea—it's a local phenomenon. Funding is necessary, but first the paradigm must shift and the priorities must tip toward a sustainable school food environment.

SIX

FARM TO CAFETERIA

When food service directors see kids eating something, they sometimes
find more money to pay for it.

—MARION KALB, DIRECTOR, NATIONAL FARM TO SCHOOL PROGRAM

What *Isn't* in the Food?

The declining health of America's children can also be measured in the
declining health of America's soil. According to recent USDA data, you
would need to eat five apples to get all the same nutrients that were contained in one apple in 1965! Synthetic fertilizers, pesticides, herbicides, and
large-scale mono-cropping have led to depletion of topsoil and loss of a host
of soil-borne nutrients. A significant loss of vitamins and minerals has been
measured in most of today's conventionally grown fruits and vegetables.
Healthy soil contains good bacteria, enzymes, and other microbes that are
essential for the transportation and uptake of minerals and other nutrients
into the roots of the plant. While chemical additives may boost crop production in the short term, they kill the good organisms along with the bad, and
prevent proper growth and development of crops over time. A Canadian
study of potatoes reveals that the once mighty spud has lost 100 percent of its
vitamin A (necessary for good vision), 57 percent of its vitamin C and iron
(needed for healthy blood), and 28 percent of its calcium (a major building
block for strong bones and teeth). The story is similar for twenty-five fruits
and vegetables that were analyzed. A child has to consume a whole lot more
fruits and vegetables today in order to get adequate vitamins and minerals,

and most health professionals now recommend a daily whole-food vitamin supplement for all children, even those who follow a proper diet.

Modern farming methods may result in cheap food, but Americans are paying the price by sacrificing our children's health and the economic sustainability of family farms. According to the folks at SustainableTable.org, every week as many as 330 farmers are forced out of business, unable to make a living doing the work they love. There's just one farmer left for every two hundred Americans and half of America's farmers are between the ages of forty-five and sixty-five. Only 6 percent of our farmers are under the age of thirty-five. In 1950, an American farmer received 41 cents of every dollar spent on food; today that figure has dropped to 19 cents. Yet there's a small but growing sector of the farming economy that is working to reverse this trend by revitalizing farmland, challenging the "bigger is better" mentality, and developing sustainable farming practices.

Organic farmers, biodynamic farmers, and many small farmers without organic certification are using both traditional and innovative farming methods to replenish and enrich the tilth of their soil. It can take many years to reclaim land that has been treated with chemicals, compacted by machinery, and eroded by wind and rain. Dina Brewster, a young farmer friend of mine, has brought her family farm, the Hickories, back to life by top dressing the fields with layers of organic matter—municipal leaf mulch and compost from her flock of laying hens. Over the course of several seasons, these living nutrients and conditioners have worked their way into the soil that was once so hard she couldn't get the leaves to turn into it. Dina now holds up a handful of soil that is teeming with life—worms, tiny insects, and a network of rhizomes are visible to the naked eye, indicating a thriving microscopic environment that now can support, nourish, and protect her crops without chemical controls.

A 2007 study found that yields from organic farming on average equal those of conventional farms in the United States, and in developing countries organic methods can produce up to three times as much food as conventional farming. These findings contradict arguments that organic farming practices are not as efficient as conventional techniques. The study looked at 293 different examples and concluded, "Organic methods could produce enough food on a global per capita basis to sustain the current human population, and potentially an even larger population, without increasing the agricultural land base."

The makers of pesticides, herbicides, and fertilizers are working hard to prevent the public from believing that message, insisting that farmers need to have these inputs to reliably produce food.

My farmer friend Dina grows healthy food in healthy soil for healthy people and in order to do so, she needs to maintain a healthy bottom line. The farm's CSA (Community Supported Agriculture) program sells farm shares to four hundred participating families. These families share the bounty of the farm, but equally share the risk of a failed crop, something that most school districts can ill afford either financially or logistically. I wonder if it's possible to connect small farmers like my friend Dina with local schools? Is her produce too expensive, or limited for the school cafeteria? What are the logistics that make a Farm to School program work? I've seen great Farm to School programs in some private and charter schools, and out on the West Coast, but many of the public school programs that get the attention of the media are really just featuring a day or week of local produce in the fall, or a shipment of local apples with a big poster in the cafeteria. These are terrific first steps, excellent educational tools, but I wanted to know how the Farm to School program integrates into the colossus of the National School Meals Program. I asked Debra Eschmeyer, program outreach and communications director of FarmtoSchool.org, if she could point me to some model programs.

Farm to School

All fifty states now have operational Farm to School programs—there were just a handful a little over a decade ago. Debra tells me, "There are models everywhere. It's not easy but often we make it more complicated than it needs to be. Most things start with a simple conversation. Parents that are going to farmers' markets talk to their favorite vendors. They invite them to the classroom to demonstrate planting seeds or composting. A good time to ask them to come in is January when they're slow. They introduce the farmer to the school. Eventually that leads to a taste test. Then the farmer becomes the one to supply potatoes or other vegetables to the school. It's like building any relationship, like dating; it's a slow process. The farmer gives a face to the food, and brings a relationship with the food. So procurement is related to education and gardens. The model can be with a small farm or a large farm but the idea is it all starts off the same way. Whether it's a small school or LAUSD [Los Angeles Unified School District], we all have that power to pick up the phone."

I asked Debra how the economics work for the farmer. "A farmer in Connecticut versus a farmer in Washington, D.C., or Dayton, Ohio, is going to be different. Everyone is charging a different penny per pound for those tomatoes. They've got to pay for seeds, land, feed, and fuel. Is the school system their best outlet, or restaurants and farmers' markets? A farm that is healthy and diversified can do all of that. Farmers now are doing season extension with row covers and hoop houses. The school feeding system is a $14 billion market and the USDA is now encouraging Farm to School and they're trying to have 100,000 new farmers a year. You have to see this as a marketing value, you're reaching out to all these children who go home and tell their parents about the delicious food they ate and they got it from this farm. Then the kids want their parents to go to the farmers' market and join a CSA. So through the schools, the farmers are able to share their products with a larger audience. We're even seeing locally grown at the grocery store. Even Walmart is approaching small farmers now. The kids are a new generation and they are next year's customers, and in many households, the children make the purchasing decisions."

In many areas, there are both demand and supply for Farm to School but a lack of infrastructure for connecting the farms to schools and other institutions. To fill the gap, there's a burgeoning network of nonprofit and low-profit regional distribution hubs developing, funded in part by federal and state grant monies. These groups, like the FoodHub at Ecotrust in Oregon, and Fresh Fork Market in Cleveland, aggregate produce from small farms in a forty-or-so-mile radius, and distribute it to various institutions including schools, hospitals, restaurants, and prisons. The distribution coop-eratives, sometimes known as co-packers, are also working to make the pro-duce more user-friendly for the school cafeterias. Minimal processing, such as precutting and even fresh frozen produce are some of the value-added services they are offering. Debra from Farm to School says, "The local move-ment is maturing in a distribution format that is not only benefiting schools but is benefiting everyone. It's community based." She quotes Iowa farmer Michael Nash, who says, "We are cultivating more than just food here. This is about community; this is about relationships."

APPALACHIAN SUSTAINABLE AGRICULTURE PROJECT

In and around Asheville, North Carolina, federal subsidies are helping tobacco farmers transition to vegetable production. Emily Jackson is the pro-gram director for the project, and the southeast regional lead for the National Farm to School Network.

I asked Emily how the farmers got connected to the schools. She explains, "Burley [cigarette] tobacco was the backbone crop for our farmers. When we saw the tobacco buyout coming, we used the grants to find alternatives and new strategies. It's not about crops, it's about markets, and Farm to School was one of those, and a more appropriate one for farmers in rural areas that might not have access to other markets but there is a school system. We used the last of our small $5,000 grants for farmers to think of what innovations they could do to get out of growing tobacco. One farm asked for funding to increase their hydroponic system. Somebody in the school district's food service was talking about the price of lettuce going through the roof and the conversation was over-heard by a friend of the farmer and so the connection was made. The beauty of hydroponics is it's year round. For us, an important component of Farm to School is education, so we have these open farm days. Another farmer, Dewain Mackey, came to a farm day and went back and started hydroponics for his

(continued)

school system and local hospitals. Dewain hooked up with other farmers who grew other crops. They're a loosely affiliated group and they have a couple of people who do all their marketing for them. A lot of the farmers in that setup are former tobacco farmers. The way we work with many farms with Farm to School is through a produce distributor. Not many farmers in our area have formed a co-op and they don't want to drive around to forty or fifty schools."

I wondered if the farmers could make as much money growing fruits and vegetables as they did with tobacco. Emily says that the farmers are very pleased. She relates, "Schools are a dependable market, there's volume, and the alternative of buying things out of season costs quite a bit. We don't want our farmers to go out of business. We have the dubious distinction of leading the country in loss of family farms and around Asheville we don't encourage farmers to sell to schools if they have access to other (more lucrative) markets. Around Asheville they have tailgates, CSAs, restaurants, hospitals, colleges, and other institutions that can pass along the cost of local food."

I wondered also if there's an incentive for the local farmers in North Carolina to grow food using organic methods. Emily replies, "Sustainability for us is economic. Organic, for us, is up to the markets to decide. We don't recommend farmers grow any particular way unless there's the market to back it up. We're not anti-organic . . . we think it's real important to establish relationships, get to know the farmers and ask them for what you want."

North Carolina also has a statewide Farm to School program run by the North Carolina Department of Agriculture. They are one of only three states that have trucks and warehouses. Emily explains the difference between the Asheville group and the state program. "Most of the Farm to School produce comes from larger farms in the eastern part of the state. We have the fourteenth-largest apple production in the country, potatoes, and tomatoes. The way they do it, any product from North Carolina is local, even if it's trucked many hours across the state. Here, it's local co-ops or direct delivery. For us, if the kid can't see the farm and go to church with the farmers, it's not local. But North Carolina has that infrastructure."

When questioned about the visibility of the farm produce in the cafeteria, Emily is frank. "They usually incorporate one or two vegetables each month.

There aren't any of the major plate items. Parents are envisioning a plate that looks like it comes from the health food store. It's not like that. We've relied on à la carte more than most states because North Carolina doesn't contribute anything to the lunch program. We had grass-fed beef once in one system. The students had hamburgers twice from that, so it doesn't do much for the children. But it changed a lot of attitudes about that particular meat for the cafeteria staff—they learned that meat doesn't have to be gray and smell nasty. We really believe that Farm to School isn't just about healthy food—it's that whole connection thing. I know who grew my food and where it came from and learning in the school gardens and cooking with it. I've been doing Farm to School since 2002. I was a teacher before that and a farmer before that. So it all makes sense to me. I had a garden with my students and saw their passion for it so I wrote a grant to run a school-wide garden and it just snowballed from there. The value is what we're all trying to get at. If they value it, then they're going to try to hold on to it."

Emily really understands the challenges of getting the whole school community to value local food. She says, "Your kid's in second grade now and you want that change to be now and that's really hard because it probably won't be. Understand what you can about the system and don't make the child nutrition staff the problem. Make friends with them. It's funding that's the problem. We really pit children against the people who work in the cafeteria when we juggle funds for food against their salaries and benefits. Go in and find out what you can do and how you can help. Buy a CSA share for your cafeteria staff. Have parties for them and take them on farm field trips. They're the front line."

Food Sourcing and Safety

There's been a public outcry for more stringent safety standards for America's food supply. In fact, strong standards do exist, but lack of inspection and enforcement of those standards is often to blame when food-borne illnesses occur. All school cafeterias are required to have HACCP plans in place to ensure safe handling and cooking of raw products—holding temperatures below 41 degrees Fahrenheit or above 135 degrees Fahrenheit (known as the "danger zone" in food service), use of gloves, hand washing, and so on. One of the reasons many school districts insist on going the heat-and-serve route with their food service is that liability for food contamination falls on the "manufacturer," which essentially means the entity that prepares and cooks the food. Properly trained kitchen staff must know how to follow HACCP procedures.

A *USA Today* analysis of data from the U.S. Centers for Disease Control and Prevention found 470 outbreaks of illnesses due to contaminated food in schools between 1998 and 2007 that sickened at least 23,000 children. The CDC uses sophisticated methodology to pinpoint the origin of these outbreaks and oftentimes the source is upstream from the schools, and is so comingled in the food system that it's nearly impossible to determine the extent of the contamination. Over the past several years, massive nationwide recalls of hamburger, spinach, and eggs have illustrated the lack of "fire walls" in our food system.

There's a common misperception that food from local farms isn't as safe as the food from the large national vendors. Proponents of Farm to School insist that it's actually safer. The path from source to end user is short and immediately traceable, and proponents like Debra Eschmeyer point out that the face-to-face relationship between buyer and grower promotes transparency, integrity, and trust.

In 2005, when I tried to get my school district to purchase produce from local farms, I was informed that the local farms weren't certified for health and food safety. Perhaps it didn't exist then, but I've since learned that there's a program that helps small farmers meet the food safety requirements for school food. It's called GAP—Good Agricultural Practices (GAP) and Good Handling Practices (GHP), and some states, like New York and Connecticut, offer assistance to help cover the cost of certification. Many retailers, wholesale buyers, food service companies, restaurants, and schools now require produce suppliers to provide a third-party certification such as GAP or a similar standards certification. Farmers that have the GAP certification can sell to all these outlets and also through regional aggregating networks.

TIPS FOR SAFELY HANDLING FRESH PRODUCE

- Always wash your hands with soap and warm water for twenty seconds before and after preparing fresh produce.
- Wash all fruits and vegetables under running water. Check district regulations for using fruit wash solutions such as vinegar, baking soda, or hydrogen peroxide. Generally, these solutions are not required.
- Scrub produce with firm skin, such as melons and cucumbers, with a clean produce brush and rinse well.
- Discard the outer leaves of leafy vegetables.
- Peel with a clean peeler when necessary.
- Cut produce on a clean cutting board using a clean, well-sharpened knife.
- Cut away any damaged or bruised areas on fresh fruits and vegetables before preparing and discard any produce that looks or smells rotten.
- Store fruits and vegetables separate from other foods such as raw meat, poultry, or seafood. Do not use utensils that have been used for these products before washing them.
- Clean and sanitize storage areas, shelves, and bins regularly.

Procurement Restrictions

Another obstacle encountered early on in the Farm to School movement was the federal procurement regulations for the NSLP. The regulations restricted school districts and buying co-ops from stating geographic preferences in their RFPs and contracts. The 2008 Farm Bill reversed that prohibition and now actively encourages schools to "apply an optional geographic preference in the procurement of unprocessed locally grown or locally raised agricultural products." Section 4303 of the bill states, "The Secretary [of Agriculture] shall encourage institutions participating in the School Lunch and School Breakfast Programs . . . to purchase locally produced foods, to the maximum extent practicable, along with other foods." The provision also applies to state agencies making purchases on behalf of any institution participating in any of the Federal Child Nutrition Programs. As of 2011, thirty-three states now have their own legislation establishing Farm to School programs, and some even allow contracts that favor state-grown produce, even if it is slightly more expensive than competitive out-of-state produce. Federal regulations stipulate that your school district can purchase directly from a GAP-certified farmer without competitive bidding if the purchase is less than $100,000. Some states or local school food authorities set a lower threshold for direct purchasing. For purchases over the direct purchasing threshold, traditional open bidding regulations apply (see Intent to Purchase, pp. 225–26), with allowances for geographic preferences.

There's a strong economic argument for this allowance. Debra from Farm to School pointed me to data collected from her programs that

> suggests that when schools dedicate a significant percentage of their purchases to local producers the multiplier effect of purchasing locally impacts the local economy. It's good for business and for children. For every dollar spent on local foods in schools, one to three dollars circulate back into the local economy. Local farmers gain a significant and steady market. For example, the New York City school district signed a $4.2 million contract with farmers in upstate New York to provide apples for NYC schools over a three-year period. The sixty farms providing products to local schools in Massachusetts, meanwhile, are generating more than *$700,000 in additional revenue each year.* For most participating farmers, school sales represent 5 to 10 percent of their total sales.

Debra also points out that Farm to School is a bipartisan political issue because it supports agendas from the entire political spectrum. The beneficial economic impact is what got recent legislation passed that increases federal support for local Farm to School programs and proclaimed October as National Farm to School Month. And local farmers have an advantage over their distant competitors. They can deliver a fresh, high quality, safe product to schools within twenty-four hours after harvest, including value-added processing.

The Hudson Mohawk Resource Conservation and Development Council in New York State produced their own guide for Farm to School purchasing. They include some templates to help schools comply with the free and open competition purchasing regulations required by federal guidelines. The Intent to Purchase announcement should be published where all farmers will see it and have an opportunity to respond.

Below are two sample notices of intent from the Council's Farm to School Guide.

SAMPLE 1. NOTICE OF INTENT TO PURCHASE FRESH FRUITS AND VEGETABLES LOCALLY

SCHOOL DISTRICT ADDRESS

The XXX School District Board of Education is seeking to purchase the following items directly from farmers/producers/growers for the 20XX–XX school year. These amounts are per month for ten months (September XX to June XX). The district will receive quotes on the following items on [day of week] by [time] prior to the week of [date].

Full Year Cost Items—example: apples (Empire) 4 cases
Cider 8 gallons
Potatoes
Seasonal Items—example: Lettuce, Spinach, Pears

Use subject to availability of product and menu requirements. Delivery would be to the school at the above address between _____ [time] and _____ [time].

Red Leaf Lettuce (washed), Green Leaf Lettuce (washed), Spinach (washed), Summer squash, Pears

SAMPLE 2. NOTICE OF INTENT TO PURCHASE LOCALLY

SCHOOL DISTRICT ADDRESS

The XXX School District Board of Education is seeking to purchase the following items directly from farmers/producers/growers for the 20XX–XX school year. These amounts are per month as specified. The district will receive quotes on the following items weekly on Thursdays by 12 noon.

Apples, U.S. Fancy, 120 per case—50 cases, September–March

Pears, U.S. Fancy, 120 per case—25 cases, September and October

Summer Squash, U.S. #1, 25 lb.—10 cases, September

Zucchini, U.S. #1, 25 lb.—10 cases, September

Winter Squash, U.S. #1, 25 lbs.—10 cases, September–November

Tomatoes, U.S. #1, 25 lbs.—20 cases, September

Cucumbers, U.S. #1, 80 per case—10 cases, September

Green Peppers, U.S. # 1, Medium, 40 per case—10 cases, September

Carrots, U.S. # 1, 25 lbs.—10 cases, September

Potatoes, U.S. #1, size B, 50 lbs.—20 bags, September–April

Red Onions, U.S. # 1, 25 lbs.—3 bags, September–April

Spanish Onions, U.S. # 1, 25 lbs.—5 bags, September–April

Broccoli, U.S. # 1, 15 heads per case—10 cases, September–October

Cauliflower, U.S. # 1, 12 heads per case—10 cases, September–October

Use subject to availability of product and menu requirements. The district is required to obtain the products from the farmer that submits the lowest price.

Delivery would be to district schools between 7 a.m. and 12 noon. For further information, contact [name, title], at [phone number].

If your food service director insists that there are other restrictions preventing him or her from purchasing local produce, you can take a page from the USDA publication *Eat Smart—Farm Fresh!*, a guide that offers tips to work around their own regulations:

> SFAs (School Food Authorities) can: identify and encourage local farmers to submit bids; look into alternative pack sizes and distribution methods that reflect product availability, using pricing structures such as fixed delivery charges with product prices that respond to the current market price; and explore new and different products that are available through local farms.
>
> SFAs also need to develop specifications that reflect the characteristics of the products they seek. For example, local farmers grow a specific lettuce variety that students prefer, but that the SFA cannot get through their broker or distributor. The SFA can write its specification requiring this lettuce variety. However, just writing the specification alone will not be adequate to ensure local farm participation. The SFA must have "laid the groundwork," that is, identifying and encouraging local farm participation for the procurement to be successful.

And this from the same guide:

> Can SFAs split up large purchases into smaller amounts and thereby fall under the small purchase threshold?
>
> SFAs cannot intentionally split purchases in order to fall below the federal small purchase threshold. For example, if a SFA will be purchasing $150,000 worth of lettuce for the salad bar they cannot split the purchase into two purchases of $75,000 each. However, the SFA can specify different varieties of lettuce that must be provided and be willing to award its lettuce bid to more than one supplier.

Another approach, when an adequate number of suppliers exist, is for the SFA to conduct a procurement action for a specific item, for example, apples, instead of conducting a procurement to obtain a single supplier for all of its fruits and vegetables for the school year. This approach could allow local apple growers to compete for the SFA's apple contract.

The guide also explains that funds cannot be "set aside" for Farm to School programs, but that nutrition education and Farm to School projects are allowable as line items in the school food budget.

There's no question that it's easier to create a model program in a single school, especially if it's a public charter school where all the parents share an educational philosophy of sustainability. The Unity Charter School in Morris Township, New Jersey, is just such a school, and their chef, Judy Mancini, is also a parent of a student at the school. I caught up with Judy just as she was about to move into a new kitchen in a new school facility.

GARDEN STATE

"We've rescued old lockers destined for the dump, recycled desks, and given everything a fresh coat of paint," says Judy. "We're moving into a building that has a gorgeous, huge cafeteria that shares a space with a common room with a skylight. There have been in-school and alumni fund-raisers for the new kitchen. We're able to pay for it because there was money left over from the school construction, and some money was donated from a private corporate foundation."

Because the school doesn't accept commodity food, and because they don't want to waste milk by giving every child the required eight-ounce carton, Unity doesn't qualify for the National School Lunch Program, nor were they eligible for federal funding for their kitchen. "And we're serving organic milk, so we can't afford to waste it," says Judy.

She explains that the kids pay $3.75 for hot lunch, which includes a fresh fruit salad, vegetables, and a glass of milk. "We do run at quite a deficit. That's covered by other fund-raising and grants. The school does that. The lunch fee pays just for labor, not food cost or overhead."

Judy is hoping that an increase in the student population will help make up some of the deficit next year, but she emphasizes that her mandate is about the food, not about breaking even. She says, "What they care about is keeping it to a manageable cost. What they care about is having an organic vegetarian lunch program that uses local ingredients and is run by a professional chef because our mission is sustainability. They specifically do fund-raisers for the lunch program because they are invested in keeping the lunch program going. Other schools that want to do this have to understand what they're not going to get and hard choices have to be made about what that lunch program is going to cost each student and how much they're going to have to fund-raise.

"These children are in our care for six hours a day and it's not only their minds we care for. We need to nourish them so what they're doing the rest of the time gets into their brains." Judy's passion is clearly shared by the parents in her school. She tells me, "While others were sitting around waiting for the government to pass this bill or that bill we have taken action. Now they're pushing vegetables and whole grains but no kid is going to eat it if they don't have the education. We have tasting days where every child gets a small cup of whatever we're testing that day. The fortunate thing about my program is that I know every kid. I know who I can push to try this, and who is never going to eat it. You're never going to get every kid to try something. But the difference is I take the time to cook it, season it well, serve in glassware, use tongs, make it pretty, and I know every single child. I can ride them. If they want to come up for more pasta I say please eat a leaf of lettuce! It's important to teach them why we're eating lower on the food chain, because meat is not very sustainable. And parents can send their children in with anything they like. We do request that they send in reusable containers."

The Unity school received a grant from Slow Food for a garden. As part of the curriculum, the middle school students designed the garden and are researching what grows in each season. They're also learning how to compost and the curriculum was revised to include the garden and a season-extending hoop house.

The Way In

Approaching your school food service director or wellness committee with a complete overhaul of your district's food environment may be intimidating for you and for them. A Farm to School program is a manageable, and often very popular place to start. The focus is on adding some fresh food to the meal program, and not about banning and policing, which may be helpful in finding support from students, staff, and parents. Begin with a phone call or letter of inquiry to your food service director.

SAMPLE FARM TO SCHOOL INQUIRY

Dear [Food Service Director],

The USDA's Child Nutrition Services and the First Lady's "Let's Move!" campaign are encouraging school districts to include more fresh and locally grown produce in the school meal program. I'm writing on behalf of a group of community members who are advocates of local food, supporting local farmers, and raising healthy kids. We're interested to speak with you to learn about existing Farm to School efforts in our district, and to offer our services in developing or extending the program. In addition to speaking with you, it would be helpful to visit the district's school food facilities in order to help determine what steps might need to be taken. I look forward to meeting with you and will follow up to set up a time that is convenient for you in the coming weeks. Please feel free to call me at: [your phone number]

Sincerely,
[your name]
Chair, [your organization's name]

Farm to School programs also help cut down on waste from food packaging, so if your school has a green club, those students may want to take the lead. My daughter's high school has an animal rights club that is researching sources for humanely raised meat and poultry products. They intend to approach the food service director with a list of farms they've visited and approved.

Foraging

Before approaching your food service director and administrators, you should do some research. You will want to be equipped with answers and solutions when you engage them in the conversation, so you need to have an understanding of the local food and agricultural system. I've recently seen want ads posted for "forager"—organizations, restaurants, and school districts looking for a person who can connect them with affordable sources of local food. You will need to either become a forager or find someone who has this knowledge. Your local farmers' market director, agricultural extension agency, farm bureau, CSA, or feed store are good places to start.

The agricultural resources you can forage for include:

- local and regional fruit, vegetable, eggs, or livestock farmers interested in working with the schools—these may not be the same farmers at the farmers' market who charge top dollar for their products; you may need to forage farther afield
- local food grading, washing, processing, and packing facilities
- locally sourced and produced value-added products like honey, syrup, pickles, breads, etc.
- local distribution and delivery options

Once you begin your dialog with the school district, you'll also want to forage for allies and find out who are the skeptics and what their specific concerns are.

From farmtoschool.org: "The Massachusetts Farm to School project noted that Worcester Public Schools have seen a 15 percent increase in school lunch purchases since the district began buying locally. Student lunch participation in one school in Southern California increased by over 50 percent in the first two years the Farm to School program was in place."

Needs Assessment

"Farm to School in the Northeast" is an online toolkit developed by Cornell University, the New York State School Nutrition Association, and New York Farms. It contains information applicable well beyond the Northeast, plus a very thorough survey you and your food service director can use to assess the missing links needed for a farm-to-school program in your district. I've included the survey and a sample summary worksheet on my website.

Connecting with Farmers

The idea of a food hub is a relatively new innovation based on old traditions of local market development. I expect we'll see more of these hub-and-spoke systems popping up around the country. They are not the only models for local procurement. Depending upon your region and the type of food service your district has, there are other options that might be more practical for your district.

Transportation is often the most challenging issue for both farmers and schools; delivery logistics to consider include the number of kitchens in the district, school storage capacity, staff availability, and delivery frequency.

Buying directly from farmers is usually the most cost-effective method of purchasing Farm to School since there are no broker fees involved. This method requires the time and energy to create relationships with farmers and to track multiple orders and deliveries if buying from more than one farmer. One creative solution to direct buying from multiple farmers is arranging to purchase products at the local farmers' market. Food service staff makes arrangements in advance with participating farmers. The farmers bring the school's orders to the market and then a driver from the district picks up the orders from the participating farmers.

In addition to food hubs and cooperatives, more and more traditional wholesalers and food brokers are getting into the local food market. Food service directors already deal with these distributors, so they may prefer to maintain the system they are accustomed to, although it means that the relationship with the farmer isn't direct. In this scenario, it is incumbent on the food service staff to request proof of the provenance of the products, and it is also recommended that the district have a contract with the broker that stipulates proof of local purchases.

The Department of Defense (DOD) Fresh Program has been expanded to nearly every state. States are now coordinating partnerships between local farmers and school districts to provide fresh produce using existing DOD brokers and/or nonprofit food and farming organizations for pickups and delivery. This program directs federal or state payments directly to the grower or distributor, with school district funding determined by reimbursement rates in the school meals program. Eligible schools districts must claim their DOD shares; not all eligible school districts are taking advantage of the program.

LOVE YOUR FARMER

Jane Slupecki runs the Connecticut Farm to School program as well as Farm-Link, all on a part-time budget. She knows a bit about conserving local resources; she is one of them! I asked her how to get a Farm to School program going in a local district in Connecticut. Her reply: "My basic line of attack is that after you've been nice to your food service director and they know you and you've been having trouble sourcing, then you need to call me. If you're going to be a good PTA mom, you get rid of the chocolate bars at the fund-raisers and sell local apples. Have bedding plant sales in the spring. Have a holiday wreath sale in winter. It's just a mind shift away from traditional items to move

(continued)

it toward something that's Connecticut grown. Every time you shift it back to your local agricultural economy you're helping your farmer sustain his farm."

In Connecticut, the Department of Agriculture awards $500,000 each year for Farm to School programs. It can't be used for buying food and the funds must go to a municipality. Jane tells me that traditionally it gets used to rewrite agricultural legislation, or it's used to build a shed in town or to put up a barn on town-owned land to store hay or put the cows in. "That funding could be used for creating a food hub," she says. "Connecticut already has a few small hubs but in Connecticut it's more about farmers working with a wholesaler. They can't be everywhere. They're one-man or one-woman organizations."

Jane's job is to work with the farmers. "I love the farmers!" She explains, "My main job is to try to get those farmers' goods into the food service repertoire. Success stories don't have to be perfect. There's micro success. You have to walk a mile in the shoes of the food service director. The biggest thing is farmers need to learn 'food service speak' and vice versa. When you get those two talking to each other—farmers think in acres, food service directors think in pounds and portion sizes. If you need a bushel—this is how many pounds in a bushel. Farmers need to know that little kindergarteners only need four ounces of applesauce. We used to have little apples that we couldn't get rid of and now we have a little-apple shortage because the schools love them. The chefs and restaurants are using Connecticut Grown and all that competes with how much schools are going to get in a little state like Connecticut. It's all about the pressure that's being applied on the food chain that goes to the schools. They have to listen to the pressure."

When I last spoke with her, Jane was busy trying to investigate all the hurdles of getting locally raised hamburger into school cafeterias. She puts it quite simply, "A cow needs to be fed well and happy and grow up and then it needs to be slaughtered into steaks and ground beef," and then she explains the complications. "On the other side is the USDA National School Lunch Program. Children's safety is very, very front and center. Most schools get the commodity beef. I affectionately call [the commodity program] Monopoly money. You have to apply for it and get it and use it. After all the rules have been followed could a Connecticut producer still make a profit? Connecticut has partnered with the Vermont Farm to School program and we are just about to put out an RFP for a regional beef study to see if it's feasible on a regional basis. Here we hope to do it at the regional level. I can encourage the beef producers if it's feasible. We have to make sure if we want to sell beef to the lunch program that all those people have to be happy. You always have to talk about critical masses, price point, and economies of scale. My definition of sustainable is that that farm will be here in another generation."

In Connecticut, the demand for local produce far outstrips the supply, which makes it even more difficult to get it into the schools. Jane says, "It's a good-bad problem to have not enough farms. We're trying to get more production going in the state. If I can get more acreage into production, that will give schools more opportunity to work with farms."

Jane credits the parents in our state with charting a new direction. She explains, "In Connecticut, most of the food service directors cannot work directly with farmers. In Massachusetts, it's just the opposite. There they get rid of the middleman. We recently had a meeting with the Department of Defense Fresh Program. Part of the agenda for the DOD meeting was "Know your farmer, know your food." The food service director in Hartford was buying from a wholesaler. Now she's branching out into buying direct because she went to the meeting and met the farmers and loved them and realized that it wouldn't be impossible or hard. These are all new relationships. We have woken up the behemoth. It's you guys asking and asking. And then, 'Oh my gosh we have to do our jobs!' Start asking questions. It all comes back to that. Sit on the wellness committee even if it drives you crazy. There's value to sitting through that whole process. And the pain. If you work in the government that happens to you every day. It's a big huge scary system of rules and there are certain ones I just cannot fix. But there's ways to change things. I have to follow the rules that are in place. I believe in the American system. If you want those rules changed then you have to do something about it. I can't fix all that but I can try to get you some more farmers!"

Jane jokes, "I blame the parents for this whole thing! You as parents make my job a lot easier. The schools know and the wholesalers know that the parents want it. These people want this stuff!"

Farmers are not the only ones forming cooperatives. School districts are saving money by taking the "cooperative agreement" procurement approach—where several school districts jointly negotiate contracts with local vendors and procurers. This strategy works well for smaller districts and it's a win-win for the schools and the vendors. The buying co-op can influence the market by creating a greater demand, school districts can share procurement resources, and the vendors can keep costs down by dealing with fewer customers and bids and consolidating products and deliveries.

Social Justice

Is fresh local food a pipe dream for districts struggling with issues of access, hunger, and poverty? Debra Eschmeyer tells me that in New Mexico and Arizona, it's the food banks that host the Farm to School programs. She explains, "A lot of this is cross-pollination. The way the local food movement is articulated is by a lot of elite white people on the coasts, but that's not reflective of the people on the ground. There are people of all colors everywhere doing it."

I can count myself among the coastal white articulators, but two of the earliest and most successful examples of Farm to School in action are located in primarily minority communities.

GREEN IN THE DESERT

In 2006 I heard about a farmers' market salad bar program in Santa Monica, California. By the time I caught up with him, I learned that the program's initial director, Rodney Taylor, had since relocated to Riverside, a sprawling community of some 300,000 citizens located about sixty miles east of Los Angeles, on the edge of the Southern California desert. Rodney's new position as Riverside's food service manager put him in charge of school meals in a district that serves 43,000 students, more than half of whom are from at-risk families. Rodney invited me to visit him in Riverside to see how he was building a cost-effective Farm to School program in this economically challenged school district.

I learned that an eager parent advocate first pushed Rodney into the Farm to School movement. "In 1997 I was approached by a parent. His comment to me was, 'Rodney, I was happy to find out that you had salad bars in all your schools but a little dismayed to find out that my daughter wouldn't eat it. The lettuce was brown and the carrot sticks were white and filmy looking.' And his question was simple. 'What if we bought from the local farmers' market?' And I thought, 'This is another affluent parent with a little too much time on his hands. It wouldn't work.' But I had learned in working in Santa Monica that parents don't go away easy when they come to you with these kinds of things. So what we decided at that time was to have a two-week pilot. We would set up a salad bar using the fresh produce. And the first day I walked in there and I saw the kids making their choices and they were eating. That changed me and my feelings about the farmers' market salad bar forever."

The day my crew visited, we watched as one of the local farmers arrived with a truckload of beautiful produce. The produce was catalogued and inspected and loaded by forklift into the district's huge central warehouse, which was equipped with giant cold storage lockers and floor to ceiling shelf storage that would make my local Home Depot look like a dollhouse.

We toured the salad bars at several schools and saw teachers coaching kids to "take something green and something orange on your plate." Every child happily helped him or herself to the fresh produce and other salad bar items. I often hear people voice concern about kids making a mess at elementary school salad bars, but with the monitors and coaches, there was minimal mess and the line moved quickly. My favorite frame of video was captured that day in Riverside: a young boy eagerly munching on a raw broccoli tree, smiling and giggling with his classmates.

At the time I visited Riverside, there were salad bars in just three of the district's forty-three schools. Rodney was dismayed that his food service was only feeding 51 percent of the kids in the district, up from 47 percent when

(continued)

he had arrived two years earlier. "So there are 20,000 kids that aren't eating with us each day. So how am I going to get that revenue, so that I can provide healthier food to the kids? And it's to change perceptions and the salad bar does that thing."

His passion and tenacity have paid off, and after almost ten years in the district, Rodney now has a salad bar in almost every school. The district spends about $250,000 per year with local farmers. Lunch participation is now up to 65 percent and half of those children are choosing the salad bar for lunch.

Rodney says, "Most people don't think of school food service as a business and it's exactly that. The food service program in a school district is the one department that has to be self-sufficient. We not only need to break even, we need to generate excesses so that we can compensate for increasing cost of living and all those other things that affect businesses." His background is in hotel catering and marketing, so he understands that slimy looking carrots won't sell. "Fresh fruits and vegetables have been in school for a long time. The problem is you give a kindergartener a whole orange and what happens? It gets thrown in the trash. The same with the large apples. Over the years what I've learned is you'd better merchandise the food. You need to make it user friendly. So that when we have grapes they're pulled off the stem. If we have strawberries, they're cut in half. Oranges are always quartered. It's pleasant to the eye and it's a much better taste. Yes, in fact it's more labor intensive, but it will pay for itself because it's gonna improve your participation, it's gonna reduce your waste, so you've got more revenue coming in that will offset the increased labor."

Rodney is pleased that they've succeeded in bringing about a change in perception of the school meals. He's attracted more staff to the salad bars in addition to the students. As a result, the program has grown by an additional million dollars in revenue every year since he started in Riverside. His central kitchen also provides food service to other local nonprofits. The Meals on Wheels program was on the brink of bankruptcy when Rodney brought it in-house. He rescued the program and brought in extra revenue at the same time.

Rodney is philosophical about the salad bars, noting that they may not make money, or even break even, but they absolutely accomplish his goal of teaching kids to be lifelong healthy eaters, and to him, that's worth the extra work.

Go Greens

Founded in 1995 by group of innovative African-American farmers, the New North Florida Cooperative based in Gadsden, Florida, provides marketing and packing services for member farmers, and sells their produce to local school districts and other institutions.

I spoke with Vonda Richardson, the Farm Management Specialist from Florida A&M University's Cooperative Extension Program.

Vonda explains, "When we started, the schools were an alternative market for farmers. Our background was not nutrition. The product that the farmers could grow really well in this area was leafy greens and here in the Florida panhandle we can grow them year-round."

Greens are a staple of the traditional southern African-American diet, and kids like them. With a focus on curbing childhood obesity with more fruits and vegetables, fresh greens were a natural fit for the schools in the region. Greens are considered a specialty crop, so the Cooperative had a niche product that no one else was providing. "As a small, minority organization we don't want to butt heads with our competition," says Vonda. The Farm to School website tells their story like this: "In order to help secure their first customer, the Cooperative donated 3,000 pounds of washed, chopped and bagged leafy greens to Gadsden County schools as a free sample. The gesture helped to solidify the business relationship and in the 1996–97 school year, the Cooperative began selling farm fresh produce to thirteen schools in Gadsden County, Florida."

With some financial assistance, including an initial grant from the USDA, the Cooperative was able to purchase equipment to automate the work of cleaning, processing, packaging, and storing fresh products. Most of the deliveries to the school districts are done with the Cooperative's own trucks, although they do work with some produce vendors as well. Vonda says,

> We work with farmers so they're not getting shortchanged. It's to their benefit because they grow it and they're done, we do the rest. We group the school districts together so they know when they're going to receive the product. We try to secure the school district before the school year starts. We stay in constant contact with the food service directors. They give us an estimate of the volume they will need. Then the farmers can plant what they need to. NNFC grows on-site as well and since we get several plantings during the year with greens, our farmers have a little bit of flexibility. We have one farmer growing as few as four acres, which might not be enough for a school district, but because his volume is aggregated with other farmers he's able to make a profit.

The produce is labeled with a logo and nutritional analysis. Deliveries are made two to three days per week, depending upon school menus. All Cooperative members go out of their way to be helpful and courteous when delivering the produce; they unload the boxes and stack them neatly in district or school storage facilities.

Word has spread of the Cooperative's high quality produce, prompt deliveries, fair prices, and courteous professionalism, which Cooperative members refer to as relationship marketing. Positive word-of-mouth publicity, including enthusiasm among schoolchildren, has lead to a high demand for their products among school districts.

As part of its marketing and promotion, the Cooperative has developed posters showing the life cycle of a crop from production to consumption. These posters are displayed in school cafeterias, and serve not only as an effective promotion for the Cooperative, but also to promote awareness of agriculture and small farms among schoolchildren. Although an educational component of this program does exist, its main success lies in the creation of a sustainable business relationship between farmers and school districts.

The Cooperative has grown into a larger networking organization. Now they serve on average over 300,000 students in fifteen school districts, some in neighboring states. Their staples are collard greens, sweet potatoes, and green beans and they've expanded their offerings to include field peas, muscadine grapes, turnip greens, strawberries, blackberries, and watermelon. Vonda say the New North Florida Cooperative delivers to districts as small as 1,300 students, and as large as Fort Lauderdale with 250,000.

Over time, well-managed Farm to School programs increase participation rates in school meal programs, bringing in new revenue and enhancing the overall financial viability of participating school food services. It's a win-win-win situation for the farmers, the school food service, and the kids. Which is why the USDA funds Debra Eschmeyer and other regional heads of the Farm to School Tactical Team working to link local farms to schools. Their research shows that Farm to School meals result in an average increased consumption of one or more servings of fruit and vegetables per day.

Menu Planning

How does Farm to School work for the food service department and staff? First of all, someone needs to have real cooking experience. I saw a tragic photo of a Houston Farm to School meal with a side of limp, steamed bok choy. This Chinese cabbage is delicate and flavorful when braised or chopped and stir-fried with rice, but from the looks of the picture, I can only image the smelly, bitter-tasting slime the Houston kids confronted that day. A school chef with a culinary school degree would be overjoyed to obtain a shipment of surplus bok choy, but prepared without culinary experience, or at least a good recipe, the stuff is destined for the garbage. I've met wonderful school cooks whose only prior experience was making meals for the family—what's important is knowledge of basic cooking techniques and a passion for produce. A little butter, olive oil, homemade dressing, or dipping sauce can make those veggies much more exciting for the kids. Your district's wellness policy would do well to define "scratch cooking." In my district the food service director insisted they were cooking from scratch. When we asked for an example, she told us they made their own tuna salad by mixing prepared mayonnaise with canned tuna. Okay, but . . .

School food service operators must plan menus twelve to eighteen months in advance because of the commodity food procurement system. That type of planning may seem to contradict the spontaneity of incorporating seasonal ingredients, but with some consultation with local farmers or crop calendars it's easy to learn what fruits and vegetables are available in a given month in your region, and to create menus that are flexible enough for substitutions. You don't have to wait eighteen months to get a Farm to School program started, either, but you may have to compromise some of your goals until current commodity items are used up. There are great resources for menu planning and recipes for school food. In Beaufort County, North Carolina, the cooks are going retro, returning to scratch cooking using old USDA recipes from the 1960s and 1970s. Based on my childhood memories, some of those recipes were winners, and some could use a little updating. Chef Ann Cooper has a terrific online resource at thelunchbox.org that lists 120 simple school meal recipes portioned for school groups based on serving sizes required for particular age groups. For example: "ingredients—27 pounds broccoli for 133 elementary school children."

It's a good idea to meet with farmers over the winter to plan for crops for the coming season. When farmers have a guaranteed customer, they can plant according to required yield. In order to avoid shortages, a farmer would want to plant in excess of the request, with the option of selling the excess to another customer, and lessening the risk of falling short.

BUDGET TIPS

Cost is always a factor, but food service directors suggest the following:

- Purchase produce that is plentiful and in season.
- Purchase directly from farmers.
- Offer locally made value-added products à la carte.
- Introduce new items in small portions at first.

FOR THE RECORD

From the *Los Angeles Times*, Wednesday, September 15, 2010:

"Correction—School lunch: An article in the Aug. 26 Food section quoted Liz Powell, director of food services for the Santa Maria-Bonita School District, as saying that buying 80 percent of its produce locally had added to food costs. After publication, Powell said the costs had actually gone down, with one analysis showing a $3,000 savings over four months."

HOW TO HOLD A TASTE-TESTING

Find out which foods are available locally.

Make a green salad, a fruit salad, a composed salad, a salsa, a smoothie, or roast vegetables.

Put small portions in little tasting cups—paper condiment cups or Dixie cups.

Invite students at lunchtime to taste the recipes.

Display the raw ingredients—ask students if they can identify them.

Ask students to rate the dish.

Add top-rated items to the lunch menu.

The main purpose of Farm to School is not to just feed children better, but to connect them with their food and food choices. The program I visited in Peterborough, New Hampshire, did that by enlisting students to design a month's worth of healthy menus that were tested, tasted, and implemented in the lunch program. Similarly, the USDA's Recipes for Healthy Kids Challenge calls for teams of students, parents, and school cooks to submit recipes in the categories of whole grains, dark green and orange vegetables, or dry beans and peas. Winning recipes receive cash prizes.

Limit Options

Kids are human. When offered broccoli or a Pop-Tart, a lot of them are going to choose the Pop-Tart. Especially if they're really hungry—the temptation of that sugar rush will win out. Most kids don't really think about "good choices," no matter how much nutrition education they've had. Farm to School programs do require more labor, which means less time to prepare a variety of meals. Fresh produce has wonderful eye appeal, and if it's part of a meal that's not competing with à la carte pizza and burgers, there's a much better chance that the kids will choose it. While it's nice to have "treats" now and then, habituating kids to meals that are less salty, fatty, and sweet than the foods they are already conditioned to takes some time, repetition, and reinforcement. Rather than begging or demanding that they make a healthy choice, offer them a limited amount of choices that are all healthy.

Stealth Health

Several popular cookbooks promote hiding vegetables in popular treats like brownies. Purists decry this as trickery. I don't consider something hidden if it's an ingredient in a tasty recipe. When my kids were little, I always added lots of vegetables to my tomato sauce, and then partially pureed it for a smoother consistency. The kids loved the sauce, and it was a great way for them to experience the flavors that carrots, onions, celery, and herbs imparted without the fear factor of strange chunks and leaves in the sauce. Kids generally like simple food. When introducing a new fruit or vegetable, it can be either added in small quantity to a familiar dish (like bok choy in fried rice) or nicely prepared and presented on its own (like roasted broccoli). Tread carefully—you don't want to ruin a favorite dish by adding something that changes it too much.

Who's Going to Chop
the Rutabagas?

That's the headline of an article about the challenges of Farm to School in Minnesota. It tells the story of one frustrated food service director who has access to fresh potatoes, carrots, and rutabagas but doesn't have the staff hours to cut up the vegetables, or a food processor to do the work for her. She's got 1,800 kids to feed. A mom wrote a comment below the article, suggesting that perhaps a group of parents could volunteer to prep the local harvest. The director might also ask the PTO if they could fund a commercial-quality food processor—these cost from $1,500 to $3,000 and can quickly pay for themselves in labor savings. Someone still has to wash those veggies and operate the machine, so in addition to a trained cook or chef, school kitchen staff needs to be trained not only in food safety, but also in basic culinary skills, like how to handle knives and measure ingredients.

Culinary boot camps offer training at local culinary institutions, or on-site for larger districts investing in Farm to School programs. In Colorado, a consortium of state health foundations and agencies have coordinated week-long boot camps led by Cook for America. The training provides immersion in food system history, sanitation, culinary math, basic knife skills, menu planning, time management, and the basic cooking techniques required for proteins, grains, legumes, vegetables, sauces, and baked items.

BEHIND THE SCENES

John Turenne, the consultant behind the scenes in Jamie Oliver's West Virginia television series, reveals some of the secrets to introducing the kitchen staff to scratch cooking. He says, "Nine times out of ten, when we walk in with our chef coats on, the look in their eyes is fear or anger. If we go about it

(continued)

in the right context with support and empathy, we can melt the ice and then we show them the technical tips and processes. We have to convince people we're not Jamie Oliver. That was a reality show based on drama. We're the reality behind the reality." The reality isn't always pretty, either. He says, "They sat me down and said 'Let us tell you why we can't do that.' They'll say there's not enough time, but that's a knee-jerk reaction. Anybody who sees them sees they have a lot of time—but I can't accuse them of taking two hours of breaks. We suggest we'll just try a few things and get your input and see what works."

John confesses, "There are times I want to grab some of these ladies by the collar and say snap out of it but you can't do that. We take the attitude that we're going to work with you, we're not against you. It's about collaboration."

John has developed an approach to that collaboration that has paid off. He explains, "We are training from two perspectives. Number one is the how—the technical—it's our hands. Number two is why and it's the emotion or the heart. If we're going to try to show how to make a better tomato sauce from scratch with some different vegetables blended into it, we'd better show them why. We teach them to read ingredients. Michael Pollan's book *Food Rules* is a great training guide. We put his rules on index cards that we'll hand out. Don't eat blue food, etc. We get the ladies talking. Many are not young. And in the end, they were all very supportive, especially the cooks. Every time we left the kitchen on Friday afternoon they were hugging and thanking us."

John consults for hospitals, schools, and corporate customers. He observes, "I've never met an institution that says it's okay to increase their costs. These are one-time investments because our changes do not increase operational costs. Funding is just for our services, or training, or small equipment. Advocates have to find local funding to cover these costs."

One of the most important things I learned from John is the power of building a team of people invested in nurturing and nourishing children. He's creating a community in the school cafeteria by bringing people on board with the emotional context of food as life force. This bond among workers makes the workplace feel like a safe place, and once they are able to relax and feel good about their work, they are eager to participate. I witnessed this transformation when John took a staff group on a tour of the Yale Sustainable Farm. As they tasted cherry tomatoes and fresh-picked basil, their eyes lit up, they recalled family meals from childhood, they asked questions about the crops and discussed how the fresh produce could be used in the cafeteria. Laughter and smiles replaced fear and anger as the group shared the powerful feeling of being part of something extraordinary.

Salad Days

Several years ago, my mom sent me a newspaper article about my former elementary school's lunch program. The article, with photos, proudly touted the success of a salad bar filled with fresh broccoli, lettuce, cherry tomatoes, chickpeas, and cottage cheese. The kids loved it, but the food service director complained about the time it took to prepare the ingredients for the salad bar. In conclusion, the article said that the salad bar would next appear at another elementary school in a few weeks. Sadly, I realized that all the hype was about a salad bar that materialized for only one day.

Chef Ann Cooper and her LunchBox team at the Food Family Farming Foundation have partnered with Whole Foods Market, United Fresh, the National Fruit and Vegetable Alliance, and First Lady Michelle Obama's Let's Move! campaign to see to it that salad bars become a permanent fixture in our lunchrooms, particularly those in high-poverty areas. The Great American Salad Bar campaign aims to award 6,000 child-sized salad bars to needy schools by 2013. The program will only benefit a fraction of the eligible districts, but like all the other models—it's a start.

In the Kitchen

Most schools are able to rearrange the cafeteria to accommodate a salad bar, ideally front and center in the lunch line. Finding the space to prepare the ingredients for the salad bar can be more of a challenge. Most public schools built for the baby boomers between 1950 and 1970 had fully equipped commercial kitchens. Many of the schools built since then do not. As heat-and-serve became the norm for school food, school kitchens fell into disuse, so as those older schools became overcrowded, kitchen space was converted to classroom space. This leaves some school districts with a patchwork of semi-functional kitchens equipped with ancient appliances. I've also seen well-equipped, underutilized school kitchens in both urban and suburban districts. A number of forward-thinking school districts took advantage of federal stimulus funds to update kitchen facilities in 2009–2010.

Switching to fresh produce, raw ingredients, and cooking from scratch requires about twice the space of a heat-and-serve setup, because you need room to store, sort, wash, and prep. The Center for Ecoliteracy's "Rethinking School Lunch Guide" suggests a good rule of thumb is one square foot of kitchen space for every meal served, with a minimum of 1,000 square feet to serve between 200 and 1,000 students. The guide recommends a 50-50 rule: allow 50 percent of kitchen space for food preparation and 50 percent for storage.

School chefs agree that centralizing food preparation and cooking saves time and money. Program directors in Baltimore, San Francisco, and other large cities cite the lack of a large, centralized kitchen as a major obstacle to incorporating more Farm to School products into their menus. Ambitious school chefs are making do with limited facilities and adjusting recipes based on availability of equipment. "My central kitchen doesn't have a stove. I'm doing 2,200 meals out of this place and there's not even a stove in it," was one of the first revelations shared by Ann Cooper on my visit to Berkeley. Somehow, she was managing to cook from scratch using a giant steam kettle and ovens in lieu of a stove.

If you are planning to renovate or build a kitchen, consider building excess capacity into your blueprint. Better meals will mean increased participation. Perhaps your kitchen could serve a neighboring district that might be willing to share in the investment. Eliminating disposable packaging can save money by eliminating both the cost of the packaging and the cost of disposal. The "Rethinking School Lunch Guide" says that the average American child generates 67 pounds of trash from school lunches every year—that's 18,670 pounds per year from the average elementary school. Plastic and foil on individually wrapped items, cardboard trays, plastic utensils, and Styrofoam bowls and cups all add to the cost of a meal, as much as 50 percent of the food cost according to the guide. An investment in reusable trays, plates, and utensils can save money down the road, but requires planning space for a dishwasher and washing area.

The "Rethinking School Lunch Guide" offers a financial calculator for food service directors and business managers. The calculator is an Excel template that allows them to try out different scenarios for food cost, labor hours, and meal uptake to track assumptions about income and expense for making the switch to Farm to School meals.

FARM TO SCHOOL FINANCES

Chef Peter Gorman from the Unquowa School has embraced Farm to School practices throughout his program. As the chef for a small, private school, Peter has been able to develop his program in harmony with the school's philosophy of sustainability and educating children to be stewards of the earth. The minimum specifications laid out in Peter's Food and Health Policy for the school require all food to be fresh, local, and seasonal. Specifically, the policy pledges to:

- Serve organic food to the maximum extent possible and to constantly look at ways to manage total costs to achieve this goal.
- Cook food from scratch and serve it fresh.
- Satisfy the health and diet needs of all clientele—i.e., vegan or vegetarian requests, attention to specific dietary/allergy needs.
- Serve homemade desserts no more than four times per week and with a portion size no larger than one ounce.
- Use only fresh, whole eggs from chickens raised in a cage-free environment.
- Use only milk, grass-fed beef and all-natural poultry from animals raised without the use of growth hormones and non-therapeutic antibiotics.

(continued)

- Use only natural oils in cooking (no hydrogenated or trans fats).
- Completely avoid any ingredient containing high fructose corn syrup.
- Never serve deep-fried foods.
- Serve only organic yogurt.
- Offer only homemade and low fat or organic salad dressings.
- Use only dolphin-safe tuna.
- Serve only Applegate Farms brand (or the equivalent) deli meats. Salami or other processed meats shall not contain nitrates or nitrites.
- Use only Barilla Plus pasta or a whole-wheat pasta equivalent in nutritional profile or organic.
- Use only unbleached flour.
- Serve only organic rice.
- Bake all breads in-house

In addition, Peter has to keep the food affordable. His costs are certainly higher than the federal reimbursement rate for a school meal, but not as much higher as you might expect. In order to provide a model for his policy, Peter shares his financial analysis with us:

FINANCES: OUR WORK SO FAR

From the start, it has been our expectation and goal that the changes to the dining program at the Unquowa School not increase our overall food service budget. A significant challenge, considering the average cost for locally produced and organic food generally costs more than conventional food. After two and one half years, we can say that we have truly succeeded in achieving this goal and have not increased our food budget until 2009–10. This is how we strategically implemented the program:

The first year, we realized that we would spend our time and energy just trying to implement upgraded small changes in items that could have cost neutral effect, like organic milk in large containers instead of conventional milk in individual containers.

The second year brought the real evidence of cost savings. We began significant food cost monitoring and control methods, thus eliminating waste and high cost, processed foods. Some of our progress:

- Created a budget based on projected food costs per meal (fcpm) ($1.90), overhead, and labor.
- Incorporated formal weekly inventory, invoicing, and operating report systems.
- Measured the actual operating costs ($1.50/fcpm) against our projections and adjusted staffing and menus accordingly.
- Realized significant savings in food costs due to these controls and fresh, whole food.
- Added staffing to support additional production needs.
- Currently operating at combined all costs per meal served at $4.25 and a fcpm served at $1.80.

In year three, we have invested our savings in food costs into an increase in our labor costs to hire an assistant chef who understands and aspires to the sustainable food movement in order to support additional fresh, whole scratch cooking and to be mentored for future leadership.

Year four we performed a study for Hobart Corporation using their 40-quart mixer (to make our own bread). We found significant savings of $4,500.

Because of our fiscal success, the school increased the food budget by $5,000 in year five. The result has been an organic salad bar and a new purveyor, Albert's Organics.

OUR GOALS FOR THE FUTURE

Manage and adjust our budget to anticipate additional increases in the cost of food and continual improvement in food specifications so as to incorporate even more organic and sustainable food into our menus.

Peter reports that a number of overweight students have lost weight after several years on his healthy meal program.

The Gleaners

Though it runs on biodiesel, the delivery truck I spent a morning in is really fueled by the efforts of the Glean Team, a group of volunteers organized by a local organic farmers' cooperative, Marin Organics. Six months of the year, these folks gather on Mondays to harvest leftover produce from the fields of Marin Organics' farms, enabling 10,000 kids in about half of the county's public schools to eat local organic foods. The gleaned food isn't old or rotten, it's just food that would normally be left in the field because it's not pretty enough for sale to local restaurants or at farmers' markets. According to their website, "This can account for up to 20 percent of what is grown, and throughout the year may include potatoes, squashes, spinach, leeks, beets, carrots, arugula, lettuces, meats, eggs, yogurt, ice cream, and more!" Instead of tossing it, the food is delivered to the schools along with their regular orders from the co-op, effectively offsetting the higher cost of ordering local organic produce.

Results

Schools that utilize the cafeteria as part of the curriculum seek the same quality in the food and in the food service that they demand from teachers and from textbooks. Where school districts are able to purchase meat and vegetables from local farmers, I observed that food service directors, administrators, parents, and even students all join in taking responsibility for the quality and taste of the meals. Deb Eschmeyer cites the following results collated from various Farm to School research:

- The choice of healthier options in the cafeteria through Farm to School meals results in consumption of more fruits and vegetables (+0.99 to +1.3 servings/day) and at home. For example, studies in Portland, Oregon, and Riverside, California, have found that students eating a farm-fresh salad bar consume roughly one additional serving of fruits and vegetables per day.

- Better knowledge and awareness about gardening, agriculture, healthy eating, local foods, and seasonality. In Philadelphia, the percentage of kindergarteners who knew where their food came from increased from 33 percent to 88 percent after participation in a Farm to School program.
- Demonstrated willingness to try out new foods and healthier options. In one school in Ventura, California, on days in which there was a choice between a farmers' market salad bar and a hot lunch, students and adults chose the salad bar by a 14 to 1 ratio. Reduced consumption of unhealthy foods and sodas; reduced television watching time; positive lifestyle modifications such as a daily exercise routine.
- Positive gains in phonological awareness of the alphabet, increased social skills, and self-esteem.

There is now a Farm to School program in every state, and as these programs expand they are generating some striking models. What we need now is an army of farmers, teachers, and cooks to implement the models on a larger scale.

FoodCorps

Gathering and deploying that army is the mission of FoodCorps. It's a division of AmeriCorps and a project of the National Farm to School Network. FoodCorps places young adults in high-need communities to help improve the quality of cafeteria food and teach children about food in the classroom and in school gardens. Funded through a Kellogg planning grant, Food-Corps came about in response to calls for help from all over the country. Farm to School's Deb Eschmeyer is one of the project's founders. She writes:

[FoodCorps] members will work in school districts suffering disproportionate rates of childhood obesity. The program will at once serve vulnerable children, improving access to healthy, affordable school meals, while also serving its AmeriCorps members by training a cadre of leaders for careers in food and agriculture.

She goes on to explain the rationale like this: "I consistently hear from parents and school staff, 'Oh, we love Farm to School and we love school gardens, but our budgets are tight. We just don't have the sweat equity and the labor to pull it off.' That's what FoodCorps is here to do. Help improve America's school meals and give our kids a fighting chance for a passing grade in health."

FoodCorps is launching in the fall of 2011 with about eighty volunteers in ten states. The locations were chosen, she said, "through a competitive proposal process that identified the places service members are most needed and best able to make a difference."

FoodCorps intends to supplement and weave together the network of food reform organizations that are already working to improve school food by offering "boots on the ground," and extra hands in the dirt.

It's Not Nutritious if They Don't Eat It

In my travels, I hear the obvious stated repeatedly. Food isn't nutritious until it is eaten. Adults can suggest that students "choose a rainbow" or "grab five," but if it gets dumped in the garbage, it isn't healthy. The food has to be attractive, tasty and most of all, kids have to choose it, and then choose to eat it.

Special events, salad bars, grab 'n' go fruit baskets, fruit or veg on a stick, colorful posters, and tastings are all great ways to introduce new foods to kids, and marketing healthy food is the subject of many a workshop at school nutrition conferences.

The philosophy of Farm to School runs deeper than the choices in the cafeteria, though, and the food itself is just one facet of a program that connects students and their families to their food at its source. These programs not only lead to better food choices, they also promote an appreciation for food quality, agriculture, and the environment, all of which adds up to students who enjoy healthy food and choose it without coercion. Farm to School pro-grams create a learning environment that connects healthy food marketing messages with meaningful experience. And when the kids get that, they bring it home. Debra Eschmeyer says, "Incorporation of a parent-education component through a Farm to School program can ensure that messages about health and local foods are carried into homes and reinforced there by parents and caregivers. Farm to School education inspires parents to incor-porate healthier foods into their children's and their family's diets and better equips them to do so through both shopping and cooking tips." In a project in Vermont, 32 percent of parents with participating children believed that their family diet had improved since their child's participation in the pro-gram. In another project in Philadelphia, 78 percent of parents with partici-pating children reported that their children ate more fruits and vegetables.

In restaurant parlance, there's the chef and kitchen staff overseeing the chemistry, artistry, and controlled chaos that goes on in the kitchen, which is referred to as the "back of the house," and there's the maitre d' and waitstaff in charge of the customer service, décor, presentation, and degustation that takes place in the dining area, the "front of the house." In the world of school food, the back of the house, which has everything to do with procurement, food ser-vice staff, and government compliance is under the jurisdiction of the USDA's Child Nutrition Services. Connecticut's Jane Slupecki pointed out to me that in Connecticut, our Farm to School statutes are split down the middle, with the USDA handling the back side and the Connecticut State Department of Education handling what I would call the front side. Jane's jurisdiction is Part A of the state's regulations—she works for the Department of Agriculture and her job is to connect schools with farmers and ensure that the produce meets the needs of the school districts in terms of safety, quantity, quality, variety, and delivery. Part B of Connecticut's Farm to School statutes is in the hands of the Department of Education—they're the front of the house. Part B states:

> The Department of Education, in consultation with the Department of Agricul-ture, school food service directors, and interested farming organizations, shall (1) establish a week-long promotional event, to be known as Connecticut-Grown

for Connecticut Kids Week, in late September or early October each year, that will promote Connecticut agriculture and foods to children through school meal and classroom programs, at farms, farmers' markets and other locations in the community, (2) encourage and solicit school districts, individual schools, and other educational institutions under its jurisdiction to purchase Connecticut-grown farm products, (3) provide outreach, guidance, and training to districts, parent and teacher organizations, schools, and school food service directors concerning the value of and procedure for purchasing and incorporating into their regular menus Connecticut-grown farm products, (4) in consultation with the Department of Agriculture, arrange for local, regional, and state-wide events where potential purchasers and farmers can interact, and (5) arrange for interaction between students and farmers, including field trips to farms and in-school presentations by farmers.

The Connecticut State Legislature, in their wisdom, determined that Farm to School should be an educational program for students, parents, and school staff in addition to creating an economic stimulus for local farmers, and they charged the Department of Education with carrying out that mandate. Not all teachers are comfortable or familiar with the subjects of farming, gardening, media, and eco-literacy. As advocates, we can help connect our educators with the materials, knowledge, and skills they need to teach principles of sustainability, land, water, and air stewardship. There's a wealth of learning experiences that can be taught through farming, gardening, growing, and harvesting, and they can readily be incorporated into existing lesson plans and curriculum objectives.

SUMMARY: HOW TO START FARM TO SCHOOL IN YOUR COMMUNITY

Research

Contact your state Farm to School program and local organizations to find farmers and other sources of locally grown and locally produced food.

Contact your state office of child nutrition, the American School Food Service Association or the National Food Service Management Institute to find out what training is available for food service staff.

Outreach

Coordinate a farm-fresh tasting, invite a farmer to school for a demonstration, or organize a field trip to a local farm. Organize a meeting to present Farm to School to stakeholders in your school community.

Assess

Meet with your district business manager and food service director to identify needs, build trust, create a strategic plan, develop a budget, and identify staff or volunteers to support the program.

Implement

Introduce local products one or two at a time. Test recipes. Build relationships and get comfortable with the process of ordering, preparing, and cooking with farm fresh ingredients.

SAMPLE FARMER SURVEY

Name: _____

Title: _____

School District: _____

Street Address: _____

City: _____

Telephone: _____

State: _____

Zip: _____

Fax: _____

E-mail: _____

Date: _____

1. Are you currently supplying produce to the schools in your area? If yes, skip to number 8. If no, go to number 2.
2. Is there excess capacity on your farm that you could plant specifically for a Farm to School program?
3. Do you currently have extra product that you could sell to schools?
4. Do you do value-added processing? If no, skip to number 6.
5. Do you have the capacity to do additional processing to make your product acceptable for sale to your school or district?
6. Are you a member of a cooperative?
7. Do you have the infrastructure (e.g., trucks, driver, cold storage) to deliver product to schools or a central processing location?

If you are currently participating in Farm to School

8. Please describe the products and quantities you are selling to schools.
9. Do you sell to Dept. of Defense Fresh program?
10. How did you become involved in selling to schools?
11. Is this project economically viable from your perspective?
12. Do you sell to other institutions?
13. Are there policies at the school, district, local, state, or federal level that support or undermine selling to schools?

Transportation and Delivery

14. Who delivers your products to schools? How?
15. How often are pickups made?
16. How often are deliveries made?
17. Are they picked up from your farm?
18. Are they delivered on the same day?
19. Are deliveries made to a central location or to individual schools?
20. How did the transport mechanism evolve?

Supply

21. How many schools are you supplying?
22. Are you able to consistently meet demand?
23. Are you able to provide products to schools year-round? What, when?
24. Do you sell processed products, e.g., apple juice, dried fruit?

Pricing

25. How is the price for your product determined?
26. Are you selling at or below the standard wholesale price?
27. Are you selling at, above, or below the retail price?
28. Are you making enough profit to continue selling to schools?
29. If you deliver your product washed, pre-cut, packaged, or processed in any way, do you charge extra for that service?

Outside Support

30. Are you part of a group that has helped organize this project?
31. Do you or the organizing group receive outside support for this project such as grant funds, donations, or services?

(CREATED BY THE COMMUNITY FOOD SECURITY COALITION AND THE CENTER FOR FOOD AND JUSTICE, OCCIDENTAL COLLEGE, AND REPRINTED BY PERMISSION FROM THE NATIONAL FARM TO SCHOOL NETWORK)

SEVEN

TEACH FOOD

Imagine teaching school food as if it were an academic subject.

— ALICE WATERS

I wasn't raised on a farm but until I was four our suburban backyard shared a fence with a dairy farm. I have fond memories of pulling up fresh grass from my yard and feeding it to the gentle giants through the fence wires. Often when we would drive to our local shopping center, known as Bishop's Corner, my dad would say, "I remember when all this was farmland." Farms just seem to invoke some kind of collective nostalgia—most of us have farming not so far back in our gene pool. Although our parents or their parents' parents may have struggled to see their children "get a good education" so they wouldn't have to break their backs farming, the pull of the land evokes a romantic yearning for a connection to nature.

Farming is the result of humankind's efforts to tame nature in order to serve our need for food. Without it, we'd still be hunter-gatherers, spending our days as nomads in search of food. To tame nature, we must understand it, and a large part of that understanding comes from living in nature and observing our environment. Most of our children won't grow up to be farmers, but they all will be stewards of the earth, and their behavior will be influenced by how they experience the natural world as children.

Nature Deficit Disorder

Our children are growing up farther removed from nature than ever before in human history. The dangers of urban streets, the pull of television, video games, and hand-held communication devices, the lure of the mall, over-scheduling, lack of open space, and a fear of germs, bugs, dirt, weather, and wildlife have all conspired to drive kids indoors. Many kids now experience some sort of ersatz, Disney-fied version of nature more often than the real deal. In his 2005 book *Last Child in the Woods* Richard Louv coined the term Nature Deficit Disorder, linking this disconnection from nature to a wide range of behavior problems. Learning in nature and from nature is a form of kinesthetic learning that integrates experience with understanding. Children learn more rapidly and lastingly in a multi-sensory environment, particularly children with so-called learning disorders. The congruency of multi-sensory experience and observation has a measurable positive impact on learning and brain activity. Whether in the form of free play in nature, with natural materials in a classroom, or as an organized lesson in an outdoor setting, children need these types of experiences for proper growth and development.

A Taste for Health

There's only one subject that I can think of in which children learn with all five senses, and that's *food*. Incorporating food studies into the curriculum offers opportunities to taste, touch, and literally ingest lessons in virtually every academic subject on every grade level. Developing a sense of taste is not just for food snobs. That connection between healthy food, healthy soil, and healthy kids is made through the sense of taste. Teaching children to taste real food at a young age enables them to discern junk food as junk. The typical junk food combination of salty, sweet, and fatty flavors masks the lack of essential taste in processed foods. Once a child develops a taste for food with real flavor, that junk food may not taste so good.

Programs like Farm to School emphasize the experience of tasting fresh food and learning where it comes from and how it's grown so that children can develop a relationship to the environment that nurtures the food that nourishes them. In schools where Farm to School programs take place, schoolchildren visit farms, sometimes working on them as a learning experience, or bringing their acquired knowledge back to school gardens and greenhouses. They learn to cultivate healthy plants by nourishing them with sunlight, water, and healthy soil.

The variety and availability of nutrients in the soil imparts taste to the plants. A bell pepper tastes more like a bell pepper when it is grown in healthy soil. The notion of *terroir* stems from wine production, where variations in weather and types of soil cause distinctive regional and annual modulation in the flavor of grape varietals and the wines produced from them. The term is now being applied to other fruits and vegetables; those that come from healthy soils will be enhanced with flavor variations from season to season and region to region. A healthy soil need not be overly rich in nutrients and the climate need not be perfect to produce delicious, nutrient dense produce; in fact, plants that are somewhat stressed will send out deeper roots and absorb more minerals and nutrients from a deeper spectrum of soil, producing a richer, deeper flavor. Once a fruit or vegetable is harvested, its flavor will slowly fade, its sugars will turn to starch, and so the *terroir* of a tomato will be most pronounced when plucked from the vine and popped into your mouth.

The more we teach our children about their food, the better equipped they will be to make decisions about what they want to eat and where that food comes from. Isn't that what education is all about?

THE GARDEN WHISPERER

Kirk Cusick founded the Whispering Cottonwood Farm Educational Center in Salina, Kansas, as an after-school program where kids could connect to the earth, observe, journal, and record what they saw. He was struck by both their scientific and emotional responses to the horticultural plantings and acres of native prairie grasses. After seven years of spring and fall after-school programs, Kirk began wondering how he could make a larger impact on more kids. He wanted to bring nature to the kids instead of having them come to the farm. He approached teachers and administrators at his local schools; they liked the idea of school gardens, but the building and grounds director wasn't immediately sold. Kirk's first school garden was at one of the private Catholic schools. From there, Kirk says, it just kept spiraling. He connected with the Department of Education and was given a grant to get gardens started in ten more schools. The department also set some money aside to pay Kirk for his time and resources. He needs $1,800 to get a garden started. Each school has to raise matching funds of $900. Kirk now works with twenty-two schools in his area. With reassurances that Kirk would handle the maintenance, the grounds director came on board. Kansas, like most every state, has been hard hit by the long recession. When his state funding was recently cut back Kirk tells me that the local community rallied, and many of the schools have been able to fund-raise the shortfall from within.

Each garden plot is 50′ x 50′ and all the work is done by hand. The gardens operate twenty-eight weeks during the school year as well as ten weeks over the summer. Kirk is careful to plant his summer crops late for maximum production during late August, September, and October when school is in session. The produce can be used in the school cafeterias or however the community wants it to be used. The estimated worth of the produce harvested is between $1,500 and $2,000, which makes up for the initial investment and some of the labor as well. One of Kirk's goals is to help the school gardens become self-sustaining, and he's turning to the students for input. "I form a group of kids and we look at the garden as if it were a business," he tells me. "We're looking at growing flower bouquets and maybe selling summer subscription shares as ways to generate additional revenue."

Kirk went through the Kansas state educational standards and matched existing grade-level curriculum to lessons in the garden. Fourth-graders were studying the life cycle, so when tomato hornworms appeared on the tomato vines, the students were able to observe the stages of their development. Another class harvested pumpkins and estimated their seeds, then counted to see if they were accurate. After the math lesson, the children got to mash up the pumpkins and make a pie!

A School Garden

A school garden can be a great starting point for your school food advocacy. Though they have been around for over one hundred years, school gardens seem to ebb and flow in popularity. Thanks to the Edible Schoolyard, and media coverage of First Lady Michelle Obama harvesting sweet potatoes on the White House lawn with a group of Washington, D.C., fifth-graders, school gardens are popping up like weeds in a strawberry patch. In addition to learning to plant and grow food, a school garden is a wonderful place for children to experience nature and observe the life cycles of plants and insects. With a garden as an outdoor classroom, lessons in math, science, history, geography, social studies, and art can all be taught through hands-on projects and experimentation. Gardening emphasizes cooperation over competition, and is a wonderful way for children to get fresh air and exercise. You don't need to be an experienced gardener, and you don't need a whole lot of money to get a school garden started. What you do need is a core group of advocates, some willing partners in the school system, and a plan that fits your school and your natural environment. Armed with these resources, I've seen school gardens built in a day.

FLOW LIKE WATER

One of my school garden mentors is Dorothy Mullen, founder of the Princeton School Gardens Cooperative. The cooperative came about when several parents discovered that they were simultaneously working on gardens in different schools in the township of Princeton, New Jersey. To my knowledge, they are the first school district to lay claim to achieving the goal of "a garden in every school." Dorothy says that as an advocate, you must learn to flow like water. Water follows the course of least resistance. For Dorothy, school gardens offered the opportunity to flow into the school community and into the curriculum with minimal conflict and maximum results.

Dorothy says that assembling a team of stakeholders is essential to the success of your garden. The first "non-negotiable" stakeholder on her list is a superintendent, principal, or assistant principal. If they're not already on board, write a brief letter to the administrator explaining what you'd like to do. Tell them which members of the school community and which parents are working with you. Suggest some ideas of where you'd like to site the garden. Give an overview of how it will be funded, managed, and maintained. In particular, provide assurances about the health and safety of the garden and how it will enhance the school grounds aesthetically. Describe who will be using the garden and some of the lessons the garden can be used for. Dorothy got the green light for her first garden only after she provided a plan for its removal and restoration in the event that it wasn't successful.

You'll also need support from a teacher or a few teachers (they don't have to be gardeners!), a few parents, students, and community volunteers, a school custodian to discuss maintenance requirements, someone on the food service staff, a school nurse, a school librarian, and other school and community gardeners for advice and resources. With buy-in from this group you will have help solving the issues and challenges that will inevitably arise when planning and building the garden.

Dorothy and her team were able to realize their goal by making a concerted effort to involve the larger Princeton community in their mission. Being a college town, Princeton has a number of local small businesses that cater to the community. The ice cream shop donated a flavor to the school gardens. The children grew mint in the gardens and brought it to the shop where it was used to make mint ice cream. Proceeds from the mint ice cream were given to the gardens. A coffee shop donated sales of coffee during a local film festival, and a local restaurant did a fund-raiser for the gardens.

Fran McManus, another of the cooperative members, has a background in community organizing, bringing people together, and creating ownership. She describes another fund-raiser like this: "Princeton has a problem with street gangs, something we have in common with L.A. We bought soap from the Watts [L.A.] school garden project and then sold the soap here. So our gardens were connected."

(continued)

Fran insists that there MUST be a paid position for a garden coordinator. The Princeton co-op received a grant from the local garden club to help cover this part-time position. The group reached out to the community for more than just funding. They found individuals and businesses that were willing to offer materials, services, and expertise. Participation ranged from providing wood, tools, soil, and seeds to volunteering a morning of labor or publicity and PR.

Typically school gardens tie into the content that is being taught in the classroom. In Princeton, the classroom content sometimes evolves in the garden and the teacher then ties it in with the curriculum. Fran says that in this process the children take ownership of what they are creating. "Every child wants to sample their lettuce in the salad bar."

Fran gave me a sample of the lessons Princeton teachers are creating around the gardens. "The third-graders have a butterfly garden. There's an herb garden. The first and third grades created a map of the courtyard garden. The fifth-graders recorded soil and air temperature and sunlight between 9 a.m. and 3 p.m. They made a microclimate map and graph of courtyard using data collection, data analysis, and patterns. Based on that graph, they decided where to plant certain crops."

High school classes work on budgeting how much produce can be grown per square foot of garden space and what the market value of the produce is. They use Excel and QuickBooks and even develop their own software and macros for the calculations.

Fran tells me that one garden was plagued by an aphid infestation on their nasturtiums. She explains, "The bugs were too small to see so the students used microscopes, seeing on one leaf every life stage. These were second- and third-graders learning a different metamorphosis than butterflies. The third-graders study food webs and they found ladybug larvae living nearby that love to eat aphids."

Another class studies the minerals in kale to see if they are the same minerals as in a rock. The lesson has students grind kale and then test it using a strong magnet to see that the iron is the same as in the rock.

In one lesson, Fran says, "Kindergarteners learn where food comes from. Sunchokes are [the root of] a native sunflower. The kids dig them up and wash them and slice them into shoestring fries. That's what they ate at the first Thanksgiving."

Basil, garlic, onions, and tomatoes are planted by the fourth-graders and harvested in the fall when they get to fifth grade, with the kindergarteners. Then they make tomato sauce and pizza dough. "Our biggest hope is that these lessons don't stop here—they go on to home," Fran emphasizes. "The kids are asking parents to plant a garden at home."

Make a Proposal

Your administration may want a detailed, formal proposal. While this might seem like an annoyance, especially if your garden plan is a simple one, the process of writing a proposal can actually help you clarify the details of your project in a very productive way. Writing the proposal forces you to consider options, obstacles, and opportunities for your school garden. The proposal will actually be a document that reflects your planning process. It will help all the stakeholders understand the purpose and use of the garden, and it will also clarify their roles and responsibilities. If you plan to apply for grant funds, you should easily be able to adapt your proposal to fit the framework of most grant applications.

STATE THE PURPOSE

It may be obvious to your team how cool a school garden will be, but you should consider how the various parts of the school community would use it. Will culinary arts classes use the food or will it be used for school meals, sold at a farmers' market, or donated to a shelter? Does everyone agree that the garden will be organic in order to teach principles of sustainability, or do some people want to ensure "success" by using chemical fertilizers and controls? Must the garden look like a showpiece, or could it be focused more on experience and trial and error than perfection? Are there priorities for a specific department or curriculum that might impact other uses? Make sure all your stakeholders have a say in articulating the purpose of the garden. You may need to educate and negotiate with some of them to come to an agreement of purpose.

JOHNSON PARK ELEMENTARY SCHOOL (PRINCETON, NEW JERSEY) MISSION STATEMENT

The mission of the Johnson Park Courtyard Garden is to create and sustain an organic garden that will serve as an outdoor classroom for our students. The garden will provide hands-on experiences that enhance curriculum in many areas including science and math. It will also enhance awareness of healthy food choices and an appreciation of the outdoors. Students will be involved in all aspects of gardening including planning, planting, tending, harvesting, and preparing healthy foods.

LITTLEBROOK ELEMENTARY SCHOOL (PRINCETON, NEW JERSEY) MISSION STATEMENT

The Littlebrook Elementary school garden will be a living, edible classroom in our courtyard that will supplement and enhance the curriculum, provide fresh produce to the cafeteria and community and actively include teachers and students in every stage of the garden's growth and development.

SITING AND DESIGN

Even if you have an experienced garden designer on your team, it's still a good idea to visit other school gardens in your area if you know of any. Otherwise, ask around for examples of backyard, frontyard, rooftop, vacant lot, and community gardens so you can gather ideas. Garden clubs, garden stores, and botanical gardens are all good resources for design input.

The garden must be located in an area that gets at least six hours of sunlight a day (preferably more). A southern exposure is ideal for most gardens, especially those in the northern states. You'll need a convenient water source—generally a tap on the outside of a building to connect hoses or sprinklers. Size is an important consideration. It may be easier to get a project going if you keep the scale small, but if you are going to start small, try to find a location that has room for expansion. You'll also need storage for tools, either inside the school building or in a garden shed.

Locate the garden in a high visibility area in front of the school, or in a courtyard where there's a lot of traffic. You want students and staff to walk past the garden regularly, to see who's working in it and what is growing there. Depending on your location, you may need to create protection around your garden. Deer are very fond of most garden crops, often necessitating eight-foot deer fencing in suburban and rural areas. Instead of a fence around one Princeton garden, they planted a thick border of prickly shrubs that deterred the deer while preserving the natural look of the landscape. Urban districts may opt to place a garden within the confines of an existing fenced-in area to address safety concerns and prevent vandalism. Make sure the garden is located away from garbage cans and septic systems and is protected from any other potential sources of contamination including wildlife and pets.

Your school garden should be as accessible as possible. In Riverside, California, the one-acre school garden is an optional place for any child to go during recess and many kids choose gardening as their recess activity.

A school garden design must take into account the particular needs of a classroom of children. Pathways between planting beds must be wide enough to accommodate lots of two-way foot traffic, and level and smooth enough for a wheelchair as well. The beds themselves should not be too wide for small children to reach halfway across—a maximum of 3.5 or 4 feet across so that the center row can be reached from either side. Consider raising at least one bed up on legs to a height that would make it accessible to a child in a wheelchair. A sitting area with tables is a plus; straw bales are used for seating in San Francisco's school gardens (not hay because it carries weed seeds) and benches made from tree stumps and wood planks are long lasting and sustainable as well.

EDIBLE SCHOOLYARDS SPROUT IN NORTH IDAHO

Michele Murphree moved from California to the Northern Idaho panhandle, where she developed a passion for gardening. Michele says she and her group of garden friends had no experience starting a school garden club, and so they dove in with low expectations.

"Much to our surprise, thirty-three kids signed up, including all different ages and many diverse personalities," she reports. "After the students designed their garden and decided what and where they would plant, we met on a cold day to plant lettuce starts. Our garden club meeting was next to the area where students jumped onto the school buses. On that day, there was a lot of snickering about the 'garden club.' That snickering quickly turned to awe when the lettuce seeds transformed into actual plants in sunny windows at the school. The garden club was quickly becoming cool."

A local philanthropic organization gave a grant to purchase some garden tools and seeds, and the project became so cool that local businesses followed suit, donating plants, soil, manure, compost bins, and even funds for an automatic watering system.

"We thought that the students would be excited about harvesting, but had no idea about how much fun they would have building their garden. They worked really hard. They shoveled the dirt and manure, built beds, and planted like crazy without a complaint," Michele says. "In a very short time period, we saw many different kids come together as a team, laughing, getting their hands dirty, keeping garden journals, and expressing absolute joy at seeing seeds sprout."

At their first harvest, they reaped one hundred pounds of lettuce, as well as carrots, peas, green beans, squash, tomatoes, potatoes, berries, onions, peppers, and pumpkins. The students decided to share a portion of their bounty with the local food bank. The district's director of nutrition gave permission for the students to eat the produce they grew as long as it was grown organically and school staff prepared it.

Michele writes, "They were quite the heroes when their harvest was included in the school lunches and snacks. In fact, the kitchen staff reported that this was the first year that the school had run out of dressing because so many of the students were actually eating salad."

Based on the success of that first garden, the garden club has received more grant money to build gardens at other local schools. Weaving garden lessons into the district's curriculum is an important goal of their project. They've built a hoop house, which, says Michele, "serves as a great educational tool about expanding the garden season by allowing us to grow greens into October. We also integrated other school subjects into the garden. As a math lesson, for instance, students were asked how many seeds would yield how many pounds of produce. Other subjects, like biology, reading, writing, life skills, health and fitness, and social interaction were explored in the garden."

Michele hopes to put together a workbook and workshops for other schools in the area. She wants to share her experiences about gardening in the Northern Idaho climate, along with the many resources her group has assembled.

And, much to her delight, the project has exceeded all expectations. "This has been a really rewarding experience," she writes. "We are inspired by the enthusiasm of the students and how they have worked together to build their own gardens. We are looking forward to seeing the contributions that these gardens will give to our schools and communities."

MAKE YOUR BEDS

Your site and your soil type will help you determine what kind of beds you want to grow in. Have the soil tested for heavy metals and other contaminants by a reliable lab. Your state USDA Agricultural Extension Office will either provide soil testing or can recommend a reasonably priced lab. If you've got decent soil, you may only have to amend it with some natural conditioners like leaf mulch, compost, potash, lime, or peat moss. Kids love to be part of the groundbreaking and everyone will enjoy a good cardio workout digging and turning the fresh earth.

If there is any doubt or evidence of contamination, you can still use the site, but will have to plant in raised beds that don't come in contact with the soil underneath. Raised beds are also a great alternative to rocky soils, hard-packed ground that is difficult to till, or heavy clay soils that have poor drainage. I've started many a garden with a rock-picking party, and it is possible to condition these types of soils but that process can take several years. A drawback of raised beds is that they may dry out faster that the surrounding ground, or they may retain moisture leading to mold more readily. They also have to be filled with good-quality soil. Make sure you know where the topsoil will come from and then test it to make sure it's free of contaminants.

Raised beds are also a solution when siting a garden on a blacktop area. They can be made from hardwood (we use white birch), but it must be untreated. Pressure-treated wood is impregnated with chemical preservatives that can be toxic if they leach into the soil. A great resource book, *How to Grow a School Garden* by Arden Bucklin-Sporer and Rachel Kathleen Pringle, recommends using stamped metal livestock watering troughs with drainage holes drilled in the bottoms, bender board (plastic wood from recycled milk jugs), urbanite (chunks of recycled sidewalk), and wattle (burlap netting filled with straw), as alternative and cost-effective materials for raised beds. The wattle is interesting because you can create beds with curved borders in all sorts of shapes; the drawback is the wattle will decompose and need replacement after a few years. They caution against using plastic wood made with wood fiber or any recycled wood of unknown origins. Other materials that are unsafe to use for food production include railroad ties (creosote), old tires, plywood (formaldehyde), and bricks with old paint that may contain lead.

The growing season can be extended further into the school year with a cold frame incorporated into your garden design. A cold frame is simply a raised bed that is deep enough to cover with a plastic or glass top to allow plants to mature past the fall frost season. A greenhouse, especially in the northern states, enables gardening to be part of the curriculum year-round. Children can plant seeds in January or February and then transplant them into the garden in the spring.

Composting can be a source of controversy in your proposal, so be prepared to discuss, educate, and possibly compromise or revisit this at a later date. Make sure there is a composting area in your garden design, and perhaps an area for a chicken coop, although that too will probably be an add-on after you've had some proven success.

Involving students in the garden design is a great way to initiate excitement about the project. The plan can be drawn up by hand on graph paper. On my visit to Princeton I met a high school sophomore who had designed his school garden using an architectural design program on the computer.

GABBY'S GARDEN

Over her school's winter break, eleven-year-old Gabby Scharlach wrote a proposal for an Edible Garden Classroom for her San Rafael, California, middle school.

In the proposal she says, "this type of project helps in combating childhood obesity through good health education and fights global warming/cooling the planet in many ways such as growing of local produce, reducing waste, creating habitat, storing of carbon, and in creating a beautiful, social and educational place for students and the community."

Gabby's school principal, Greg Johnson, was so supportive of her proposal that he quickly arranged to present her idea to the school site council, the school district board, the parent–teacher association, and several community nonprofit organizations. Greg says, "It's critical that kids understand where their food comes from, how it's grown, how it helps their growth and attitude. I also think the idea of growing, preparing, and enjoying food builds community." Gabby's dad, Gary, adds, "The fact that Gabby approached the school

(continued)

board just asking for the land, and promising to find the funding outside of the school system, made it hard for them to say no. And at her age, she doesn't understand no." In short order, Gabby raised close to $30,000, all through private funding sources impressed with her proposal.

By midsummer, the site was graded and drainage, deer fencing, raised beds, a shed, and water cistern were installed by parents and other volunteers. In the fall Gabby entered seventh grade and with her group of volunteers erected a greenhouse, installed a drip irrigation system, a brick and board walkway, an outdoor kitchen classroom, and a vertical garden of " 'woolly pockets'."

The $30,000 was enough to fund the garden as well as a garden coordinator. Gary says, "She'll have to fund-raise a bit every year, but the funds will be generated by the garden." The community envisions a summer camp using the garden, cooking demonstrations in the outdoor kitchen, cooking classes, and parties.

By November, the garden was ready to plant. Gabby wrote about the first planting day in her blog: "It was really fun and exiting. The seventh-grade classes were chosen to be the first students to plant in the garden . . . We stood in a semi-circle in the central gathering spot and Katie, our garden coordinator, explained what we had to do. My class began the seed plantings in the woolly pockets, which is our vertical garden. Other classes did the plantings in the raised beds . . . We had many different types of seeds such as little gem lettuce, carrots, and other herbs. We only had about half our science period to do it, but it was really fun to plant. Our garden is looking more like an Edible Garden every day!"

Gabby's next effort is forming a Project Lunch team at her middle school to get more of the student community engaged in the healthy food movement. When asked what kind of food she'd like to see in the lunch program, Gabby's response was, "Don't change the menu, change the food." Her goal as a Project Lunch leader is to tie the garden's harvest to the middle school's lunch program.

Budgeting

A school garden can cost as little as a few hundred dollars to as much as half a million (see "A Greenhouse Effect" on page 287). Include a rough start-up budget in your proposal and another for anticipated annual expenses. Your big-ticket start-up costs might include paving removal, grading, fencing, materials for raised beds, soil (if building raised beds), drainage and irrigation systems, gravel or paving stones, shed and/or greenhouse construction, and garden tools. Any of these items on your list are well worth a bit of research. Westport Green Village Initiative learned that they could save about two-thirds the cost of what they spent on the fencing for their first garden by using different suppliers and materials. This kind of budget research can get time consuming, so ask members of your committee to each research or get bids on one particular item. Alternatively, you can hire a garden or fencing company to bid on the entire job. Once you've created a budget based on real costs, you can probably cut it in half by asking for in-kind donations from local businesses. That farm nostalgia I mentioned earlier will work in your favor when you approach potential garden sponsors—everyone wants to help out with the garden! Lumber, bricks, gravel, topsoil, tools, seeds, and even fencing may be donated by local garden and hardware stores, lumberyards, paving companies, and utilities in exchange for a nice mention in the local paper, a credit in your PR materials, and maybe a logo on a garden sign. Be sure to include any in-kind donations you receive in your proposal so that you can show support from the entire community.

Annual expenses include a garden coordinator (this could be someone already in the school system), repairs and tool replacement, seeds and seedlings, soil amendments (if necessary), library and curriculum materials, and outdoor classroom expendables (paper cups, art materials, sign-making materials, etc.).

Your budget should also reflect plans for growth. If you anticipate that funding will be a big challenge, and you want to get going quickly, plan a very small sample garden for the first year and use it to promote your full-scale plans.

The Fun in Fund-Raising

It's not in the budget. That's usually the first thing you hear when you bring up the idea of a school garden. Ultimately, your goal should be to have garden maintenance included in the school district budget, because that would ensure continuity and integration with other curriculum-related activities. Capital expenses are different, so it's usually up to the garden committee to raise funding for the start-up. If you're very lucky, you might find a philanthropist in your community who happens to be a passionate gardener, foodie, or children's health advocate. For a local family foundation, a school garden is a perfect-sized project that can really maximize the impact of their giving. Selling garden-themed T-shirts, seed packs, herbal soaps, and plants and hosting local food dinners are also a great way to raise funds along with raising visibility for your garden. Ask your PTO or PTA if some of their funds could be allocated to the school garden; they may want to help with a fund-raiser specifically for the project.

Garden Grants

There are garden grants that cater to special needs populations, gifted and talented education, urban agriculture, rural development, and other special populations. The grant applications will generally ask how many children will participate in the school garden program, how many hours a week of instruction they will receive in the garden, the duration of the gardening program, which subjects will be taught through gardening, and which state and national educational standards will be linked to the garden program. Some of the garden grants are from organizations that are funded by pesticide or junk food manufacturers, so your group should determine a position on potential conflicts of interest.

GARDEN GRANTS

There are probably more than this out there, but here's a list I compiled from searching around online:

Children's Garden Network http://www.childrensgardennetwork.org—
  Great teaching, grants list, and seasonal resource
USDA People's Garden School Pilot Program http://www.fns.usda.gov/fns/
  outreach/grants/garden.htm
National Gardening Association www.kidsgardening.org—A really comprehensive list of school garden grant opportunities
The Foundation Center www.foundationcenter.org—A resource for finding
  grants
AeroGrow Growing Kids Award
Hansen's Natural and Native School Garden Grant
Healthy Sprouts
Heinz Wholesome Memories Intergenerational Garden Award
Hooked on Hydroponics
Mantis Award
Mantis Adopt a School Garden
Midwest Adopt a School Garden Award
Syngenta IPM in School Gardens Grant
Welch's Harvest Youth Garden Grant—$250 to $1,000
Lowe's Charitable & Education Foundation—ongoing, no deadline $5,000 to
  $25,000
Box Tops 4 Education—Cash for box tops
American Honda Foundation—Youth Education and Science Grants
America the Beautiful Fund—Operation Green Planet—free seeds
The Fruit Tree Planting Foundation—Schoolyard Orchards
Schoolyard Habitat Program—up to $8,000
Annie's Grants for Gardens—Grants for garden tools and seeds
Captain Planet Foundation—Grants for hands-on environmental education
Fiskar's Project Orange Thumb—$5,000

(continued)

Herb Society of America—Grant for Educators—total of $5,000

ING Unsung Heros—$2,000 to $25,000

Muhammad Ali Center Peace Garden Grants

Welch's Harvest Grants—$500 to $1,000

Toyota Tapestry Grants for Science Teachers—$10,000

A TALE OF TWO TOWNS

We held a school garden workshop in my county that drew parents, teachers, and students from all over the county and beyond. The biology teacher from Wilton High School, in a small suburban town, described the lengthy process he was subjected to in trying to get a school garden approved. Meetings with the school board were delayed by prerequisite meetings with the town's planning and zoning board and conservation commission, and so on. Proposals, plans, and budgets were submitted and amended; the entire process took more than a year to reach a final approval. An incredulous teacher from urban New Haven shared a very different version of the process in her city. "We spent a couple hundred dollars, we put our shovels in the ground and started digging. It's really not that complicated!" she exclaimed.

Who Will Manage the Garden?

Plants need regular care so your garden proposal should include a plan for garden maintenance. You may have a willing parent, teacher, groundskeeper, school cook, or administrator who is willing to provide the necessary maintenance or coordination of volunteers. The garden coordinator will need to perform or organize a regular watering and weeding schedule as well as organize other activities as necessary: staking or caging tomatoes, training vines, fertilizing, pruning, bug picking, turning compost, mulching, harvesting, succession planting, and fall cover cropping.

If your regional agricultural extension service offers a master gardener certification program, they may require their trainees to fulfill a certain number of community service hours. A master gardener can help set up a maintenance program and schedule, he or she can troubleshoot problems, train your volunteers, and lead classes for students. Ideally, your district will fund a part-time garden coordinator who can act as a liason between the community, school staff, students, and school administration, as well as coordinate class schedules in the garden and after-school garden clubs or other garden-based activities.

Who Will Teach in the Garden?

Ideally your garden will be so popular that teachers will be vying for time. Along with the maintenance schedule, your garden coordinator can work with the teachers to create a class schedule and activities that mesh with the garden cycle and chores. However, not all teachers are enthusiastic at first. They may have little or no garden experience, they may be intimidated by the garden, they may not want to get their hands and clothes dirty (a complaint often heard from middle school kids as well), and they may be too busy to see how the garden could fit into their schedule. Some schools begin with a voluntary after-school garden program for interested students and let it grow from there. Your school garden plan should include teacher training workshops, either as part of ongoing staff development or as a voluntary supplemental program after school a couple of times per year.

Teachers need to learn that the human food cycle is the life cycle and that nearly every aspect of the K–12 curriculum can be taught in the garden. When my daughter heard about the Princeton lesson using a magnet to find iron in ground-up kale, she told me that her class had done that lesson by grinding up breakfast cereal that must have been fortified with iron. Ironic!

We created a school garden workshop for teachers and school staff that specifically addressed curriculum integration. We discussed ways that lessons in the garden could be matched to state standards. It's essential to consider the curriculum needs of the teachers when planning the garden, and then to collect and distribute successful lesson plans among teachers in your district and in your state.

An important aspect of the overall school food environment is the food IQ and behavior of the teachers. As role models for students, when teachers are excited about learning in the garden, tasting new foods, and making the connection with their own health and lifestyle, they will pass that excitement on to their students. When a teacher trades in her Diet Pepsi for an herbal tea grown in the school garden, the kids take notice, and when that personal choice becomes a lesson on the healing and digestive properties of herbs, everyone benefits.

GARDEN THEMES

- Herbs
- Historical
- Science lab
- Shade garden
- Flower gardens
- Food production
- Square Foot Garden
- Native plants and grasses
- Butterfly and pollinator garden
- Companion planting and beneficial insects

Curriculum Links

Every state in the U.S. has academic content standards that define what students need to learn by completion of their K–12 education. These standards ensure consistency of content, and they may determine what and when specific concepts will be taught in every grade. The standards do not dictate how that content will be taught—whether by lecture, by rote, by reading, research, experimentation, or other means. Local school districts and the teachers themselves select the instructional materials and techniques they feel will best achieve the grade-level standards most effectively. Teachers are encouraged to tailor their strategies to their students' learning styles and to the culture of the school and its values. You can encourage your teachers to use the garden by sharing lesson plans for garden education with them. In the resources section for this chapter you will find links to New Jersey and California school garden curricula that are tied to their state standards.

Curriculum standards are fairly similar state to state. You can find yours by a simple online search for "(your state) education standards." The standards are often expressed as a series of goals for the various subjects. It's a fun exercise for a workshop or garden committee to come up with lessons that tie into specific standards for grade levels and subjects.

SAMPLE GOALS AND LESSONS

As a result of education in grades K–12, students will:

- describe how people organize systems for the production, distribution, and consumption of goods and services. Students can grow a crop of lettuce, potatoes, or herbs and sell them to their peers, at a fund-raiser or at a local farmers' market.
- recognize the continuing importance of historical thinking and knowledge in their own lives and in the world in which they live. Students can learn the importance of knowing how to grow their own food for food security in times of war or other crisis.
- use geographic tools and technology to explain the interactions of humans and the larger environment, and the evolving consequences of those interactions. Students can learn about climate zones in different regions and how certain foods grow better in certain climate zones and regions.
- seek arts experiences and participate in the artistic life of the school and community. Students can paint colorful signs for the different areas of the garden, create markers with names of plants in English, Spanish, Chinese, and other languages, study ads from junk food marketing, and make their own ads for garden food.

(continued)

- understand the connections among the arts, other disciplines, and daily life. Students can create a mosaic on a garden wall, build a garden gate, or design a garden for a special purpose.
- recognize and practice health-enhancing lifestyles. Students can taste new foods they've grown in the garden and learn about the vitamins and minerals in different colored vegetables and fruits. Chart the glycemic index of junk foods vs. foods from the garden.
- establish and maintain healthy eating patterns and a physically active life. Students can learn to prepare a salad, a soup, or other healthy dish from the food they've grown.
- demonstrate an understanding of the traditions, products, and perspectives of the cultures studied. Students can grow vegetables from a specific part of the world, or grow a Native American "Three Sisters" garden of corn, squash, and beans and write about how traditional foods connect people with their culture.
- understand how organisms are structured to ensure efficiency and survival. Students can study the plants and insects in the garden to learn how they interact with one another. Research the vitamins, minerals, and micronutrients in organic food vs. junk food and study the digestive system.

The Garden Secret

Even if you do everything just right in your garden (and nobody does!), some things won't grow, some will wilt and die, others will be plagued with insects. I've learned far more from my garden failures than my garden successes, though I don't brag as much about the failures. One year an infestation of bindweed was choking my beans, so I went after them with a vengeance, hoeing and yanking the weeds at their roots, only to discover that three more vines would sprout back up for every one I pulled out. Exasperated, I asked a farmer friend what to do for bindweed and her counsel was, "Do nothing. The more you pull, the more you cause it to spread." Over the winter, I covered the bed with thick mulch, and the bindweed hasn't been much of a problem since.

There are lessons to be learned about people as well as weeds in the garden. Who shows up when they're scheduled, who doesn't, and who is responsible when things go wrong (and they will!). You'll have to consider summer care as well; those summer weeks that school is out are often a crucial time for long season crops like tomatoes and eggplants. One way to manage the summer schedule is to find a volunteer family for each week of the summer. That family is responsible for watering, weeding, and harvesting for their assigned week—this can usually be taken care of in two visits to the garden.

A rainy season, hungry critters, and scorching temperatures will all conspire to offer young gardeners real-world challenges. They will have to learn to flow like water to deal with the challenges and solve problems. A garden changes from year to year. The secret of the garden classroom lies in learning to let it teach you.

TOOLS FOR THE GARDEN

Baskets
Books
Buckets
Clipper
Cultivators
Hoe
Hose
Live traps (for gophers and woodchucks)
Mallet
Measuring tape
Rakes
Scissors
Shovels

(continued)

Spade
Sprinklers, timer
Thermometer
Trellises
Trowels
Twine
Weeding forks
Wire clipper

School Garden to Cafeteria

Health and safety concerns are front and center for everyone involved in creating a sustainable school food environment. As much as we wish to protect our children from the hazards of our industrialized food system, we also must beware of the safety and sanitation of everything we bring into and grow in the garden. Food-borne microorganisms can exist in organic gardens as well as those using so-called "conventional" chemical treatments. The safety of your school garden's produce begins with the soil and also with your seed sources. Look for seeds that are untreated, non-genetically modified, and preferably organic. Children must be shown the do's and don'ts of safely handling garden tools to avoid injury, and they must learn to wash their hands thoroughly before and after tending the plants and the produce they harvest. Garden gloves are a good protection for everyone working in the garden. Sanitation protocol requires that children with cuts or open wounds refrain from harvesting until they have healed.

I've heard many stories of school districts that don't allow the produce from their school gardens to be used in the cafeteria because of fear of contamination. After some investigating, I discovered that there are no actual regulations that prevent the produce from going to the cafeteria, and many districts are now allowing and even encouraging garden-to-cafeteria programs, provided basic health and sanitation rules are followed. In fact, a USDA school garden memo from 2009 states that school food service funds may be used to purchase seeds, tools, and other materials for a school garden. The food service may purchase produce from a school group that is managing the garden, and the food service may even sell produce grown in the garden provided all profit goes back into the school food service program.

The rules for school garden produce in the cafeteria are the same for Farm to School and any other fresh produce. Tools and baskets used for harvesting should be "food grade" and should be washed regularly in hot soapy water and dried. Produce coming from the garden should be inspected, washed, and refrigerated according to the same standards as all other produce.

For our school garden workshop, I asked Lori Romick, a sanitarian from our local health district, to share her thoughts on school gardening safety:

Natural soils must be thoroughly tested for pesticides and other pest control chemicals (for termites)—especially those that are currently banned but may have been applied to the property many years ago.

Soils must also be tested for lead if the grounds have/had any pre-1978 buildings and also for hydrocarbons.

There should be a layout with locations of wells, septic systems, and in-ground oil tanks on the property.

Raised beds with pretested and approved soils would be best. They should be protected from animals and animal feces.

Many parts of fruits and vegetables may be poisonous, such as the leaves of rhubarb and the tomato plant itself.

Many insects will be attracted and consideration must be given to students that have allergies to stings.

Levels of added nitrogen should be monitored so that elevated levels do not accumulate in leafy greens such as spinach.

Good drainage in the garden areas will be important to prevent ponding and mosquito breeding.

Only potable water should be used when watering.

If food material for composting will be piled on-site, then only plant
materials should be included to prevent the intrusion of rats and other
problematic wildlife, creating a nuisance or safety concern.

The Poop on Compost

Americans throw away about half their food. A 2002 USDA study estimated
a direct economic loss of $600 million a year in food waste in the National
School Lunch Program. A sustainable school food environment must
endeavor to reduce waste by providing food that kids actually eat, but also
by recycling fruit and vegetable parings and uneaten organic matter. Our
culture is quite phobic about discussing the dirty business of waste management, whether in the form of hydrocarbon emissions, garbage, food waste,
or poop, and that phobia is at least in part to blame for the environmental
and health crisis we are in the midst of. Perhaps the most valuable lessons
our children can learn from school gardens and Farm to School cafeteria
programs are those on this end of the food/life cycle.

There are many different types of compost. If you are using composted
manure, it should be fully rotted in aerobic conditions reaching temperatures of at least 130 degrees Fahrenheit for a year for cow manure and two
years for chicken manure. If compost is purchased for your school garden,
you should ensure that it comes from a reliable and traceable organic source.
I was horrified to learn that the "organic" compost I was purchasing at my
local hardware store was actually composted human sewage from a big city
sewage treatment facility. The thought of dressing my veggies with all the
excreted pharmaceuticals of modern humanity, no matter how organic, was
a dealbreaker.

Of late, compost is becoming a more acceptable subject of polite conversation. San Francisco and Halifax, Nova Scotia, are both leaders in municipal
composting. Worm composting, compost tea, and lasagna gardening (layers
of mulch and compost) are trendy topics among young farmers and gardeners, and if you're lucky enough to have someone with this knowledge

in your area, I would encourage you to bring them to school for a compost workshop. You might make some compost converts. With an understanding of the subject, school administrators might agree that school cafeterias and school gardens make wonderful living laboratories to learn about the different methods of composting and the conditions needed to produce a clean, safe product that will nourish the crops of future seasons.

A GREENHOUSE EFFECT

When Nancy Easton, founder of New York City's Wellness in the Schools, asked me if I wanted to pop up to her kids' elementary school to visit the rooftop greenhouse that had just been installed, I eagerly agreed. My expectation was that I would see a plastic-covered frame lined with potting benches and grow-lights tethered to a tar paper roof. Instead, Nancy ushered me into a living science laboratory the likes of which I had never encountered.

The 1,420-square-foot steel and glass greenhouse is controlled by a computer that senses variations in temperature and humidity, opening or closing roof and side vents to let in a breeze or keep out the rain. If it gets too hot, the low-energy consumption air-conditioning system sends water through a wall of corrugated cardboard to cool the plants and the students tending them.

Nancy invited me to return for the grand opening of the greenhouse. City officials and media swarmed around the pairs of K–5 students posted at the various stations in the greenhouse who were eager to share their knowledge of the greenhouse systems. A kindergarten girl in a frilly dress grabbed chunks of growing medium and explained to me that it was light and spongy because it was made from exploded rocks. Another group of children were picking aphids off of the tomato plants. They told me that the plants had arrived infested, but their vigilance was keeping the bugs under control. I was shown a stack of plastic trays in which worms were digesting cafeteria waste, and two large cisterns painted with colorful murals for collecting rainwater. A series of pipes running across the ceiling and down the sides of the greenhouse

(continued)

funneled the water to the various growing areas, and through an aerator into a round tank the size of a large hot tub. Two boys jubilantly described how the plants growing in a floating disk on the tub's surface were getting nutrients from the fish poop generously provided by the tilapia swimming in the tank below. A fifth-grader charged with demonstrating a solar-powered toy car provided this caveat: "You have to think about how much energy it takes to make these solar panels. This panel doesn't generate much energy at all, so I wonder if it took more energy to make the panel than it can make from the sun."

After the speeches, the students harvested their first crop of delicate greens, and shared them with the guests. The rooftop greenhouse is expected to grow 8,000 pounds of fruit and vegetables a year for the school cafeteria.

Nancy says the project cost about $750,000, but could be replicated for about $500,000 now that they have a template. She and two other moms raised the money through grants and fund-raisers. The construction was done in partnership with the city's school building authority and New York Sun Works, a nonprofit devoted to urban sustainability through science education. The city hopes to create another hundred rooftop school gardens in the near future, several of which are already underway.

Brag About It

Maintaining the school garden requires TLC from students, staff, and volunteers and in order to sustain interest from the community you need to keep them updated on garden news. Use school bulletin boards, the school newspaper, and PTO e-mail communications to publicize seasonal garden events, and share recipes, stories, and tips about what students are learning in the garden. Designate a student or volunteer to take photos and publish them on the district's website, a Facebook page, or in the local paper.

Making the Grade

Need to convince your administrators of the educational value of a school garden? There are several good studies that show the effectiveness of garden-based education. A 2005 study done by Texas A&M University has shown that third-, fourth-, and fifth-grade students that participated in school gardening activities scored significantly higher on science achievement tests compared to students who did not experience any garden-based learning activities.

A 2004 study focused on a youth gardening program in Detroit. The study found that after gardening, kids have an increased interest in eating fruits and vegetables, possess an appreciation for working with neighborhood adults, and have an increased interest for improvement of neighborhood appearance. In addition, they made new friends and showed increased knowledge about nutrition, plant ecology, and gardening.

The Effects of School Garden Experiences on Middle School–Aged Students' Knowledge, Attitudes, and Behaviors Associated With Vegetable Consumption, a 2009 study by the Society for Public Health Education, indicated that students who had experienced school gardening demonstrated improved recognition of, attitudes toward, preferences for, and willingness to taste vegetables as well as an increased variety of vegetables eaten.

Along with the studies, offer skeptics some fresh garden produce, or something you've just made from the bounty of your own garden. I once brought zucchini bread to a prison superintendent when I went to ask permission to film there. She had never let a film crew in before—we were the first to gain access.

Homeroom Grown

When I toured with *Two Angry Moms* in 2008, I had the pleasure of meeting parents and educators all around the United States who were as passionate about food education as the moms I had met closer to home. In Salt Lake City, I met Patricia Messer and her business partner, Heidi, who were working toward expanding their farmers' market, heirloom seed and spice business into a food-in-the-classroom educational program. They'd been holding classes at the market, and gave me a little booklet they had published on how to save tomato seeds. It's a fascinating process that involves fermenting the tomato innards for a couple of days to produce a fungus that protects the seeds from rotting and even prevents diseases in the future tomato plants. What a great science lesson that would be. From the booklet, I was able to track Patricia down three years later to find out how her program was progressing.

Patricia reports that it's taken three years to get involved with the school district and now they're just weeks away from launching the program. They'll be starting off with "growing carts" in nine of the local elementary school classrooms. Patricia and Heidi use these carts in their business, so they will be advising and training the teachers on how to use them. The carts have five tiers, each with a grow-light on its ceiling, and five removable racks on which the students will grow micro-greens for their cafeteria's salad bar. "The kids get to sow the seeds and the micro-greens can be used in the salad bar in two to three weeks. They'll bring the greens to the lunchroom, where they will be carefully washed and put out on the salad bar for the whole school." Why micro-greens? "Not only because they grow fast indoors in the winter, but because at the micro stage the plants have twenty to fifty times the nutrition compared to the mature vegetable," explains Patricia. Though young broccoli shoots don't have the same crunch as the adult plant, the assortment of pea tendrils, lettuces, mild mesclun mix, red amaranth, Swiss chard, oak leaf lettuce, red romaine, green and purple mizuna, and radishes will add an enticing zing to the typically bland salad bar fixings.

A grant from Slow Food for $2,000 seeded the project and an article in the local newspaper attracted interest and a sponsorship from an insurance company affiliated with the Farm Bureau. The stainless steel carts cost $90 each, plus the lights, seeds and soil. Patricia believes the investment will more than pay for itself in short order, and the ongoing costs will be minimal. When the program is rolled out, they will introduce it with a school-wide assembly for students and parents.

She's pragmatic about the launch. "Some of the teachers are excited and some could care less because they're already totally overwhelmed with over-crowded classrooms in the district's public school system." The carts are on wheels so they can be moved out of the way to accommodate other activities when space is at a premium.

"We're conservative out here, so we're going slowly, but I believe Providence was involved in making this happen. We've built friendships over the years, because you can't just go in there angry, making demands. The school principal now grows food in a garden, and last year I took our vegetables to the district's nutritionist and wouldn't you know, she happened to be the one who got an earwig in it!"

In spite of the earwig, Patricia says the nutritionist is changing things a little at a time. They're baking their own whole-wheat bread and incorpo-rating more locally grown food into the menus on a regular basis. "She's changing because we invited her, so she's on board."

For now, it's a pilot program in one school, but Patricia and Heidi's vision includes bringing the garden carts to other schools in the district, teaching students and staff how to compost with worms, and turning an unused play-ground into a school garden. Gardening teaches patience. Patricia says she has plenty of that.

"We try new things every year in our half-acre market garden. This year we grew sweet potatoes and I learned you can eat the sweet potato greens—they're a poor man's vegetable. We made chili powder with a yellow pepper we grew, and that turned out to be a premium item at the farmers' market because no one had ever done that before."

She hopes to share her excitement about these discoveries with the stu-dents. "It's a love thing. I'm a great-grandma. My kids and grandkids went to that school."

Food Literacy

A school garden is not the only resource for teaching food literacy. I have visited many school-based programs, and after-school programs that are teaching students about food from a cultural, scientific, economic, historical, and artistic perspective without a garden. Chefs Move to Schools, the program coordinated by Michelle Obama's Let's Move! initiative, brings chefs into the classroom for a weekly lesson about food that may include tasting new foods, a chemistry lesson about baking, or, in the case of one chef I met recently, a classroom calf adoption that will culminate in a field trip to the farm in the spring when the calf is old enough to milk. Food field trips to community gardens, organic farms, green markets, grocery stores, or a local restaurant offer many opportunities for students to interact with the food environment.

Teachers tell me that they like to have simple, one-page lesson plans that integrate food studies into the curriculum they are teaching. There are a number of food curriculum resources available—some are based around garden projects, others take into account that not every school has the resources for a garden (yet!). School chef Lisa Suriano has created her Veggiecation Curriculum as a tool to integrate new recipes at lunchtime with regular classroom activities. Lisa's kit includes recipes, Veggie of the Month posters, a lunchtime ballot box for kids to vote on the new recipes, "I tried it" stickers, and lesson plans about the vegetable's nutrition, growth, and origins. The lesson plans are standards-based and include games and exercises teaching literacy, math, science, and social studies from a veggie perspective. Full color veggie counting cards can be printed and laminated, and there's even a take-home recipe booklet for families.

Jane Marie Siemon teaches Nutrition and Foods at the Youth Initiative High School in Viroqua, Wisconsin. Her curriculum, "The Whole Plate," has four fifteen-lesson units for all grade levels. Each unit is composed of lectures, readings, field trips, study questions, recipes, and homework assignments—including preparation of a family meal. The curriculum approaches food from a holistic perspective: It provides lectures on adolescent nutrition, agricultural practices, and herbs and spices; readings from Michael Pollan's *The Omnivore's Dilemma* and Rachel Carson's *Silent Spring*. There's a Weston A. Price DVD, a PowerPoint on reading labels, and hands-on experiences that include canning tomatoes, making homemade pasta and chocolate cake, and a field trip harvesting wild foods.

The Center for Ecoliteracy is a wonderful resource for teaching the principles of sustainability in our food systems. They offer strategies, tools, essays, and downloadable activities such as the "Needs and Wants" activity to teach students to distinguish between things that they need to live a healthy life and things they want. Their book *Big Ideas: Linking Food, Culture, Health and the Environment* offers a conceptual framework for integrated learning based on food and food production.

Offer your teachers a gift of one of these curriculums or books as a class present—it may give them a whole new perspective, and you may win another advocate for your team.

EIGHT

OUTSOURCED

First they ignore you, then they laugh at you, then they fight you, then you win.

—Gandhi

ood Service Management Companies (FSMCs) operate food services for hospitals, prisons, stadiums, colleges, universities, corporate cafeterias, and increasingly K–12 schools. The largest of these management companies are multinational conglomerates with familiar names and are publicly traded on the stock exchange—Aramark, Sodexo, and Chartwells (a division of the Compass Group). In 1969, the USDA's Food and Nutrition Services first permitted school food authorities participating in the National School Lunch Program to contract with outside management companies. Since that time, the prevalence of FSMCs in school food service has slowly risen and some USDA literature even recommends that school districts go this route. Most school food advocates strongly disagree, although some are finding these companies to be increasingly cooperative and interested in reform. Eighty-five percent of school districts in the United States remain self-operated districts, meaning the district runs its own food service program, with school administration hiring a manager and staff and purchasing food with the district's food service budget. A minority 15 percent of school districts have opted to outsource their food service to a food service management company.

Why choose an outside food service vendor? FSMCs market their expertise in the business and their ability to manage costs, and they often entice potential customers with a guarantee that they won't lose money for the school district. The expertise these companies offer is a business model for procuring, managing, and serving food that meets the minimal federal guidelines cost efficiently but with little assurance to the actual wholeness and freshness of the ingredients or the health impact of that food. This lack of regard for food quality is borne out by lengthy contracts that make no mention of the sourcing or quality of the actual food being served. More than anything else, the management companies offer convenience. Once a school administrator has signed the contract, the day-to-day operations of school meals are in the hands of the management company. School administration is obligated to oversee the contract and maintain and report all required information to state agencies, but that information (meal counts, etc.) will be supplied by the FSMC.

There seems to be a correlation between wealthy districts and outsourcing. This works in two ways—the wealthy districts have the means to pay a management fee over and above the cost of the meals program, and the management companies can reap greater profits selling competitive foods in the wealthy districts. The poorer districts can't afford those management fees and most prefer to seek discounts by directly dealing with suppliers.

In regard to cafeteria staff, the district may employ food service staff on their own payroll, but managed under the direction of the FSMC, or the management companies may hire their own staff, which may or may not be unionized. Using a management company is sometimes seen as a way for hard up school districts to avoid paying benefits to these employees.

If you are part of a wellness group advocating for meaningful reform in a district that's outsourced, you will not only be working locally to win community support, you will also have to deal with the corporate practices of your FSMC. These companies often claim to be locked into making purchases from large national vendors, although due to pressure from parent groups, some are now making attempts to source more foods locally.

Types of Contracts

There are two types of contracts allowed between a school district and a management company. One is known as a fixed price contract. Originally, the only allowable form of payment to a food service management company was a fixed price per meal served. The food service management company was required to purchase food for the school food authority and send invoices directly to the school district for payment. The cost of these food purchases was limited to the fixed price agreed upon between the food service management company and the school food authority. The danger of a fixed price contract is that when costs go up, the FSMC will use lower quality ingredients in order to fulfill the contract.

Over time, the limit on costs and the direct invoicing were abandoned. A small minority of outsourced school districts still adheres to some type of fixed price contract, but most are choosing a more flexible contract known as a cost reimbursable contract. Cost reimbursable contracts mean that the FSMC will incur costs on behalf of the school district. These expenses will be billed back to the school district with an additional monthly fee or fee per meal served, so there's a fixed cost component over and above the cost reimbursement. These cost reimbursable contracts protect the management company from losing money and don't fix costs for the school district. The other danger here is that the district must trust the FSMC to make purchases and sell foods that are in the best interest of the children of the district. And there's the rub.

National Volume Discounts

In the movie *Two Angry Moms*, Kate Adamick, a school food consultant and an attorney, charges that "food service management companies do not make their profits off their monthly fees that they're charging the district. Their real profit comes from National Volume Discounts, or NVDs, and those are rebates from the manufacturers of the junk food that you see sold in the schools today. Based on how many cases of potato chips, for example, that they sell to all of their accounts across the country, then the food service management companies will get a nice big check back at the end of the year from the manufacturer of those potato chips. That's why they're so resistant to adapting to these new changes that are being demanded by the wellness committees across the country. . . . They don't want them to work because they stand to lose a lot of money."

There are no volume rebates on broccoli, carrots, peas, or peaches because farmers don't have vast warehouses of shelf-stable inventory to sell. So the management companies have an incentive to sell more processed food than fresh food, which may explain why many districts with management companies aren't signing on to state and federal incentive programs promoting healthier school food standards.

The NVDs enabled management companies to offer attractively low management fees to the school districts, while keeping rebates that amounted to as much as 150 percent of the management fees they were charging. A USDA audit uncovered this practice and a 2007 ruling attempted to close the loophole by declaring that ". . . contractor costs paid from the nonprofit school food service account be net of all discounts, rebates, and applicable credits."

USDA regulations don't govern food service companies so their ruling applies only to the nonprofit school districts, although the regulations do state that contractors must "provide sufficient information to permit the school food authority to identify allowable and unallowable costs and the amount of all such discounts, rebates, and credits on invoices and bills presented for payment to the school food authority."

Regulations place the burden of these cost-reporting requirements squarely on the school food authority. All large government contracts are required to go out to bid in a manner that provides "full and open competition" and "a level playing field." The convoluted scheme of rebates prevented competing management companies from making more honest bids that included reimbursing the districts for anticipated rebates and therefore charging a higher management fee.

A second government audit found that "the failure of a school food authority to describe its cost reporting requirements fully in its solicitation document undermines full and open competition by placing unreasonable burdens on potential contractors. Without adequate details on how it must report costs to the school food authority, a potential contractor lacks the information needed to properly establish the fixed price component (management fee) of its offer. In addition, school food authorities cannot determine whether nonprofit school food service account funds may be used to pay all or only part of the costs billed by the contractor."

The government auditors concluded that allowing the FSMC to keep the discounts and rebates results in the net affect that "... excess charges are made against the food service account, thereby diminishing food service resources." Prior to these updated regulations, state agencies were required to review all contracts between the local school food authorities after the fact with little recourse if irregularities were identified. The new regulations require a state review prior to signing the contract. These regulations went into effect in 2009, but because districts are only required to bid out their food service contracts every five years, your district may still be operating under an old contract without these updated provisions.

RE: REBATES

In July 2010, Sodexo agreed to pay $20 million in settlement of claims by the New York attorney general that the company had fraudulently retained rebates from food manufacturers that were owed to school districts in New York State. In a public statement, New York Attorney General Andrew M. Cuomo said, "This company cut sweetheart deals with suppliers and then denied taxpayer-supported schools the benefits." The lawsuits were a result of a five-year whistle-blower investigation prompted by a pair of brothers who were general managers for the company and were "outraged when they discovered Sodexo's practice of pressuring food and beverage vendors to kick back huge rebates and then secretly pocketing the savings rather than passing them on to government clients as required by their contracts," according to their attorney's statement.

In August 2010, attorneys for District of Columbia Public Schools refused to release a full accounting of the rebates the district received through purchases by Chartwells, the district's food service provider. The decision was based on the claim that details of the rebates constitute trade secrets that might hurt the competitive position of Chartwells. School food investigative reporter Ed Bruske, who made the request, calculated that the district had received more than $1 million in rebates over two years, based on monthly invoices he was able to obtain. He reported that "D.C. schools have come under steady fire in recent months for the dubious quality of industrially processed convenience foods Chartwells routinely serves to schoolchildren here."

According to a researcher, a group of forty-five self-operated districts in eastern Connecticut ordering through a buying co-op pay, on average, 25 percent less for food and supplies than districts operated by the Big Three food service management companies.

Request for Proposals

If your school district is looking to contract with a management company on a fixed-price basis, they will put out an Invitation for Bid, which is a simple announcement seeking a low bidder on a per-meal basis. The fixed-price contracts are exempt from reporting discounts, rebates, and reimbursements, as stated in the following regulations:

Fixed price contracts are not subject to the provisions of the rule requiring that allowable contractor costs paid from the nonprofit school food service account be net of all discounts, rebates and applicable credits because contractors have already taken into consideration factors such as discounts; rebates and other credits when formulating their prices for fixed priced contracts.

For a cost reimbursable contract, the district must post a Request for Proposal. The standard RFP makes no specifications for the types of meals to be provided, other than a mention of Compliance with Program Regulations requiring the meals to comply with federal regulations. Usually the template will contain a clause stating that the FSMC will provide a twenty-one-day meal cycle menu that will represent the first twenty-one days of food service.

For districts working with an outside vendor, the RFP is where the rubber meets the road. Everything in your wellness policy that has to do with food should be specified in the RFP, and again in the final contract. The RFP should be publicized to ensure fair competition, and should allow ample time for competitors to visit the district and compile a bid.

READING REQUEST

On my school food trip to England, I was escorted to the city of Reading, to visit the lunch program. Our group arrived a bit late for lunch—the students had already been through the lunch line but there was enough left over for us. Though the menu was limited to just one or two choices, I was treated to a tasty meal of curried vegetables over rice, a green salad, cut-up fresh fruit (ripe and delicious), and a pudding for dessert. I was surprised to learn that the district's food service management company was the same company that provides meals for my district in Connecticut—Chartwells.

How'd they do that? I asked Colin McIntosh, the Reading Borough Council's school district business manager. It turns out that Colin takes his job very seriously. Growing up poor in England meant Colin didn't have enough to eat and suffers chronic health problems from childhood malnourishment. Though he's in charge of much more than the lunch program, feeding kids well is his passion. He wrote the specifications for his RFP, which was bid on by many of the same food service management companies operating in schools around America, Europe, and elsewhere. Colin has given me permission to share excerpts of his specifications as a guide for your district's RFP and contracts. Note that several of the specifications reflect the culture of his school district, which is quite ethnically diverse.

1.1. The Council is committed to providing a high-quality, nutritious catering service to schools that meets the local needs of schools and pupils. This Specification sets out the nature of the Services to be provided. Where quality standards are set out, they are the minimum acceptable level to be achieved on a consistent basis.

2.1. The Council considers that the need for nutritious school meals to improve the health and well-being of school-aged children is essential. The school lunch is the main meal of the day for many children and provides an opportunity both to provide good food for young people and to encourage the development of good eating habits and other social skills. It should allow pupils to become acquainted with a wider range of foods and to practice food choices. The Service should be an integral part of the school day and all children should be able to take a nourishing meal in a pleasant, orderly environment.

2.2. All meals should be adequate in quantity and quality so as to be suitable as the main meal of the day and reflect the new National Nutritional Standards (NNS), which are to be introduced by 2008 in primary schools and 2009 in secondary. Menus should be developed that are appetizing and appealing to young people.

2.3. The Contractor's arrangements for the Service shall incorporate due diligence in all aspects of purchasing policy, food delivery and storage, preparation and handling of food, health and safety, cleaning, care and operation of equipment, and transport of hot meals.

GENERAL

7.3. The Contractor shall provide the Authorized Officer with standard recipes including recipe preparation, cooking method, and nutritional analysis of all menu items. The Contractor shall also advise, and signify by color coding, the menus in their tender submission whether items on the menu are fresh, dry, tinned, or frozen products. Locally sourced fresh ingredients, country of origin, and food travel miles shall also be indicated.

(continued)

7.4. Menus in primary, nursery, and special schools shall be based on a three-week cycle. The core menu should be changed at least twice per year in September and April.

7.5. Once in each menu cycle a public analyst shall carry out an actual nutritional analysis. The cost of this analysis shall be met by the Council if the standards meet fully the Caroline Walker Trust recommendations. If the standards are not met, the cost of analysis shall be paid by the Contractor.

7.6. An alternative list of main course protein and pudding items shall be available for use as menu cycle replacements when it is considered more appropriate to meet the needs of an individual school. All alternative menu items shall be nutritionally analyzed in advance to provide an equivalent nutritional alternative in accordance with NNS.

7.7. Once a menu is agreed, the Contractor shall only alter it in exceptional circumstances. Valid reasons would be, for example, product quality inadequacy, published food warning, or short-term inability of a supplier to supply. Any changes in the menu which are necessary because of exceptional circumstances shall be notified to the school and Authorized Officer by 10 a.m. on the day concerned. An explanation shall also be given for the change. The Contractor shall ensure that despite product changes the menu continues to meet minimum nutritional standards.

7.8. A choice of menu shall be maintained throughout the Service. A meal suitable for vegetarians must be available throughout the service. Presentation and service shall enhance the attractiveness of dishes.

7.9. Once the menu cycle has been agreed the Contractor will produce photographs of all meals and agree upon presentation of dishes.

MENU CONTENT AND QUALITY OF INGREDIENTS

7.10. All raw materials and ingredients used in food production shall be of a high quality and in all respects safe, wholesome, suitable, and acceptable to pupils.

7.11. With the exception of beef burgers, sausages, and fish products, no manufactured items will be used on menus. Should Tenderers propose any other items these must be detailed in their tender. Any manufactured items shall comply with the Government's minimum specifications for manufactured foods. Beef burgers will only be allowed once per menu cycle.

7.12. No main course dish shall be repeated more than twice in the three-week cycle.

7.13. A traditional Christmas lunch with appropriate vegetarian alternative shall be provided at the same price as the core menu. Individual schools may also request a food service that replaces one of the menu choices on certain other religious/cultural feast days. These shall be provided at the same price as the core menu. If schools request it, a Christmas buffet may be provided in place of the traditional Christmas lunch. Christmas lunch must be available for all children entitled to free meals, which will be reimbursed by the Council/school.

7.14. Appropriate sauces (gravy, mint sauce, etc.) shall be served with the main courses. This is particularly important when the meal consists of mainly "dry" items.

7.15. The serving of tomato ketchup shall not be permitted. Salt shall not be used in the cooking process and no added salt will be available in the dining room.

7.16. A minimum of one roast meat dish shall be on each week.

7.17. Main course halal meat (lamb and poultry) dishes shall be available on the menu for those schools that have requested a halal service.

7.18. Pre-peeled potatoes may be used, provided they are of a high quality and have not been dipped in a holding solution. Dried potato shall not be permitted except in the event of an emergency. It should be noted that potato rumblers will be available in all kitchens.

7.19. Pizza toppings shall be made using fresh ingredients. Brand-name sauces will be permitted. The Contractor shall be permitted to use pre-prepared pizza bases.

7.20. All vegetables, fruit, and salads shall be of Class 1 standard.

7.21. Fresh fruit pieces shall contain no less than four types of fruit daily.

(continued)

7.22. All homemade flour dishes shall contain at least 25 percent wholemeal flour.

7.23. All eggs shall be of Lion Quality "Class A."

7.24. Low-fat vegetarian cheese shall be used.

7.25. Good-quality, low-fat, brand-name margarine, suitable for all cultures, shall be used for all homemade pastry and sponge dishes.

7.26. Bread with low-fat vegetable spread shall be served daily.

7.27. Packet mixes for biscuits shall not be permitted.

7.28. No nuts or nut derivatives shall be used.

7.29. Drinking water shall be available for all children having a meal, including those children who have brought their own packed lunch.

7.30. The Contractor shall be encouraged to source produce locally wherever possible.

Your school administration may fear that no contractor will bid on an RFP with these types of specifications, but RFP's based on specific wellness policies are becoming more prevalent and management companies are now competing to stay abreast of new policy requirements. Holding the companies to the terms of the RFP and contract is yet another challenge for districts that have outsourced their meal programs. Ask your administrators who in the district is responsible for auditing the FSMC's provisions. Your group may need to conduct your own audit (see chapter two), and request copies of invoices to ensure the management company is complying with the specifications.

Freedom of Information

You are entitled to see the RFP and the contract your district has with the management company. The Freedom of Information Act (FOIA), Title 5 of the United States Code, section 552, provides that any person can file an FOIA request to obtain access to federal public records or information.

SAMPLE FOIA REQUEST
(FROM THE NATIONAL SECURITY ARCHIVE)

Agency Head
Name of Agency
Address of Agency
City, State, Zip Code
Re: Freedom of Information Act Request
Dear _____:

This is a request under the Freedom of Information Act.

I request that a copy of the following documents [or documents containing the following information] be provided to me:

[Identify the documents or information as specifically as possible.]

In order to help to determine my status to assess fees, you should know that I am **[insert a suitable description of the requester and the purpose of the request.]**

[Sample requester descriptions:]

1. a representative of the news media affiliated with the _____ newspaper (magazine, television station, etc.), and this request is made as part of a news gathering and not for commercial use.
2. affiliated with an educational or noncommercial scientific institution, and this request is made for a scholarly or scientific purpose and not for commercial use.
3. an individual seeking information for personal use and not for commercial use.
4. affiliated with a private corporation and am seeking information for use in the company's business.

[Optional] I am willing to pay fees for this request up to a maximum of $____ . If you estimate that the fees will exceed this limit, please inform me first.

[Optional] I request a waiver of all fees for this request. Disclosure of the requested information to me is in the public interest because it is likely to contribute significantly to public understanding of the operations or activities of the government and is not primarily in my commercial interest. [Include a specific explanation.]

Thank you for your consideration of my request.

Sincerely,
Name
Address
City, State, Zip Code
Telephone Number [Optional]

Review the Contract

If you haven't studied law or business, reviewing contracts is pretty much like trying to read a foreign language that uses the same alphabet as your own. It looks familiar but is impossible to comprehend. If possible, find a friend with contract experience to look it over and explain it in plain English.

I've heard many stories of improprieties regarding RFPs and contracts. For example, your food service director is required to be a member of the district wellness committee, but if the wellness committee is meeting to discuss the food service RFP, and the food service director is employed by the FSMC, the director must not be allowed to have input or even attend the meeting. Advocates from a number of districts have reported that their food service directors helped write the RFP. Likewise, a number of districts use contracts that were originated by their FSMCs, although federal regulations specify that potential contractors may negotiate contracts but are not permitted to draft contract terms and conditions.

Contract Contradictions

Alice Smith, a holistic nutrition coach and PTA representative to the Redding, Connecticut, Wellness Committee, spent some time going over her district's contract with Sodexo. She raised a number of questions and found several contradictions between what she had been told by administrators and what she actually read in the contract. For example, Alice had been under the impression based on what she'd been told by district administrators that Sodexo received no payment from the district, that they made their money from food service sales alone. Yet she discovered an article in the contract referring to a "General Support Services Allowance" of $37,336 per year.

Another article in the contract stated that there should be regular meetings with a Sodexo representative and an advisory board composed of parents, teachers, and students in which they would plan menus. Yet Alice, who is a representative to the wellness committee, had no knowledge of such meetings. In a presentation she demanded, "Who is doing this? The Wellness Advisory Board isn't! If they are, then it is not transparent to the entire wellness group nor to the school district. There has been no invitation put out there by Sodexo to meet and actually do menu planning. And menu planning means creating a menu that is unique to the site! Not what is universal around the country. Our district should [for the next RFP bidding process] request more open-minded, transparent, and creative practices— meaning a service that cooks real food on-site and allows community to view ingredients. This needs to get in the next RFP."

A big sticking point in outsourced districts is that PTOs and other nonprofit school groups complain that they are forbidden to use the cafeterias for school-related activities. This is one area that could be more clearly articulated in the contracts with the management companies, but in fact federal regulations state that the school kitchens and cafeterias belong to the school district, and the contracts must reflect that. School groups wishing to use the school kitchen facilities for after-school programs, community dinners, or to prepare food for athletic events must assert this right. You may consider asking one of the food service staff to assist at the event, or offer to have a ServSafe-certified person on-site when you are using the facility.

A common misconception about school food service contracts is that they only come up for renewal every five years. Although the contracts are required to be rebid every five years, the contract actually must be renewed annually and can be terminated by either party without cause at the end of every school year. Any substantial changes made to the contract would require that a new RFP would have to be posted whether the five-year rebid was due or not.

KIDS FIRST, RHODE ISLAND— DOROTHY BRAYLEY

I saved Dorothy's story for this chapter on management companies, although her story really exemplifies everything to do with school food advocacy. She's been at it a long time, and has been flexible enough to work through many changes.

Dorothy is a trained chef who got involved with school food when her daughter's elementary school teacher asked her to come and do some demonstrations on healthy food for the kids. Dorothy says, "That was the experience that shocked me the most. I went into the fourth-grade class with real fruit and Fruit Roll-Ups and other fake fruits. These kids were from a middle-income, educated community. They couldn't identify grapefruit. They argued with me. They thought it was a lemon because, they said, 'We've seen the picture on Starburst!' They could identify a Fruit Roll-Up from the back of the room by color and flavor. That was nineteen years ago."

After that Dorothy took a job teaching at Johnson & Wales, a prestigious culinary school in Rhode Island. At Johnson & Wales, her supervisor was a

Team Nutrition leader (USDA). To Dorothy's dismay, the supervisor "walked in with a super doughnut."

Dorothy explains that a super doughnut is a vitamin-fortified doughnut that the USDA offers for its school breakfast program. "So I quit Johnson & Wales and became a lunch lady in our town. I worked my way up to lead cook in the central kitchen in two years. Our district was a self-op. We could cook and the kids liked it. Eventually I moved up to the state level, advocating."

She got a grant and formed the nonprofit group Kids First, Rhode Island, in 1998. One of her first programs was a series of food demos in the schools. Eventually the program expanded to encompass many more initiatives. Now her mission is: "Every place where kids learn will be a place where they will learn and practice healthy eating. These places use our public money, why can't they be the place? We can't get into people's homes, so it's got to be a community effort."

Rhetorically, Dorothy asks, "Who sits in the gap between all the wonderful ideas and all the results that actually help spark the work in the community? It's not based on research because you change every day. We're always looking for where the energy is and building off of it and adapt to that."

Rhode Island is rather unique in its school meals programs, in that nearly every district in the state is run by an FSMC. She's identified a big gap between the management company practices and the need for RFPs that specify food quality, as well as enforceable contracts. She's now become the go-to authority in her state for writing RFPs and working on contracts that will get better food into the programs.

I wondered why most of Rhode Island had outsourced their food service. Dorothy explains, "For many years, the state was running the food service program and state employees were working in the cafeterias. The change-over occurred in the early 1990s. The state cut food service programs out of the budget one year in late spring for the coming September school year. The schools had no idea how to [run a food service program]. When this happened, the management companies swooped in with their contracts that they wrote themselves. The districts that tried to do it on their own struggled.

(continued)

Thirty-four of thirty-six went to FSMCs. The districts had no budgets. Aramark, Sodexo, and Chartwells ran into our state and divvied it up. So my work is now focused on working with FSMCs to deliver better service and in teaching the state oversight in their role in managing contracts. My staff and I are developing the knowledge and capacity to understand and transmit all this and provide technical assistance. We are rallying the community, training staff, bringing them peelers, pushing Farm to School, and we're working the competitive forces to bring the quality up. All three management companies are on my board of directors. They come to the meetings knowing their competitors have just started a Farm to School program, so they'd better do it too."

She emphasizes, "It's the district itself that has to enforce the contract, but they don't read it. It's written at the state level. It's got to be monitored because you cannot rely on the companies to provide the service; they're always continuing to find a work-around and they always push back on it. The key is the wellness committee. Members must go out and visit the schools. We're still trying to figure out what works and what's going to be sustainable. How much does the committee take on? How much can they battle with their management company?"

I wondered about the finances of the school meals programs in these districts.

Dorothy is skeptical. "For the most part our districts are at break even. Some management companies are returning money to the districts. How real those numbers are I can't say. The management companies seem to have a lot of money. When they can go in and buy out a district and promise a million-dollar return, where does the money come from?"

Meanwhile, funding for her organization is always a challenge. She says, "The money is targeted toward national organizations, but it's the smaller groups like ours that are doing the work on the ground. But it can't be about us. The hardest work you have to do is not making it about you, even though it's hard to get money if people don't see your name all over the place. If we own it, it's not sustaining community change. So you hardly hear about us because we believe it's got to be people making their own decisions because they have a vested interest."

Take It Back

Once your district is outsourced, it may seem impossible to take back the food service in-house. When school budgets are being cut to the bone and teachers are getting laid off, districts are understandably reluctant to take on any financial liability or new staff members. However, several districts are doing just that. Dissatisfaction with meal quality, increased loss of revenue, and lack of appropriate bids are some of the reasons school districts revert to self-operation.

NEW HAVEN, REVISITED

I wrote about New Haven's chef Tim Cipriano, the Local Food Dude, in chapter three, but Tagan Engel, a chef-educator who chairs New Haven's Food Policy Council, told me the story behind the story. Tagan credits the success story in New Haven to a combination of good luck, good community organizing, goodwill, and good connections in high places. I also believe that the particular structure and hierarchy of the New Haven Food Policy Council had a great deal of influence on all those factors. Tagan explains that New Haven has a board of aldermen that functions much like a city council. Within that board, there are a number of councils that citizens can serve on, the food policy council being one of them. In 2008, the food policy council chose to focus on the school food issue because of the effect better food in schools would have on a huge amount of the city's population. The council worked with the school district's wellness committee, which had already been focused on school food reform. The group organized a coalition of community organizations that are all involved with children's health, including New Haven's food bank, local restaurants, the Chamber of Commerce, composting businesses, Yale University's Rudd Center for Food Policy and Obesity, and Cityseed, a nonprofit that organizes the city's farmers' markets.

(continued)

Tagan headed up a working group that met once a month in a public school classroom. "Our goal was to establish better communication between the community and the school district, and the school district and the community," says Tagan. The group studied and published a food policy primer that among other goals challenged the city to transition to a self-operating school food service program that "optimizes existing resources, infrastructure, and expertise to economically serve fresh, healthy food."

The policy challenge came about because, says Tagan, "The custodial and food services were very unhappy with their treatment under the management company [Aramark] as well as with the quality of the food. We used both of those things to bring out parents and students. We did a great deal of organizing and got enormous visibility. There was a huge protest in front of city hall. We held meetings at the central kitchen with the company people just trying to make it better with the FSMC."

Ultimately the district made the decision. The school food service had a $2 million deficit. They terminated Aramark and put the contract out to bid for another management company. Tagan says, "A lot of people said we couldn't just bring in another management company. They're going to just keep giving us the same junk. We were fortunate in that Will Clark, the COO of the board of education, is a parent in New Haven. He went and searched out Tim. The position was for a manager, not a chef, but they knew there was enormous and very visible support."

Tim Cipriano had to deal with all the commodity foods that had already been purchased the year before. And, "A lot of it is getting rid of the competitive foods," says Tagan. "He only offers one choice, so he can afford it, and there's more vegetarian food on the menu. The vegetarian meal is often very inexpensive and he can use the extra money to buy roasted chicken on the bone. He knows Connecticut farms and is able to purchase local and regionally grown foods."

Tagan and Tim both complain to me that breakfast is still sugar cereal. She says, "Tim's hands are tied and there are still places we'd like to see it grow, but there's been no push back. The deficit went down and the food is better. The unions still had some issues over pay and hours. They're expected to operate unlike any other city department. What if we took that money and paid just for food?"

Tagan reiterates, "The piece that we put together is this very formal working group on school food that had a logo on it and we took it seriously and we were organized. We had an actual agenda and kept minutes and we put our meetings on the district calendar."

In fact, that's how I found Tagan—the minutes of their meetings stamped with an official-looking logo were all published online—a very good tip for visibility and giving credibility to your council.

While outsourcing to a large FSMC may appear to take advantage of economies of scale, much of the food costs saved is on highly processed bulk foods.

Every school food expert I consulted concurred that the numbers are in favor of self-operation. The same staff, with the same expertise, can be hired without the additional management fee. Hidden costs of working with a management company include staff hours for supervising and auditing the bookkeeping, as well as supervising and auditing the kitchen and cafeteria to ensure that the management company is sticking to the contract.

Kate Adamick opened my eyes to the fact that the balance of power with the management companies has evolved into a dysfunctional dynamic. The companies are hired to work for us, but somehow the hierarchy of decision making has been inverted. A civics class would teach that as citizens of the school district, we choose our board of education members to represent our priorities to the school administrators, in this case in the form of input on the RFPs. In turn, the school administration is obligated to manage the FSMC and see to it that they are meeting the terms and conditions that the contracts put forth. In the topsy-turvy world of school food, the FSMC wields the power, dictating to the administration what they can and cannot do, and the board of education generally goes along with the administration's obsequiousness, ignoring the health impact the poor quality food has on the kids, and ignoring the entreaties of parents who dare to speak up.

Without equivocating, Kate tells me, "I get calls from lots of people in outsourced districts, not just parents. I tell them that they need to take the food service back. I tell them that children learn every waking moment of their lives, and just because the school has abdicated its responsibility to teach students during the lunch hour, it doesn't mean that the students aren't still learning. Consequently, what the students are learning are all the wrong messages. . . . In the twenty-first century, concerned parents have to be constantly vigilant that industry is not profiting at the expense of their children. That is the bottom line."

The bottom line with FSMCs is the bottom line. They exist to make money for executives and shareholders, whereas school districts are non-profit entities. Yet as more parents put pressure on their school districts and management companies to provide real, whole food, there are managers within these companies beginning to work with wellness councils (as mandated) and attempting to offer meals that meet specific wellness policy requirements.

ALTERED STATES, PART 2

In chapter three I told the story of how Beth Loveridge, a mom from Port Angeles, Washington, helped pass Farm to School legislation in her state. I got back in touch with Beth a couple years after the bill was signed, to ask her how it had impacted the food in her school district. She reported that after the legislation, not much changed. Beth reluctantly continued her advocacy, attending a national Farm to School conference in March 2009.

Beth tells me, "I didn't want to go. Our committee had a bit of funding and I wanted our assistant superintendent [Michelle Reid, see chapter four] to go. I'm the choir already, and I didn't want to get sucked in deeper." But the committee chose her to represent the district. She says, "There were six hundred people and lots of young people and we talked about the need to focus on what Farm to School does for the local economy, and how we need to get the government, and the school board, and the community on the same page. Win-win-win. We're constantly trying to attract people up here and our schools are not high-quality schools. One thing we could do is to have a high-quality food system."

Since she couldn't get the school leaders to go to the big conference, Beth, reinvigorated, partnered with a local nonprofit, the North Olympic Peninsula Resource Conservation and Development Council, to host a regional conference nearby to get them on board. She figured that from there they would know the right path to take to make this work. Beth's conference drew 163 key decision-makers from the Olympic Peninsula—mayors, city council members, superintendents, county commissioners, farmers, and the food service director from the self-operated Olympia School District, Paul Flock, who has an organic salad bar.

"The conference was a *huge* success," reports Beth. "There were five different school districts represented at the conference. One is already buying locally and has a garden that is growing food for the lunchroom. We have a lot of people who care. We got together in small little groups and there was lots of enthusiasm."

One of the mega management companies, Sodexo, has been the food service provider in Port Angeles for thirty years. Their five-year contract was coming up for renewal, Beth tells me. "We couldn't get answers to where the money goes. We made a huge effort to get Chartwells to come for a competitive element. We had been working on something that we called the Jefferson Lunch Project. I met with the food service director. He said to me, 'You know what, Beth? You get me an alternative menu and I'll run it for three weeks at one of the schools next year. We'll see if we can make money on it.' I said, 'Okay, but we want to run it for six weeks.' I pulled together people and resources and we came up with some really lofty goals. We were asking him to cook from scratch for this six-week period, eliminate junk food, and have a real vegetarian option."

They chose one elementary school with a kitchen. The big bosses came to see. Beth believes they put so much effort into it because their contract was coming up. A month before it started they did taste-testings with volunteer

(continued)

parents during lunch hour. She describes a minestrone soup with big chunks of vegetables, a stir-fry, and hummus.

Lunch participation went up, trash was reduced by two-thirds. She tells me, "The kitchen staff went from sitting in on meetings with arms crossed and aggressive body language to smiling and saying how much more they are enjoying their jobs. We ended up running the program until the end of the school year."

Then, she says, "We petitioned the school board with over six hundred signatures from our small community. We wanted to require that bids include scratch-cooked whole foods. The kids spoke to the school board and they put all these requirements in the RFP. So when they went to bid, Chartwells had pictures of the Jefferson Lunch Project in their proposal. They proposed an improved breakfast—no more cinnamon rolls, no more waffles on a stick. Our food is still sort of crappy because of the commodity thing but the image and symbolism has changed."

If I'd known Beth before I made the movie, I probably would have followed her crusade in Washington. She exemplifies the Angry Mom spirit, and she's still frustrated, but proud. "I am so sick of everybody telling me to take small steps. I spent years trying to figure out what other people were doing and in the end we did our own thing and had great results. Trying to follow the steps of other people might not be what works in your district. We always took advantage of patting the district on the back and making them look good. Who's going to want to look like they don't support healthy kids? Now the district is taking it on themselves. This year, with the support of the assistant superintendent who has been on the committee the whole time—I've always been irritating to her although she has always treated me with respect—we have a whole plan of rolling this out district-wide based on proximity and resources."

As if there weren't enough obstacles, Beth points out, "Every five years the USDA audits all school districts to make sure they meet the standards. Our new program doesn't meet the requirements. The assistant superintendent was incensed that they would have to add bad calories to meet the requirements. She wants to write a letter to Michelle Obama and state policy makers. Now it's not just me. It's really beautiful to watch. They are taking the initiative. They will pass the audit with the old food, then change over to the new menu. That's like an idea that a radical parent would come up with!"

In the new contract with Sodexo there's now a clause that says 5 percent of the produce budget must be spent on local food in the first year. There's a 5 percent increase each year until 25 percent the fifth year. Now, says Beth, "The manager meets with farmers every year to plan what they will need for planting. The FSMC is going to be held accountable in terms of reporting to the committee. They promised to post all the ingredients on their website. Our committee got a lot more power from this contract."

The same Sodexo manager is in twenty-two districts in Oregon and Washington. After the Port Angeles contract was signed, he put out a challenge to his other districts to make changes based on what happened in Port Angeles. Beth says, "If there's a district where parents want it, it will be easier now. If you can make changes in a food service company that big, then it's going to bubble up through that system."

The lunch war isn't over in Port Angeles, but many battles have been won. "What has inspired me through this whole thing is anger at being manipulated by the system," Beth confesses. "There's a fire in your belly. It takes time away from my family and I've become obsessed and I can't really stop now because here we have really changed. Our contract that was drawn up and the new menus are all because of the moms and dads who have worked on this. The hugest thing we proved is that kids will eat something besides hamburgers and chicken nuggets!"

The RFP that Beth and the Port Angeles wellness committee wrote was the basis for a contract that contained actual food specifications. Your RFP can be as specific as your wellness committee demands. Companies bidding on the RFP will know that those specifications will be written into the contract, so it's important to avoid language that is vague or open to interpretation.

PORT ANGELES MENU MAKEOVER

BEFORE	Chicken Nuggets with Mashed Potatoes
AFTER	**Beef Shepherd's Pie, Black Beans and Rice**
BEFORE	Beef and Cheesy Nachos
AFTER	**Nacho Bar—Meat, Beans, Lettuce, Cheese, Salsa**
BEFORE	French Toast Sticks with Oven-Browned Sausage Links
AFTER	**Baked Potato Bar—Chili, Cheese, Steamed Broccoli, Whole-Wheat Roll**
BEFORE	Baked Meatloaf with Mashed Potatoes
AFTER	**Chunky Turkey, Mashed Potatoes, Roasted Root Vegetables**
BEFORE	Teriyaki Dippers with Steamed Whole-Grain Rice
AFTER	**Assorted Meat and Vegetable Pizzas on Whole-Wheat Crust**

Alternative Food Service Vendors

Many private schools contract with smaller, local catering services. There are local caterers that are willing and eager to provide food services to public schools as well, and there are no regulations that prevent districts from contracting with a local catering service, but the RFPs, which are borrowed state to state, all require experience in the public school food service business. Though it's not a law, these businesses are often thwarted by the RFPs. A typical RFP stipulates: "Contractor must have successful prior experience providing similar contracted food service activities with school districts of similar volume and enrollment."

Dorothy Brayley from Kids First in Rhode Island says that her organization is trying to help districts to put out an RFP that would encourage a smaller local catering service to bid. But she asks, "Who's going to sit in that gap to help that chef navigate the school meals program? You need someone who's going to be able to educate and train." Schools that outsource their meals most often do so because they want a guarantee of service without dealing with training and other support. So the local caterers must get their school food experience before competing in the public school arena. There are some companies doing just that; they're participating in the NSLP by providing catering and management services to after-school and summer programs, nursery, private and parochial schools, as well as public charter schools. Once these companies have been able to establish a track record, they can viably compete for public school meal programs with the big multinationals.

Two examples of recent start-up companies are Revolution Foods and Freshlunches. Founded by a pair of women, Kristin Richmond and Kirsten Tobey, who met in graduate school, Revolution Foods has grown from serving three schools in 2006 to now providing meals at over one hundred locations in California, Colorado, and Washington, D.C., schools. Their food philosophy is simple—they believe in using real food, cooking with few ingredients, and making sure the ingredients are recognizable and close to their original state. A sample menu features honey-glazed chicken with roasted potatoes and garlic braised collard greens.

Freshlunches, Inc., is also committed to scratch cooking and high quality ingredients—natural and organic fruits and veggies, hormone- and antibiotic-free meats and poultry, no hydrogenated oils, HFCS, or artificial colors or flavors. Also founded in 2006, Alan Razzaghi and Winnie Tong developed recipes with a team of nutritionists, parents, children, and chefs and began delivering boxed lunches on-site to kids who had opted into their program. They now also have a division that provides meals that meet the USDA guidelines for reimbursable meals, and they've expanded from their home base in Southern California into New England.

Pressure from parents, new federal mandates, and competition from start-ups are all bringing about positive changes in the way food service management companies work with school systems. Some are now actively purchasing from local vendors (although mostly on a limited basis), whereas in the past we were told that was against company policy. Yet the traditional FSMC model still relies on sales of competitive and processed foods, which ultimately undermines the incentive to provide the highest possible quality school meals. The added layer of management forces administrators to choose sides when advocates and wellness committees ask for input into RFPs and contracts, and many would-be advocates are intimidated by all the legal documents involved. Though it's more daunting to navigate a school food revolution through the management company maze, your success with these companies, as Beth Loveridge says, may "bubble up through the system."

NINE

SCHOOL FOOD FROM SCRATCH

If we can fix school lunch, if we can change how we feed kids and teach them about food, we might be able to save the world.

—ANN COOPER

Thanks to supportive federal and state legislation and mandates, lots of media coverage, and a groundswell of popular support, active advocates are replacing angry moms. The school food revolution is underway, and the vision that the revolutionaries, angry moms, and advocates have is coalescing and converging. As we move forward with innovations, projects, and programs large and small, we can move past the tipping point by measuring results and reporting them in all media.

Performance Measurement

The term "performance measurement" sounds like something out of Sociology 101—and it probably is. If your school food revolution has the backing of the district, a nonprofit organization, and/or a college or university, you may be able to collect and analyze data that can have an impact on the continuation and expansion of your projects and those of other districts as well. Data reports that show improvements in test scores, attendance, food IQ, behavior, BMI, and athletic performance can drive decision-making and long-term adoption of policies, curriculum, and programs. Though it takes some resources to obtain the data, it can really pay off in the form of grants and investments down the road.

If possible, design an appropriate measurement system into your initiative. Choose a few simple parameters that you can assess before and after exposure to the program. If the results from a first round of new menu items, or new curriculum, aren't stellar, it's a good indication that you need to revisit the components of your program. You can learn from what worked and what didn't work.

Performance reporting can also be anecdotal. Stories from teachers, students, food service, school nurses, parents, and administrators, while not statistically measurable, can help to reinforce data from other studies if your project hasn't been measured.

Your school food initiative may be a result of changes to local wellness policy. School districts are required to establish a plan for measuring implementation of the wellness policy. Schools must report on how wellness policy impacts the school food finances and how has it impacted students, parents, teachers, and administration. The evaluation and report need not be elaborate. It should outline the changes that were made in the policy and the resulting changes in the school's food environment—curriculum, food access, food quality, food sourcing, drinking water, time to eat, and so on. Increases in student participation in the meals program, and any behavior and performance outcomes, should be noted. The report should describe what is working and what needs work. This periodic assessment is intended to encourage districts to update their policies as necessary, and celebrate success as well!

Process and Progress Report

Michelle Reid, assistant superintendent from Port Angeles, shared her detailed report on the inner workings of the Nutrition and Physical Activity Advisory Committee. The report exemplifies the way an action plan can be charted and implemented over time. With her permission, I've included excerpts from Michelle's report.

PORT ANGELES SCHOOL DISTRICT NUTRITION AND PHYSICAL ACTIVITY ADVISORY COMMITTEE REPORT, JUNE 9, 2008

In addressing the need to implement and evaluate the Nutrition and Physical Fitness Policy, the advisory committee decided first on a meeting schedule. Given this task had a finite timeline for study and recommendations, the group agreed to meet on six Monday afternoons from 5 p.m. to 6:30 p.m. . . .

The committee spent a significant amount of time outside the regularly scheduled committee meetings with subgroup assignments. Committee members chose to work in smaller research groups, which then reported to the whole group. . . . The student surveys garnered 1,754 responses district-wide. The advisory committee considered this a strong response. . . . In general, students responded that they did eat healthier foods at school this past year, particularly those at the elementary and middle levels. Further, the majority of students polled indicated that they also ate healthier foods at home this year. While no causal effect can be confirmed, we would like to believe that the new policy and procedure implementation has aided in this behavior.

Another clear message is that the significant majority of students responded that they knew there was a new policy and procedure surrounding nutrition and physical fitness this past year. While on the surface this does not seem like such a big deal, it is reassuring that students would have such firsthand knowledge about a new policy and procedure. . . .

The teacher/staff surveys completed had 154 respondents. Overwhelmingly, they were aware that there was a new policy and procedure surrounding physical activity and nutrition this past year. Most of the support and resources the staff had to implement the policy and procedures came from meetings and/or handouts.

Several of the most significant data points teachers and staff note are positive changes in student behavior and ability to learn. In general, staff

(continued)

overwhelmingly reports that students' health is changed for the better. This is good news as the committee continues its work in the coming year.

[This report] highlights those areas we have made progress in and those we have work yet to do within. Teacher and student evaluations will continue to inform our conversations and inform our work in the upcoming academic year. We will also be surveying parents in the coming year and will adjust our implementation of the policy based on an analysis of the data we receive. . . .

On the nutrition side of the policy, the implications of the new policy and procedures have been significant in both content of items sold and those no longer sold. Nutritionally sound items are now the exclusive choice for students of the district. The policy and procedures are clear on the nutritional guidelines for both food and drink in the schools.

At least two of the subcommittees charged by the advisory committee have been in the nutrition program area. A subcommittee was charged to review the high school gymnasium vending machine food options. This work was undertaken in response to Ms. Kreider's concerns raised about the need for availability of quality snacks, particularly for those student athletes who go right from a full day of academic classes to late afternoon practices without any intervening nutritional opportunity. Also, those students who are not eating breakfast often could benefit from a late-morning, nutritious snack.

This subcommittee came back with the recommendation that the gym snack machine needed to be reinstated with healthy snacks to meet this need. The advisory committee supported this recommendation. This is an example of the successful iterative process the advisory committee has engaged in for the past year and plans to continue for the upcoming year.

Another subcommittee charged by the advisory committee was the subcommittee to meet with the new food service director and explore the organic food possibilities available for district students and staff to partake of. This committee will continue its work in the upcoming academic year. A particular possibility from the work this subcommittee did was the plan to work with at least one school in the district to integrate local organic food into the regular meal menu. This conversation will continue this coming year. Also a number of interesting food suggestions arose from the evaluation survey data. These will be looked at in terms of their possible integration into menu planning.

Clearly there has been a fiscal impact for schools' Associated Student Body budgets as the vending machine item selections are different than those currently available. At the high school level, there has also been some impact on the student store with the items available for sale needing to meet the new nutritional expectations. . . . Nutrition program conversations will continue as we look at the survey evaluation information from students and teachers. Parents will also have an opportunity to weigh in on surveys during the coming year.

Appendices to Michelle's report include graphic charts and tables illustrating results from each school's surveys.

School Food Outcomes Report

Jamie Oliver received tons of media attention for his *Food Revolution* TV series, much of which consisted of rumors, commentary, and opinion about his project's impact. A lot of it was hearsay and not necessarily based on actual reporting.

In 2009, a report from the Institute for Social and Economic Research summed up the actual results from Jamie's original "Feed Me Better" initiative, which took place in school year 2004–2005 in the school district of Greenwich, England. The program was taken up in eighty-one schools out of the eighty-five in the district and involved retraining school cooks (in a three-day boot camp), providing them with new kitchen equipment, and replacing all the processed, junky food in the schools with nutrient-dense menus cooked from scratch and designed by the chef.

It was noted that when the new healthy meals were originally offered alongside the original junk food, most children preferred to stick with the junk food. When the strategy changed to complete replacement, there were some children who refused to try the new food, but overall the new menus were well accepted within a few weeks.

The report addresses a potential placebo effect that might have been induced by the attention received by the schools that were filmed for Jamie's original *Food Revolution* TV series. An assessment of only those schools actually revealed a negative effect on test scores, implying that the disruption of TV crews counteracted any potential positive placebo effect. Nevertheless, average test scores for all the participating schools improved significantly, with increases of 3 to 8 percentage points in English and Science. The district also documented substantial decreases in absenteeism.

. The authors claim, "These effects are particularly noteworthy because they measure direct and immediate effects of improvement in children's diet on educational achievements only. There could be additional benefits (in particular in terms of health), beyond the improvements in educational achievements, which we are unable to measure because of lack of data."

The school district increased the budget for school meals for the experiment in order to cover costs for training, equipment, and promotion to the parents. The report concludes, "Even if we only take these short-term benefits into account, we find that the campaign was very cost-effective."

Other measurements of the success of the Greenwich transformation are reported on the website of the Health Education Trust. Consumption of fruit and vegetables as part of the school meal has increased fourfold as a result of the new menus and uptake of meals has increased.

The Health Education Trust website also quotes positive teacher feedback from the head teacher at Kidbrooke School (the first school on the program): "Because the children aren't being stuffed with additives, they're much less hyper in the afternoons now. It hasn't been an easy transition, as getting older children to embrace change takes time." Another teacher comments, "Children enjoy the food and talk about it more than they did in the past. They seem to have more energy and can concentrate for longer."

Edible Outcomes

The long-awaited performance report from Berkeley's School Lunch Initiative was published in the fall of 2010. The three-year study of children who participated in the initiative's garden education, cooking and nutrition classes, and locally sourced, cooked-from-scratch meals program revealed that elementary students increased their consumption of fruit and vegetables by one serving (one half cup) per day, and also ate more fruit. The report notes that these positive changes took place at schools where students had more exposure to the School Lunch Initiative and that these schools were chosen first because they served more low-income students.

Results for middle schoolers showed that "students who had attended the middle school with the most highly developed School Lunch Initiative components (where students spent more time in cooking and gardening programs), had increased their nutrition knowledge scores by 5 percent over the previous year, while students attending the other two middle schools with lesser-developed School Lunch Initiative components had decreased their knowledge scores by 6 percent and 14 percent, respectively." One of the report's conclusions is that "The need for continued exposure to the School Lunch Initiative into middle school is further supported by the observation that at the one middle school where seventh-grade students showed a mean decrease in fruit and vegetable consumption of about one serving per day, the cooking and garden programming was offered only as an elective." Despite the regression in some of the middle schoolers, the students reported enjoying the food served in the cafeteria, and they demonstrated knowledge of how their food choices affect the environment.

Students from schools with highly developed School Lunch Initiative components reported eating more family dinners prepared from scratch, and helping more with dinner preparations.

The report was performed by researchers from the University of California at Berkeley and funded by Alice Waters's Chez Panisse Foundation.

The Network for a Healthy California conducted a related photographic study of the contents and consumption of student lunches from school and from home. Their evidence showed that "students who ate school lunch consumed more than three times as many vegetables as students who brought lunch from home." And "About 80 percent of the increase in consumption of fruits and vegetables among elementary school students came from in-season fruits and vegetables."

These types of district-wide reports are picked up and run by syndicated media, influencing key decision makers in schools around the country and around the world.

Lunch Lessons from Around the World

In chapter one, I wrote about the school food in Finland, with its simple mandate for a tasty, colorful, and well-balanced plate of food. Ninety-five percent of students in Finland eat those school meals daily, which are, incidentally, free for all. For some geeky, school-food fun (or a class lesson on culture) you can do a Web search for "school food from around the world." There are numerous blogs and websites with eye-opening photos and menus of school meals that range from tantalizing to sad. One site features a big bowl of rice porridge in Honduras; small bowls of white rice and sauce in Ghana; brown rice and beans in Haiti; a whole fried fish, scrambled egg with tomato sauce, rice, spinach, cauliflower, and soup in China; and a chili dog with cheese, french fries, and milk for the U.S.A.

One of my first school food inspirations came from my family in France, and later I was awed by the newfound support for scratch cooking school food in England. In fact there is a wealth of knowledge and practical information that can be gleaned from school food programs in many other countries and there are models to be found in some surprising places. As we see the United States plummeting in global health statistics, falling behind what we used to call Third World countries like Cuba in life expectancy, we now see so-called developing countries passing ours by with the quality of their school meals standards and programs.

Childhood obesity statistics in Mexico rival those of the United States. In response, Mexican President Felipe Calderón launched a major anti-obesity campaign that banned all junk foods from public schools by the start of the 2011 school year. Soda, juice, processed snacks, candies, and some fattening local favorites like pork rinds, fried tacos, and *atole* (a sweet corn-based drink) will be replaced by tacos, burritos, and salads that are lower in fat and higher in nutrients. The regulations apply to all 220,000 public and private elementary and middle schools in Mexico.

In South Korea, a typical school lunch consists of the national superfood, kimchi (pickled cabbage), rice, tofu, chicken or fish, and soybean sprouts. The country places great emphasis on proper nutrition, and they've banned junk food advertising aimed at kids, something the United States would do well to copy.

A decade ago, 17 million Brazilians suffered from malnutrition. That number was dramatically reduced by former President Lula's school food policies. The new federal policy requires schools to purchase 30 percent of their products from local producers, many of whom use organic farming methods. My friend Leandra comes from a small city in southern Brazil. Before immigrating to America, Leandra used to teach at the school where her mom has been a lunch lady for seventeen years. Leandra explains that Brazil has a commodity system similar to the system in the United States. "We get food from the government—rice, beans, yucca—with a big government stamp on it so it can't be sold. Those are the staples. Then all the produce comes from the school's garden. It's a public school, and the gardener lives on campus. My mom cooks from scratch every day. Her kitchen is very well equipped. She makes salad, fresh vegetables, soup, and cookies, all from scratch. The teachers eat the food, too, and whatever the kids don't eat the staff brings home for dinner. It's good food! The workers—the gardener, the cooks, all get paid well; they have job security and a pension."

Leandra tells me that in Brazil, canned food, sweetened condensed milk, frozen food, and McDonald's are expensive, luxury foods. She says, "I never had McDonald's till I came here. Fresh food is cheaper. Brazilian people think they want the convenience food because it sounds good and it costs more so they think it's better, but they don't know the food they have is better for them."

Leandra's mom's only complaint about being a lunch lady: she wishes she could change to a job where she would be allowed to wear nail polish!

THE FRENCH CONNECTION

My husband's recollections of school food in France were of hearty, four-course meals. His was the post–World War II generation, and there was a great cultural emphasis on proper nourishment in the wake of years of food shortages and deprivation caused by the war.

Though I haven't been to visit a school cafeteria in France firsthand, I've seen sample menus that rival menus in some of the finest restaurants. If anything, school food has improved since my husband's childhood. Meals still consist of several courses—an hors d'oeuvre, a principal plate with a side vegetable, a cheese plate, and a dessert. The hors d'oeuvre for a week in March consisted of either a couple of salads (lentils, cabbage, carrots, tomato, celery root, or grain salad like tabouli) or a soup and salad, or a crêpe filled with vegetables garnished with cheese. Main dishes were roast chicken, beef and mushroom stew, salmon filet with lemon herb sauce, and a curried pork or turkey entrée. A serving of cheese or yogurt, and then a dessert of fruit salad, chocolate mousse, cake, or compote follow these dishes. The French menus also include suggestions for a light supper at home, implying that the expectation is that the school meal is the main meal of the day.

My husband's two brothers now live in different parts of the country and both had stories to tell me about school food. One brother told me that his son's school food is so good that the school won an award for having the best food in the region. The other brother told me that his kids' school food used to be quite good, until a management company took over the food service. Within a year, the families protested against the food so loudly that the management company was removed. The French have a strong tradition of organizing and protesting that which causes outrage—messing with their food is risky business!

Clearly, food is of great cultural significance to the French, who consider fine dining as much of a pastime as Americans value their hot dogs at the ballpark.

To my mind though, the reason school food is so good in France is that not only is it valued as part of a child's cultural education, it actually *is* part of the educational mandate. In the United States, we have a separate department that regulates school food (the USDA), whereas in France, the Ministry of Education regulates school food, as is the case in much of Europe and Japan (where 85 percent of students eat the school meals). The school food budget per meal in France is roughly twice that of the United States; it's about the same as the current U.K. allowance. The school food environment in those countries is considered one and the same as the academic environment. An example of this connection comes also from one of my French brothers-in-law. Felicien is a civil servant employed as a gardener for the city of Paris. For most of the year he supervises the design and upkeep of several of the city's many public parks. For a month each year, his job is to work with students in the city's public schools, teaching them how to plant, grow, and nourish produce for the table. Felicien isn't part of a progressive model program—this has been part of his job for the twenty years he's been employed by the city.

Feed Me Better

The school food budget in England was not always so generous; in fact the quality of British (state) school food was reputed to rival some of the worst in the world. In 2005, a teacher, Jackie Schneider, began a one-woman crusade. Disgusted by the horrible school food, and outraged that her students (and her own kids) were paying for the privilege of eating that junk, she began speaking out. When that got her exactly nowhere, she started taking pictures of the lunches and posting them on a daily blog. As Jackie says, "a picture is worth a thousand words" and soon other Merton parents (Merton is a neighborhood of London) began to get angry. Despite their protests, Jackie says, "We failed miserably." At school meetings they were brushed off, told that this was as good as it could be, and Jackie was told that she would lose her job if she didn't quit her activism.

Enter Jamie Oliver, who was by then a celebrity in England. He'd been inspired by the independence, enthusiasm, and talent of one lunch lady, Jeanette Orrey, whose simple, traditional, cooked-from-scratch meals were making waves beyond her district. Jamie used his celebrity status to launch a national campaign for better food in schools via a website (FeedMeBetter. com) and a four-part British TV series, *Jamie's School Dinners*, much like the series he now hosts in the United States. The campaign collected over 260,000 signatures on a petition, which Jamie took to the country's secretary of state for education.

With school food suddenly a hot topic, the British media got wind of Jackie's crusade and made her a local hero. The Feed Me Better campaign was a success, with the ministry nearly doubling the funding for school feeding programs in England. Jackie's job was saved by the publicity, and her parents' group now has a website (www.mertonparents.co.uk) that still shows pictures of the school food—only now you can see how far they've come!

In the wake of Jamie Oliver's successful campaign, the British government did something that I as an American am truly awed by: in 2005 they funded and created the School Food Trust, an autonomous, quasi-government agency, whose mission is to provide curriculum, skills training, standards, implementation, and assessment all geared toward improving the British state (public) school food environment. In just a handful of years, the School Food Trust, headed by Judy Hargadon, a former national health administrator, has made huge strides. Their website is a model that our own local, state, and federal governments can learn much from.

Yet even with the funding, training, and other resources, the School Food Trust is struggling to get schools to change. In the U.K., the challenge is the culture as much as the cost, and the trust found that parents weren't getting on board with the changes. The British media featured stories of parents passing contraband burgers and chips to their kids through the schoolyard gates at recess time. Judy Hargadon is working with community groups like Jackie's to shift the paradigm across England. She explained to me what she considers to be one of the fundamental differences between American and British culture. She thinks that the English are complacent because they have an expectancy and trust that their government will solve problems for them. Judy admires the American tradition of advocacy and would like to encourage more of that among England's parents. Perhaps because we have a healthy mistrust of government, Judy believes that Americans take matters into their own hands more, and work harder at the grassroots level to achieve progressive goals. We both wonder if we had a bit more of each other's resources whether the school food environment could be changing more dramatically.

Here in America, we don't have a School Food Trust. The movement leaders have called for a school food czar but to date all authority still lies with the USDA, which has left us to create a patchwork network of model programs and shared best practices.

ROMAN QUALITY

The school food system that has been most highly touted, with good reason, is that of Rome, Italy. At the turn of the last century (2000), following much protest from local parents over the poor quality of school food, the city of Rome decided to confront rising rates of childhood obesity with a complete overhaul of its school meal program. The goals of the overhaul were better food quality, nutrition and safety, combating childhood obesity, and also to develop sustainable production and regulate public contracts. The underlying philosophy was one of connecting school meals to the local economy and the Italian cultural value of regionalism in food production. Banking on the success of several other smaller school districts in Italy that had made the switch to organic food, Rome's "All for Quality" school meal system focuses first on procurement, emphasizing organic and locally produced ingredients—now a whopping 70-plus percent of all the food used in the program. Ingredients from farther afield must be sustainably produced, non-GMO, and fair-trade certified. Environmentally friendly equipment and cleaning products are also now the norm in the city's school kitchens.

The structure of the school food service system in Rome also provides an interesting model for the United States. A handful of the city's 740 public schools are what we call "self-operated," with in-house staff providing procurement, cooking, and serving meals. The majority of the 150,000 school meals served daily in Rome are provided by a number of small catering firms that each operates several schools in the district. A 100-point system awards contracts based on lowest bids, but also for purchasing organically, seasonally, regionally, and with a freshness guarantee for both produce and animal products. The contracts go to bid every three years, and successive RFPs may weigh the points differently from year to year, often including fees for improving the kitchens, refurbishing cafeterias, replacing plastic utensils with silverware and dishwashers, training programs for staff, informational and marketing campaigns, and ensuring waste is properly recycled and composted. Silvana Sari, Rome's director of educational services, has been the driving force behind Rome's school food revolution. She developed the point system in order to bring up the level of food quality along with the increased financial commitment that was required from the contractors. Her job is roughly equivalent to that of a school district business manager; she oversees the food service contracts, supervises a staff that includes seventy nutritionists, and contracts with two separate companies to inspect schools for food safety and contract compliance. Schools are now inspected frequently and penalties are assessed for violations. In addition, parent volunteers are elected to a Canteen Commission that uses a checklist designed by Silvana's staff to report on the meals program to teachers and other parents.

Rather than a breakfast program, Roman students are provided a mid-morning snack, often a small sandwich. Ninety-six percent of the meals are made on-site from scratch. Teachers sit with the students at the lunch table to reinforce nutrition lessons learned in class. A sample lunch menu includes a first course of a mouthwatering vegetable stew over homemade pasta, followed by a breaded veal cutlet baked in butter and milk or an omelet. A soup of celery, carrots, potatoes, chard, and pumpkin is pureed for the younger children with cooked rice added after for texture. Silvana emphasizes that improvements were implemented gradually over a period of years, to allow for adjustments all along the supply chain. The switch to local and organic food has been a great boon to the region's farmers, but it took them some time to gear up for the increased demand. The changeover to organic ingredients raised food costs by about 21 cents per child, per day.

Every school child participates in the meal program. Roman children are not allowed to bring food from home, and there are no vending machines in the schools. Similar to the United States, Italy has a three-tiered system of meal pricing based on a family's income, but even those who pay full freight pay for less than half the actual cost of the meal, about equal to the price of a U.S. school meal. The real cost of a day's worth of food per student in Rome, including lunch and snack, is $6.56, a figure that includes all of the additional maintenance services detailed in the point system contracts. The figure does not include health care for staff, which is covered by Italy's national health care system.

Silvana also emphasizes the challenge she faced in working with management companies to bring their profits in line with the stricter demands of the program. The process took plenty of creativity, flexibility, and adjustment on everyone's part, including the students, who protested the lack of choice in the beginning.

In her briefing paper about what the United States can learn from the Roman school food system, school food consultant Toni Liquori points out, "The fact that so many companies competed in the most recent round [of bidding] suggests that school meals in Rome are an appealing market to local food companies, even with the profound changes that have been introduced." Maybe because they have so much history, the Romans take the long view, preferring to spend a bit more money on school meals now in order to reap the benefits of healthy kids and savings on health care in the future.

GOING ROGUE

Imagine if you could start from scratch and just make good food without worrying about the USDA. I tried to track down the food service director in New Canaan, Connecticut, for some time. I heard that he was doing something different, and I knew that he had attended the Institute for Integrative Nutrition (my nutrition school alma mater) on a scholarship program for food service directors and school principals. When I finally got Bruce Gluck on the phone, he described himself as "the Doctor House of school food"—in other words, a curmudgeon. He's been running the food service program in New Canaan for seventeen years. Bruce told me that the district dropped out of the National School Lunch Program thirteen or fourteen years ago because he thought the rules and regulations were stupid. Since then he's been evolving his food service program. The information and the confidence he developed studying integrative nutrition have helped him really focus on what's best for the students in the last several years. Regarding wellness committees, he said, "To tell you the truth, I don't find a whole lot of value in wellness committees. Don't talk to me about profit and loss and then tell me you want everything natural and healthy." He has little patience for committees that counsel baby steps. "In order to make change, you have to make change. You can't ease into it. Baby steps are great in certain situations but when it comes to the health of our children, you have to act now." And in reference to Michelle Obama's Let's Move! initiative, he said, "I have a problem with Mrs. Obama because she's not challenging the Tysons and the Cargills." Bruce believes these food manufacturers are too powerful and are standing in the way of policies that would enable school districts to source locally and to choose and process their own ingredients. Though he harbors some strong opinions, Bruce Gluck is a self-described shy guy. He steers clear of the limelight, but once we started talking school food, his ingenuity and his passion overcame the shyness. Apparently, I wasn't the first to notice. "I didn't think I was an advocate until somebody pointed it out to me. They said, 'You're already doing it.' So now I'm enrolled at Harvard getting a second BA in government. My goal is to make policy." By the end of the phone call, I had an invitation to meet him in the cafeteria of New Canaan High School, where his office is located. When

I walked in, he was engaged in building a new Web page for the district's school food service. Rather than promoting the traditional USDA food pyramid, Bruce was posting a variety of food pyramids based on various types of traditional and alternative diets from around the world.

He explained, "What I'm trying to do is give parents an integrated overview of everything that's out there so they can make at least educated guesses. And you know, the USDA pyramid is perfect if you want to kill your kid, not if you want to keep them healthy and happy, so I'm putting the different pyramids here so parents can see what's going on and then compare it to what we're actually doing. What we do here is—everything's fresh. At the elementary schools there is very little choice. As we get into middle school—you get more choice. And then here [at the high school] these are young adults; they really should be making good choices. But we also don't believe in taking everything away because when you make something taboo you know what happens."

He's proud that even though there is an à la carte line, most kids are purchasing the school meal. He says, "Years ago the à la carte was like 60 percent of our sales or more and now it's probably no more than 15 percent. Because now we have a fresh salad bar, fresh hot lunch, we have a Caesar salad grilled chicken bar, and a fresh deli in which we roast our own roast beefs. We're experimenting. Monday we have souvlaki, hummus, and quinoa tabouli. I roast the ducks the Chinese way, hanging in the oven. We develop our own recipes here. I use buffalo and ostrich, too. As a matter of fact, elementary kids love the duck and I'm okay with that because it's a healthier product and we cook it properly, and people say *duck*? It's the same price as chicken. Sometimes it's actually cheaper. We buy fresh turkeys and we roast them and we carve them right out there so the kids see them. And not just here, not just at the high school but at the middle school and the elementary school. We always keep a turkey on display under the lights so the kids know what they're getting and they see it and they see it being carved."

I ask Bruce if the high school students were allowed off campus during lunchtime. In response he launches into a detailed explanation of the

(continued)

cold-pressed rice bran oil he uses for frying instead of the less healthy canola or soy oil. He acknowledges that he'd rather not fry at all but explains, "If I can keep them here because they can get their chicken tenders then I can get them to try something else. And just based on my numbers it's working. We see almost every one of those students here for something. About a couple years ago I got a call from one of the delis down in New Canaan. They were offering to make our sandwiches for us and wanted our business and I said, 'No, we do that ourselves.' And I said, 'What—this is unusual?' And he said, 'Well, we're not seeing—we don't know what's wrong—we're not seeing as many kids. . . .' So I know I'm keeping them here, plus I talked to the parking lot attendants and they're saying fewer kids are leaving. So it's working."

The many students he sees with food allergies disturbs Bruce, and he's working hard to cater to their needs. "We came up with this egg-free French toast—the batter for the bread is tapioca, rice flour and we sweeten it with roasted banana and the kids love it! I do different foods from around the world. Yesterday we had Greek and Middle Eastern. We did souvlaki and spanakopita and falafel but we make the falafel with rice flour so it's totally gluten-free. Because there are kids with celiac and there are kids that have sensitivities."

A meal at the high school costs $4.00, $3.50 at the elementary. It's all-inclusive.

In fact, Bruce says, "We give them everything. I mean we'll get students at every school who will say, 'I don't want . . .' 'Well, you know what, take it,' and I make deals with them . . . 'Take it . . . try it. If you don't like that, then you bring it back and I'll give you your lunch for free,' and I haven't had anyone come back to me. Yesterday's meal we had quinoa tabouli and the kids loved it. We put up signs . . . this is quinoa and the amino acids and the protein. They really are starting to get it."

Bruce doesn't subscribe to the one-size-fits-all model of nutrition. "Not every child is the same. Not every person is the same. You may need 2,000 calories a day to survive but I surely don't. They say for K to 6 it's 600-plus calories for lunch. My menus rarely reach that. I care about the usefulness of the calories. Are these good calories? And if they're low, then that's okay with me because I am giving the student a chance to go back to class and maintain an energy level rather then spiking and falling and having twenty kids sleeping on their desks—that's what I care about. Mine are complex carbs. Are they getting the protein? Because you need protein. I hate milk. I love drinking it but I hate the idea of it. People say that's essential. But it's not. Milk is a baby food. It's not a grown-up food.".

He does serve milk, and after much searching, found a brand, Hudson Valley, that is hormone-free, grass-fed, and minimally processed. He's given this subject a lot of thought. "It's minimally pasteurized and so it doesn't kill everything; it still has some of the probiotics that pasteurized milk doesn't have, and then again it's fortified with the vitamins." Not that he's against vitamins, but, he says, "I have this firm belief that nature provides. We serve a lot of spinach, and a lot of dark green vegetables. There's a reason that in the Northeast nature provides very dark vegetables here. We do a lot of squash. Last month we did roasted pumpkin as a vegetable."

He sources his food from some of the distributors that supply organic produce to the local markets and restaurants. It's usually seasonal, and local when possible.

Bruce says, "I realized here it's like anywhere else. You can tell them how healthy it is. But if it doesn't taste like quality, it doesn't look like quality, it doesn't smell like quality . . . they don't care. I took restaurant principles. Any businessman will tell you that the best places spend more but they also sell more so they make up that excess in expenditure by an excess in sales. And that's what we do. And I've tried and tried to tell other directors and they're afraid. Here, I'll look at something and say to the lead cook, 'Let me ask you a question. Would you serve this at home?' And if they even hesitate I say throw it away. Why would you sell it here? And that's what we've been pounding into their heads. I have an amazing staff."

Bruce tells me about a call from a school district in Alabama asking for advice. "I said, 'Okay. You have a school district of almost twelve thousand kids. I have a school district of a little over four thousand. If I take your numbers, it adds up that you serve a hundred percent of your students for only

(continued)

sixty days out of the school year. I feed a hundred percent of my students for a hundred and sixty-eight days, so what's the problem here?"

Bruce says his standards are much higher than the USDA's. "When I started here we were part of the national program and I would go to the little seminars up in Middletown and I'd sit there and think to myself, *Are you kidding me? I mean really, are we serious here?* I've been a chef for many years. I have training and you can't tell me this stuff. And I stopped going. What we've done with the school lunch program is we've set up this infrastructure of fear and misinformation. And if we can't break that, then none of this is going to get anywhere." As for the commodity system, he rails, "Do you know it's cheaper to produce fresh food from scratch then it is to buy processed foods? Not only is it cheaper, it's healthier. Pork is healthy. Would I take the pork roast if it weren't pork loin? No!" He says food service directors should be able to choose between money and commodities. "And if it's only twenty cents, that's fine. I could do something with those twenty cents. Somebody said to me, 'Well, we have carrots, celery sticks, and hummus on our menu. . . . ' But where do they get their hummus? They buy it. Well, we don't buy it. We make it. Now, by the way, you're buying five pounds of hummus. Let's say you use three pounds and then it's not on your menu again for another month. What happens to that last two pounds? You can't freeze it. We make what we need. And because my staff is trained and experienced to use products, they actually have learned how to be creative. Even in culinary school I wanted to prove that you could make restaurant-quality food in the cafeteria and I've proven you can to a large extent. We have puddings. We make our own puddings from block chocolate and bittersweet chocolate and we don't buy the powdered stuff. We make our own whipped cream." (Which looked delicious, by the way!)

Like Dr. House on TV, Bruce is a very passionate curmudgeon. He insists, "When you let go of that title—the food service director stuff—and realize that you're really advocating for children and for health, your perspective totally changes. All of a sudden, things that you thought were important don't matter anymore. I use to drive my assistant director crazy with budget. She will tell you now, in two years, at least, I haven't even brought it up. I do my projections but I've told the business manager I really don't care anymore about it. And if we're serious as a district, if we're serious as administrators, whether it be their nutrition or education or health—then money shouldn't be the first thing we talk about, it should be the last thing we talk about. It takes a year or two of losing money, but are you serious about health or not?"

He advises that parents have to go first to other parents instead of going to the food service director first. Then, he says, "Parents have to go to the boards of education and say this is the way it's going to be. Do we care about the kids? Is it about what's right? In towns like ours the people that decide on the school budget are over sixty and have no children. You have to demand what you want. Tell that food service director in your district I don't want this crap anymore. Don't get angry about it—be nice. Hey, I'm a parent. It's hard because before you can be teaching them they have to want you to do it."

An Educational Mandate?

One of the ongoing debates about the American school lunch program is whether it is an agricultural program or a nutrition program. A related debate is whether it is a welfare program, a business, or an educational program. Districts that focus on those minimal federal guidelines find their meal program invariably at odds with these competing interests. Janet Poppendieck, in her book *Free For All*, asks, "Is it an interruption or an integral part of the school day?"

Since the 1960s, there has been repeated discussion among school food advocates of moving the National School Lunch Program to the CDC, or the Department of Health and Human Services. Both of these agencies have a clear public health and prevention agenda. Yet both of these agencies conform to the dietetics model of feeding children that pathologizes food rather than teaches us to celebrate it. And moving the program from one governmental agency (the USDA) to another would still keep it separate, an interruption to the school day.

Taking a page from those meal programs in other countries, what if we moved our National School Lunch Program and all school food policy from the USDA to the Department of Education? What if our educators were given a mandate to address the school food environment in the same way they are charged with playground safety, academic education, and every other policy that affects the learning environment of our children? What if we approached the program the same way we approach all other aspects of our children's public education? Such a move would not only resolve the internal conflict of interest within the USDA, it would also integrate food with education, hopefully resolving the conflict of interest between education and the current break-even business mandate for school food. Merging food into the realm of education would at least align the types of food sold in the cafeteria with current nutrition education.

Until it becomes a bona fide educational mandate, and for the foreseeable future, school districts will continue to struggle to find adequate support on the federal level for their meal programs. While we must continue to advocate for federal initiatives, we cannot wait for the ebb and flow of political interests to work in our favor. For the meantime, and probably for a long time, it's up to us. Our children's health, and the sustainability of the school food environment, lie in the enthusiasm, activism, knowledge, and creativity of our local communities.

Grassroots and Common Threads

At its best, school food can harmonize goals for local agriculture, child nutrition, and education by supporting farmers, helping children develop healthy eating habits, supplying good food to needy children, and teaching students the pleasures, etiquette, culture, and politics of our local and global food system. As a not-for-profit business it can support the local economy by employing workers from the community and serving as a training ground for young chefs while utilizing revenue to maintain a quality program. With sustainability as its focus, the meal program can provide good food to those who can't afford it, keep local dollars in the community, and teach children lifelong lessons. Across America, from Baltimore to Berkeley, there are advocates bucking the system, working hard to raise awareness, clean up the school food environment, and focus the bottom line on healthy kids, healthy staff, and a healthy planet. Communities with committed parents and administrators are creating their own guidelines, policies, and regulations and there's lots of innovation happening. Skilled chefs, and food and wellness educators are integrating cafeterias with curriculum, bringing farm-fresh products into schools, and teaching children an understanding of their connection with their food and with the planet.

A common thread among the sustainable school food programs I've seen in the United States is that what sustains them is a patchwork of revenue streams. In addition to government reimbursements and state incentive programs, food service directors and often-times dedicated volunteers are scraping together funding from public and private grants and set-asides, fund-raisers, philanthropists, and in-kind donations and services. In Minneapolis–St. Paul, a local fitness center has offered to compensate one school the balance of the cost of replacing junk food with whole-food alternatives. LifeTime Fitness wants to prove that the junk can be replaced without raising costs, and they're willing to bank on it. Nationally, the No Kid Hungry campaign spearheaded by the nonprofit Share Our Strength creates public-private partnerships between food systems and local businesses. Actor Jeff Bridges has lent his celebrity to the cause, visiting the Elsie Whitlow Stokes School in Washington, D.C., where the campaign was instrumental in obtaining donations of equipment and food from Whole Foods Market. I don't believe these types of partnerships are as insidious as the Pepsi playgrounds and Coca-Cola scoreboards; most of them don't ask for branding or credit—it's part of their community service mission.

Perception and Reality

School food has become ground zero for the convergence of so many movements that every small improvement we make contributes to a potentially huge impact. From saving our ecosystem and energy conservation to animal rights, food safety, and preserving small and mid-sized farms, from nourishing hungry children to teaching all children about one another's cultural heritage and the camaraderie of preparing and sharing a meal together, from fostering creativity and cooperation instead of competition and stress, and from protecting children from creeping commercialism to protecting farm workers from chemical exposure, the impact of 7 billion meals a year could be tremendous. Reversing childhood obesity and declining children's health is possible. The model programs add up, and over the past few years they've become more ambitious and expansive, but we haven't fixed the problems and we're not even close to finding all the answers.

New legislation may help change attitudes among stakeholders, but then it may backfire by creating a perception that school food has been fixed so we don't have to deal with the issue anymore. Additionally, legislation often takes years to go into effect, and only then do we begin to ascertain the unintended consequences. Nor should we assume that new standards guarantee better food. Without adequate funding for fresh food, food service directors will continue to look to the food industry to manufacture affordable solutions to their problems.

Still and all, as an advocate for better food in school, you have to be not only a superhero, but a magician, lobbyist, and politician as well.

The Center of the Plate

Another commonality I saw among the model programs I visited was that they were achieving success adding more fruits and vegetables to their programs, and more vegetarian entrées, but most had not made much headway improving the quality of the animal components of their meals. For meat, eggs, cheese, and poultry many of the food service directors I met and spoke with were still relying on processed government commodities. While some, like Ann Cooper and Bruce Gluck, are able to source organic and humanely raised animal products, most struggled to procure anything less processed than popcorn chicken or beef crumbles, and progress for many was serving chicken on the bone, no matter its source. Procuring these center-of-the-plate items from safe, local, and humane farmers is an area in which advocates can step up in the coming years.

Make Mistakes

Some of the best advice I've heard is that in order to create change, you have to make mistakes. Environmental and human rights activist Diane Wilson says, "I have made every mistake in the book but the thing is, I would not trade any of those mistakes because that's where I learned how to be an activist. You have to realize it's a part of your journey, it's not a weekend thing, it's not a two-day thing, it becomes a part of who you are and it's a part of your integrity. It's one of the most valuable things I have. You just have to do it with humor and with love—it's all transforming. It's not like you're just getting a law passed, you're not just getting awareness. You're changing yourself and you're changing people. I've done more stuff for my strength and inner stuff than I have made movement outside. It's been miraculous. I've never had so many people that dislike me but I've never liked myself this much."

"What we're trying to do is basically a big experiment," says environmental activist Annie Leonard. "I feel like we can't make progress if we're not willing to make mistakes. I think the biggest mistake that I made that I'm constantly trying to remind myself of is to listen more. As I learned about environmental stuff I became a missionary, basically, accosting people on the street to show them my latest chart and data and tell them all the compelling information and I didn't realize for a long time that the deeper my expertise became, the shallower my ability to communicate with others became. I alienated people in my desire to share with them the latest data. So what I've learned how to do now is listen more. When I meet someone I realize the first step in recruiting them in our cause is not to bombard them with data but to listen, to find out what they care about and to really hear what they are saying, to reflect it back to them, to let them be heard and to find the commonalities in our work because the truth is the vast majority of people out there share a lot of values in common. We all want a healthy planet, we all want security for our families and communities, we all want our children to be safe, educated, and healthy. So if we can take a deep breath and listen and then find those commonalities and then start from there, it's a much more respectful and much more effective way to build a coalition."

A Vehicle for Change

When I began investigating school food my greatest challenge was getting into the school cafeterias to see what was going on. In many cases, there was plenty to hide. I found little transparency in the culture of school food, and when my movie was released, the School Nutrition Association issued a series of "talking points" for their members to use in response to the ensuing media frenzy.

After the initial furor died down and food service directors and staff actually saw the movie, I began hearing from many of the association's members who now are embracing the movement for better food in schools; they're appreciative of the interest more parents are expressing and they are eager to work with their communities to improve their programs and participate in the curriculum. In these intervening years, I've seen school food transform from something no one was paying much attention to, to an institution that was attacked and defended, to an admitted embarrassment and complicit culprit of childhood obesity. I think we've reached a tipping point where school food has once again transformed.

In the words of leadership guru Stephen Covey, "All things are created twice. There's a mental or first creation, and a physical or second creation to all things." As a creation of a collective imagination, the school food environment has been transformed into a tremendous opportunity to create a food system that nourishes and teaches healthy kids for a healthy future. We are only just beginning to create the physical expression of this transformative vision.

NOTES

INTRODUCTION

page 2. **Advertisers spend $10 to $15 billion annually:** Marion Nestle, *Food Politics: How the Food Industry Influences Nutrition and Health* (Berkeley, Calif.: University of California Press, 2002); Kelly D. Brownell, *Food Fight: The Inside Story of the Food Industry, America's Obesity Crisis, and What We Can Do About It* (New York: McGraw-Hill, 2003).

page 3. **branding can even trump sensory input:** Thomas N. Robinson et al., "Effects of Fast Food Branding on Young Children's Taste Preferences," *Archives of Pediatrics and Adolescent Medicine* 161, no. 8 (2007): 792–97.

page 3. **"Branding food packages with licensed characters":** C. A. Roberto, J. Baik, J. L. Harris, and K. D. Brownell, "Influence of Licensed Characters on Children's Taste and Snack Preferences," *Journal of Pediatrics* 158, no. 1 (January 2011): 170–1.

page 3. **NYU's Goddard Professor of Nutrition:** Marion Nestle, Joan Dye Gussow, Kelly Brownell, and Michael Pollan, *The Politics of Obesity: Confronting Our National Eating Disorder*, University of California–Berkeley panel discussion, November 3, 2003, www.youtube.com/watch?v=WfNFjmwdAwo.

page 4. **"We're relying on the kid to pester the mom":** "How Advertisers Target Kids," Media Awareness Network, www.media-awareness.ca/english/parents/marketing/marketers_target_kids.cfm.

page 4. **"Brand marketing must begin with children.":** James McNeal, *The Kids Market: Myths and Realities* (Ithaca, N.Y.: Paramount Market Publishing, 1999).

page 4. **"The school system is where you build brand loyalty.":** John Alm, quoted in "A Lesson for Coke: Atlanta-Based CCE Takes on Critics, Defends Soft Drink Sales in Schools," *Atlanta Journal Constitution*, April 6, 2003, p. H1.

page 4. **"Reauthorizing the Child Nutrition Act this year is critical":** "America's Beverage Industry Supports Efforts to Reauthorise Child Nutrition Standards This Year," *Food & Beverage News*, August 4, 2010, http://fnbnews.com/article/detarchive.asp?articleid=28024&sectionid=3.

page 4. **Studies link the colorings, preservatives, and artificial sweeteners:** Susan E. Swithers and Terry L. Davidson, "A Role for Sweet Taste: Calorie Predictive Relations in Energy Regulation by Rats," *Behavioral Neuroscience* 122, no. 1 (February 2008).

page 5. **Kelly Brownell from Yale's Rudd Center:** Jeff Brady, "Soda in America: Taxes and a Debate Over Health," National Public Radio, May 4, 2010, www.npr.org/templates/story/story .php?storyId=126511372.

page 5. **Senator Tom Harkin criticized this monstrous scam:** *Killer at Large: Why Obesity Is America's Greatest Threat*, directed by Steven Greenstreet (Shine Box Media Productions, 2008), DVD.

page 6. **He also documented degenerative diseases:** Weston A. Price, *Nutrition and Physical Degeneration* (Redlands, Calif.: Weston A. Price, 1939).

page 6. **Our country uses 15 trillion pounds a year:** Philip Shabecoff and Alice Shabecoff, *Poisoned for Profit: How Toxins Are Making Our Children Chronically Ill* (White River Junction, Vt.: Chelsea Green Publishing, 2010).

page 7. **They found a 57 percent increase in the likelihood:** Nicholas A. Christakis and James H. Fowler, "The Spread of Obesity in a Large Social Network over Thirty-two Years," *New England Journal of Medicine* 357 (July 26, 2007): 370–79.

page 7. **Dr. David Kessler, former head of the Food and Drug Administration:** David A. Kessler, *The End of Overeating: Taking Control of the Insatiable American Appetite* (New York: Rodale Books, 2009).

page 8. **more and more of the substance to produce the same satiety:** Luke Stoeckel, "The Goldilocks Principle of Obesity," *Scientific American* (June 8, 2010).

page 9. **Americans spend $200 billion per year in diet-related health care costs:** Elizabeth Frazão, "The American Diet: A Costly Health Problem," *Food Review* (January 1996), www.ers.usda. gov/publications/foodreview/jan1996/frjan96a.pdf.

page 9. **estimated annual cost of obesity:** "Child Nutrition Promotion and School Lunch Protection Act of 2009," Bill Text 111th Congress (2009–2010) S.934.IS. http://thomas.loc.gov/cgi-bin/ query/z?c111:S.934.IS.

page 9. **Fifty percent of all cancer could be prevented:** "American Cancer Society Launches Campaign to Educate Americans about Reducing Cancer Risk," American Cancer Society news release, January 24, 2007.

page 9. **95 percent of America's health care dollars are spent on disease treatment:** Tommy G. Thompson, Secretary of Health and Human Services, April 2003, at the launch of Steps to a Healthier U.S. national initiative. In Kelley, Moy, Kosiak, McNeill, Zhan, Stryen, et al., "Prevention Health Care Quality in America: Findings from the First National Healthcare Quality and Disparities Reports," July 2004, http://www.cdc.gov/pcd/issues/2004/jul/04_0031.htm.

page 9. **The average American life expectancy:** Central Intelligence Agency, *The World Factbook*, www.cia.gov/library/publications/the-world-factbook/rankorder/2102rank.html.

page 9. **The cost of fresh fruits and vegetables:** "Food Without Thought: How U.S. Farm Policy Contributes to Obesity," Institute for Agriculture and Trade Policy fact sheet, November 2006, www.iatp.org/iatp/factsheets.cfm?accountID=258&refID=89968.

page 9. **The cost of soda, sweets, meat, dairy, fats, and oils:** "Food Without Thought: How U.S. Farm Policy Contributes to Obesity," Institute for Agricultural and Trade Policy fact sheet, November 2006, www.iatp.org/iatp/factsheets.cfm?accountID=258&refID=89968.

page 9. **Americans spend less than 10 percent of their income on food:** "Table 1. National Health Expenses Aggregate and Per Capita Amounts, Percent Distribution, and Average Annual Percent Growth, by Source of Funds: Selected Calendar Years 1980–2003," Centers for Medicare and Medicaid Services, Office of the Actuary, http://www.cms.hhs.gov/NationalHealthExpendData/02_NationalHealthAccountsHistorical.asp; and "Americans Spend Less Than 10 Percent of Disposable Income on Food," United States Department of Agriculture, Economic Research Service news release, July 19, 2006.

page 9. **Europeans spend 17 percent of their earnings on food:** "Food CPI and Expenditures, 2006, Table 97," United States Department of Agriculture, Economic Research Service, www.ers.usda.gov/briefing/cpifoodandexpenditures/data/Table_97/2006table97.htm; and "Why Germany and France Still Lead the Way on Health Care," *The Daily Mail*, April 17, 2011.

page 9. **In 1960, Americans spent 17.5 percent of their income on food:** "Table 1. National Health Expenses Aggregate," CMMS; and "Americans Spend Less Than 10 Percent," USDA.

page 9. **Only 2 percent of school-age children eat the USDA's serving recommendations:** "Children's Diets in the Mid-1990s: Dietary Intake and Its Relationship with School Meal Participation," United States Department of Agriculture, Office of Analysis, Nutrition and Evaluation, Report no. CN-01-CD1, January 2001, www.fns.usda.gov/ora/menu/published/CNP/FILES/ChilDiet.pdf.

page 9. **Nearly 30 percent of American children eat less than one serving a day of vegetables:** Ibid.

page 9. **According to the Institute of Medicine, "at least 30 percent of the calories in the average child's diet derive from sweets":** J. M. McGinnis, J. A. Gootman, V. I. Kraak, eds. *Food Marketing to Children and Youth: Threat or Opportunity?* (Washington, D.C.: National Academies Press, 2006).

page 10. **Over two-thirds of all foods consumed by schoolchildren:** "Diet Quality of American School-Age Children by School Lunch Participation Status: Data from the National Health and Nutrition Examination Survey (Summary)," United States Department of Agriculture, Food and Nutrition Services, July 2008, www.fns.usda.gov/ora/menu/published/CNP/files/NHANES-NSLPSummary.pdf.

page 10. **Children's sodium intake is 214 percent above recommended levels:** Bill Text 111th (2009–2010) S.934.IS.

page 10. **Children two to eighteen years old consumed an average of 118 more calories per day in 1996:** S. Nielsen, A. M. Seiga-Riz, and B. Popkin, "Trends in Energy Intake in U.S. Between 1977 and 1996: Similar Shifts Seen Across Age Groups," *Obesity Research*, no. 10 (2002) 370–78.

page 10. **In 2009, Americans consumed 63 percent of their calories:** "Report of the DGAC on the Dietary Guidelines for Americans, 2010," Executive Summary, United States Department of Agriculture, www.cnpp.usda.gov/Publications/DietaryGuidelines/2010/DGAC/Report/A-ExecSummary.pdf.

page 10. **Eleven percent of the calories consumed by adolescents come from soda and other soft drinks:** "Vending Machines and Competitive Food in Schools," DefeatDiabetes.org, www.defeatdiabetes.org/resource/dynamic/global/ddf_-_cap_-_vending_machine_background_briefing.pdf.

page 10. **Since the 1970s, obesity rates have tripled among children ages six to nineteen:** "Childhood Obesity," U.S. Department of Health and Human Services, Assistant Secretary for Planning and Evaluation, http://aspe.hhs.gov/health/reports/child_obesity.

page 10. **Twelve percent of American children currently have type 2 (adult-onset) diabetes:** "The Challenge We Face," Let's Move! White House Task Force on Childhood Obesity, www.letsmove.gov/sites/letsmove.gov/files/TFCO_Challenge_We_Face.pdf.

page 10. **Nineteen percent of American children are obese and 35 percent are overweight:** "Childhood Obesity," USDHHS.

page 10. **One quarter of children ages five to ten have elevated blood cholesterol:** "Prevalence of Obesity Among Children and Adolescents: United States, Trends 1963–1965 Through 2007–2008," Centers for Disease Control and Prevention, www.cdc.gov/nchs/data/hestat/obesity_child_07_08/obesity_child_07_08.htm.

page 10. **One in four children take prescription medication daily for chronic illness:** "Checklist for Camp: Bug Spray. Sunscreen. Pills," *New York Times*, July 16, 2006.

page 10. **Childhood asthma rates have more than doubled in the past thirty years:** Centers for Disease Control and Prevention Data and Statistics, www.cdc.gov/DataStatistics.

page 10. **There's been a 700 percent increase in amphetamine prescriptions for children since 1990:** Gretchen B. LeFever, Andrea P. Arcona, and David O. Antonuccio, "ADHD Among American Schoolchildren—Evidence of Overdiagnosis and Overuse of Medication," *Scientific Review of Mental Health Practice* 2, no. 1 (Spring/Summer 2003).

page 10. **Between 1995 and 1999, antidepressant use increased 74 percent among children:** Lawrence H. Diller, "Kids on Drugs," *Salon*, March 9, 2000, http://dir.salon.com/health/feature/2000/ 03/09/kid_drugs/index.html.

page 11. **American girls are beginning puberty one to two years earlier:** Sandra Steingraber, *The Falling Age of Puberty in U.S. Girls* (San Francisco: Breast Cancer Fund, 2007), http://www.breastcancerfund.org/assets/pdfs/publications/falling-age-of-puberty.pdf.

page 11. **The United States ranks near the bottom of the world's thirty most-developed countries in math:** 2006 Programme for International Student Assessment (PISA) comparison, quoted in "Educate to Innovate" White House campaign, http://www.whitehouse.gov/issues/education/educate-innovate; also search "PISA 2006 results" at OECD Programme for International Student Assessment, www.oecd.org.

page 11. **one in ten households in the United States is food insecure:** Mark Nord, Alisha Coleman-Jensen, Margaret Andrews, and Steven Carlson, "Household Food Security in the United States, 2009," United States Department of Agriculture, Economic Research Service Report no. 108 (November 2010), www.ers.usda.gov/Publications/ERR108/ERR108.pdf.

page 11. **some 16.7 million children in the United States go to bed hungry:** Ibid.

page 11. **there was an association between overall diet quality and academic performance:** "Children with Healthier Diets Do Better in School, Study Suggests," *Science Daily*, March 22, 2008.

page 13. **Significantly fewer children in the intervention schools:** Gary D. Foster, et al. "A Policy-Based School Intervention to Prevent Overweight and Obesity," *Pediatrics* 121, no. 4 (April 2008), http://pediatrics.aappublications.org/cgi/content/full/121/4/e794.

CHAPTER 1. LET'S DO LUNCH

page 15. **One should not have to be a superhero, a magician, or a saint:** Janet Poppendieck, *Free for All: Fixing School Food in America* (Berkeley, Calif.: University of California Press, 2010).

page 18. **A 1970s Environmental Protection Agency document:** Wilma R. McCarey, "Pesticide Regulation: Risk Assessment and Burden of Proof," *George Washington Law Review* 45, no. 5 (August 1977): 1,066.

page 18. **pesticides are known to disrupt a child's normal hormone balance:** "Children and Pesticides Don't Mix," Beyond Pesticides fact sheet, www.beyondpesticides.org/lawn/factsheets/Pesticide.children.dontmix.pdf.

page 19. **Livestock consumes over 70 percent of all the antibiotics:** M. Mellon et al., *Hogging It: Estimates of Antimicrobial Abuse in Livestock* (Cambridge, Mass.: Union of Concerned Scientists, 2000).

page 19. **the USDA paid $145 million for pet-food grade "spent-hen meat":** Lake Morrison, Peter Eisler and Anthony DeBarros, "Old-Hen Meat Fed to Pets and Schoolkids," *USA Today*, December 16, 2009.

page 22. **culprit for early onset of puberty in girls:** Steingraber, *Falling Age of Puberty*.

page 22. **aberrations from exposure to hormones:** Gerald A. LeBlanc and Lisa J. Bain, "Chronic Toxicity of Environmental Contaminants: Sentinels and Biomarkers," *Environmental Health Perspectives* 105 (February 1997).

page 22. **In 1998, Monsanto quashed:** Sheldon Rampton and John Stauber, "Monsanto and Fox: Partners in Censorship," *PR Watch* 5, no. 2, (1998), http://www.sourcewatch.org/index.php?title=Monsanto_and_Fox:_Partners_in_Censorship.

page 23. **confusion, diarrhea, heart irregularities, asthma, and mood swings:** "Names of Ingredients That Contain Processed Free Glutamic Acid (MSG)," Truth in Labeling Campaign, www.truthinlabeling.org/hiddensources.html.

page 30. **A 2010 Princeton study finds that consumption of HFCS:** Miriam E. Bocarslya, Elyse S. Powella, Nicole M. Avenaa, and Bartley G. Hoebel, "High-Fructose Corn Syrup Causes Characteristics of Obesity in Rats: Increased Body Weight, Body Fat and Triglyceride Levels," *Pharmacology Biochemistry & Behavior* 97, no. 1 (November 2010): 185.

page 30. **There's a strong correlation between America's type 2 diabetes crisis:** Mike Adams, "High-Fructose Corn Syrup and Diabetes: What the Experts Say," *Natural News*, June 17, 2009.

page 30. **The tumor cells were able to metabolize:** Haibo Liu, Danshan Huang, David L. McArthur, et al., "Fructose Induces Transketolase Flux to Promote Pancreatic Cancer Growth," *Cancer Research* (August 2010), http://cancerres.aacrjournals.org/content/70/15/6368.abstract.

page 30. **The food industry loves HFCS:** "Questions and Answers About High Fructose Corn Syrup," Corn Refiners Association, www.cornnaturally.com/assets/pdfs/Background_Information/HFCS%20Q&A.pdf.

page 31. **Dr. Russell L. Blaylock, author of the book *Excitotoxins*:** Russell L. Blaylock, *The Truth About Aspartame*, video embedded in "Aspartame, Brain Cancer and the FDA," International Academy of Wellness, November 7, 2010, www.academyofwellness.com/aspartame.

page 32. **Currently in the United States, about 89 percent of soy:** "Genetically Modified Crops in the United States," Pew Initiative on Food and Biotechnology fact sheet, 2007, http://uwstudent

web.uwyo.edu/L/LPETER11/Factsheet%20Genetically%20Modified%20Crops%20in%20 the%20United%20States.htm.

page 32. **It's reported that animals fed GMOs have exhibited a variety of strange symptoms:** Jeffrey M. Smith, *Genetic Roulette* (Portland, Maine: Yes! Books, 2007).

page 32. **These GMO seed companies have a history of suing:** "Goliath and David: Monsanto's Legal Battles Against Farmers," *SourceWatch*, www.sourcewatch.org/index.php?title=Goliath_and_David:_Monsanto's_Legal_Battles_against_Farmers.

page 32. **genetically modified salmon was introduced:** Emily Sohn, "Is Genetically Modified Salmon Safe?" *Discovery News*, September 10, 2010, news.discovery.com/animals/fish-salmon-genetically-modified.html.

page 34. **The American College of Sports Medicine states:** Lawrence E. Armstrong et al., "Position Stand on Exercise and Fluid Replacement," *Medicine & Science in Sports & Exercise* 28, no. 1 (January 1996): i–viii, www.acsm.org/AM/Template.cfm?Section=Past_Roundtables&Template=/CM/ContentDisplay.cfm&ContentID=2833.

page 35. **touting a study by MilkPEP:** "Changes in School Children's Milk Consumption and Nutrient Intake as a Result of Changing the Availability of Flavored Milk in Schools," Milk-PEP (Milk Processor Education Program), March 2010 report. http://media.kval.com/documents/2009-10_Flavor_Impact_FINAL_report.pdf.

page 35. **A child's brain consists of over 60 percent fat cells:** "Nutrition—Feeding Your Child's Brain!" More4Kids, www.more4kids.info/362/brain-nutrition-for-your-child/.

page 36. **Milk from cows allowed to graze on fresh pasture:** "Grassfarming Benefits the Environment," Eatwild, www.eatwild.com/environment.html.

page 36. **The USDA is working on adding substitutions for milk:** Amy Liddell, "Lactose Intolerance and Ethnicity," Livestrong, www.livestrong.com/article/388286-lactose-intolerance-ethnicity/.

page 36. **children of European descent:** Ibid.

page 36. **Both beef and milk production are a major source of global warming:** "Greenhouse Gas Emissions from the Dairy Sector: A Life Cycle Assessment," Food and Agriculture Organization of the United Nations, Animal Production and Health Division, 2011, www.fao.org/agriculture/lead/themes0/climate/emissions/en/.

page 36. **A study in the journal *Current Opinion in Pediatrics*:** Anisha I. Patel and Michael D. Cabana, "Encouraging Healthy Beverage Intake in Child Care and School Settings," *Current Opinion in Pediatrics* 22, no. 6 (2010): 779–84.

page 38. **The USDA requirements for school meals:** "National School Lunch Program [Guidelines]," United States Department of Agriculture, September 2010, www.fns.usda.gov/cnd/lunch/aboutlunch/NSLPFactSheet.pdf.

page 38. **offering french fries, Tater Tots and other potato products:** Allison Hedley Dodd et al., "Association Between School Food Environment and Practices and Body Mass Index of U.S. Public School Children," *Journal of the American Dietetic Association* 109, no. 2, supplement (February 2009): S108–17.

page 39. **A stylish graphic poster listing all fifty-plus of its ingredients:** www.boingboing.net/2010/05/26/hot-pocket-ingredien.html.

page 43. **Ninety-nine percent of public schools participate in the National School Lunch Program:** "Program Data: National Level Annual Summary Tables [FY 2008 Through January 2011]," United States Department of Agriculture, www.fns.usda.gov/pd/cnpmain.htm.

page 50. **as few as 35 percent of eligible high school students:** Carol Pogash, "Free Lunch Isn't Cool, So Some Students Go Hungry," *New York Times*, March 1, 2008.

page 50. **A typical student will consume 4,000 school lunches:** "Rethinking School Lunch: A Planning Framework from the Center for Ecoliteracy," second edition. Center for Ecoliteracy, www.ecoliteracy.org/sites/default/files/uploads/rethinking_school_lunch_guide.pdf.

page 53. **Schoolchildren who consume foods purchased in vending machines:** Madhuri Kakarala et al., "Children Who Eat Vended Snack Foods Face Chronic Health Problems, Poor Diet," *University of Michigan Medical School Journal of School Health* 80, no. 9 (September 2010), www2.med.umich.edu/prmc/media/newsroom/details.cfm?ID=1705.

page 53. **An American Dietetics Association study informs us:** A. H. Dodd et al., "Association Between School Food Environment and Practices and Body Mass Index of U.S. Public School Children," *Journal of the American Dietetic Association* 109, no. 2 supplement (February 2009): S108–17.

page 53. **Here's one from Lincoln, Nebraska:** Bree L. Dority, Mary G. McGarvey, and Patricia F. Kennedy, "Marketing Foods and Beverages in Schools: The Effect of School Food Policy on Students' Overweight Measures," *American Marketing Association Journal of Public Policy & Marketing* 29, no. 2 (Fall 2010).

page 53. **There is a growing belief among policymakers and the general public:** Annina Catherine Burns et al. *Local Government Actions to Prevent Childhood Obesity* (Washington, D.C.: National Academies Press, 2009). www.rwjf.org/files/research/20090901iomreport.pdf.

page 58. **Children who are not getting adequate nutrients have lower test scores:** "The Value of Improving Nutrition and Physical Activity in Our Schools," Learning Connection, www .actionforhealthykids.org/resources/files/learning-connection.pdf.

CHAPTER 2. GET CONNECTED

page 66. **A September 2010 study by Russell Research:** "75% of Parents Think the Food Offered at School Is Not Very Nutritious," Russell Research news release, September 2, 2010. www .russellresearch.com/filestr/09022010.pdf.

page 80. **The Organic Center reports that pesticides:** Matthew E. Burrow et al., "Scientists Estimate That Pesticides Are Reducing Legume Crop Yields by One-Third Through Impaired Nitrogen Fixation," *Proceedings of the National Academy of Sciences*, 104, no. 24 (June 2007), www.organic-center.org/science.hot.php?action=view&report_id=99.

page 81. **"All PTA members are being challenged to respond":** "Federal Policy Update and Action Alerts: PTA Takes Action, Federal Policy—October 2010," National Parent Teacher Association, www.pta.org/6025.htm.

page 82. **Since 2006, every district that participates:** "Local Wellness Policy," United States Department of Agriculture, Food and Nutrition Service, www.fns.usda.gov/tn/healthy/wellnesspolicy.html.

page 92. **"You know, Ms. Jones, Joey came home with Dum-Dums":** *The Lunch Tray*, " 'School Food Superheroes': Mrs. Q Responds!" blog entry by Bettina Elias Siegel, September 30, 2010, www.thelunchtray.com/school-food-superheroes-mrs-q-responds/.

page 93. **Mendy says, "I felt part of the reason":** *The Slow Cook*, "Mendy Heaps Answers Her Critics," blog entry by Ed Bruske, April 12, 2010. www.theslowcook.com/2010/04/12/mendy-heaps-answers-her-critics.

page 99. **Food Services Student Survey:.** "Food Services Student Survey," Greater Southern Tier [New York] Boards of Cooperative Educational Services, www.gstboces.org/ms/foodservices/studentsurvey.

CHAPTER 3. THE WONKY CHAPTER

page 117. **"The expensive machinery of education is wasted":** Mary Swartz Rose, quoted in Josephine Martin and Charlotte Oakley, *Managing Child Nutrition Programs: Leadership for Excellence* (Bloomfield, N.J.: Jones and Bartlett Publishers, 2008).

page 130. **in 2005 there were nearly two hundred individual bills introduced to raise nutrition standards:** "State Actions to Promote Nutrition, Increase Physical Activity and Prevent Obesity: A Legislative Overview," Health Policy Tracking Service, Robert W. Johnson Foundation, October 3, 2005, www.rwjf.org/childhoodobesity/product.jsp?id=15832.

page 133. **Child obesity has become so serious in this country that military leaders are:** "Too Fat to Fight: Retired Military Leaders Want Junk Food Out of America's Schools," Mission: Readiness, Military Leaders for Kids, 2010, http://cdn.missionreadiness.org/MR_Too_Fat_to_Fight-1.pdf.

page 136. **report titled *Nutrition Standards for Foods in Schools: Leading the Way Toward Healthier Youth*:** Virginia A. Stallings and Ann L. Yaktine, eds., *Nutrition Standards for Foods in Schools: Leading the Way Toward Healthier Youth* (Washington, D.C.: National Academies Press, 2007), http://www.iom.edu/Reports/2007/Nutrition-Standards-for-Foods-in-Schools-Leading-the-Way-toward-Healthier-Youth.aspx.

CHAPTER 4. LOCAL WELLNESS POLICIES

page 142. **Local school food authorities are responsible for serving meals:** "State Strategies to Help Schools Make the Most of Their National School Lunch Program," National Governors Association, Center for Best Practices, January 11, 2010, http://www.nga.org/Files/pdf/1001SCHOOLLUNCH.PDF.

page 143. **The USDA says, "The legislation places the responsibility of developing a wellness policy":** "Federal and State Laws Impacting Food and Beverages in Connecticut Schools," Connecticut State Department of Education, February 2007, www.simsbury.k12.ct.us/uploaded/District_Content/Food_Services/NutritionLaws.pdf.

page 155. **The Board of Education recognizes the positive benefits:** Kate Bowie, Alison Rowntree, and Richard Siddall, "Grab 5: A Model School Food Policy—A Practical Guide," Sustain Publications, 2002, www.sustainweb.org/pdf/G5_MFPol.pdf.

page 155. **Each school in the district shall establish an instructional garden:** "Model Wellness Policy Guide," Center for Ecoliteracy, www.ecoliteracy.org/sites/default/files/uploads/cel_model_wellness_policy_guide.pdf.

page 156. **Schools should provide nutrition education and engage in nutrition promotion that:** "School District's Wellness Policies on Physical Activity and Nutrition," National Alliance for Nutrition and Activity, Model Local School Wellness Policies, March 2005, www.schoolwellnesspolicies.org/WellnessPolicies.html.

page 169. **As many as 48 percent of girls and 32 percent of boys skip:** Gail C. Rampersaud, Mark A. Pereira, Beverly L. Girard, et al., "Breakfast Habits, Nutritional Status, Body Weight, and Academic Performance in Children and Adolescents," *Journal of the American Dietetic Association* 105, no. 5 (May 2005): 743, www.grainpower.org/docs/Breakfast%20article%20JADA-5-05.pdf.

page 171. **The Massachusetts Public Health Association offers these suggestions:** Roberta R. Friedman, "Community Action to Change School Food Policy: An Organizing Kit," Massachusetts Public Health Association, May 2005, www.mphaweb.org/documents/CommunityActiontoChangeSchoolFoodPolicy.pdf.

page 181. **And in Katonah-Lewisboro the policy commits the district to:** Katonah-Lewisboro School District Wellness Policy, 2009. Access the link below, click on "Policies," and then "5405: Wellness": http://www.boarddocs.com/ny/klsd/Board.nsf/Public#.

CHAPTER 6. FARM TO CAFETERIA

page 216. **every week as many as 330 farmers are forced out of business:** "From Today's Rose Garden Speech," Farm Aid, quoted by SustainableTable, April 29, 2008, www.sustainabletable.org/2008/04/from-todays-rose-garden-speech.

page 239. **The Farm to School website tells their story like this:** "The New North Florida Cooperative Farm to School Program," Farm to School Programs, www.farmtoschool.org/state-programs.php?action=detail&id=23&pid=32.

CHAPTER 7. TEACH FOOD

page 261. **Children learn more rapidly and lastingly in a multi-sensory environment:** Aaron R. Seitz and Ladan Shams, "Benefits of Multisensory Learning," *Trends in Cognitive Science* 12, no. 11 (November 1, 2008): 411–17, http://shamslab.psych.ucla.edu/publications/Tics2008-reprint.pdf.

page 270. **Edible Schoolyards Sprout in North Idaho:** Michele Murphree, "Edible Schoolyards Sprout in North Idaho," *Northwest Food News*, January 1, 2011, www.nwfoodnews.com/2011/01/01/edible-schoolyards-sprout-up-in-north-idaho.

page 289. **2009 study by the Society for Public Health Education:** Jeanne P. Goldberg et al., "The Effects of School Garden Experiences on Middle School–Aged Students' Knowledge, Attitudes, and Behaviors Associated With Vegetable Consumption," *Health Promotion Practice*, October 2009, http://hpp.sagepub.com/content/early/2009/10/21/1524839909349182.abstract.

page 292. **The curriculum approaches food from a holistic perspective:** "Special Offer on Curriculum and Training for Midwest Educators!" The Whole Plate: A Return to Real Food, http://www.thewholeplate.yihs.net/about/staff/.

CHAPTER 8. OUTSOURCED

page 318. **A typical RFP stipulates: "FSMC (Contractor) must have successful prior experience.":** See, e.g., Port Angeles, Washington, Food Service RFP 2010, http://www.wafarmtoschool.org/Content/Documents/PortAngelesSD_2010_FoodServiceManagementCo_RFP_4-7-10_(a).pdf.

RESOURCES

CHAPTER 1. LET'S DO LUNCH

Alpert, Barbara, and Yvonne Sanders-Butler. *Healthy Kids, Smart Kids: The Principal-Created, Parent-Tested, Kid-Approved Nutrition Plan for Sound Bodies and Strong Minds*. New York: Perigee, 2005.

Better D.C. School Food. www.betterdcschoolfood.blogspot.com.

Bock, Kenneth. *Healing the New Childhood Epidemics: Autism, ADHD, Asthma and Allergies*. New York: Random House, 2007.

Burton, David. *InGREEDients*. Directed by David Burton. Sir Rebel Films, 2009. DVD, 76 minutes.

Center for Commercial-Free Public Education. www.ibiblio.org/commercialfree/.

The Feingold Association of the United States. www.feingold.org/faq.php.

Fuhrman, Joel. *Disease-Proof Your Child: Feeding Kids Right*. New York: St. Martin's Press, 2005.

Gittleman, Ann Louise. *Get the Sugar Out*. New York: Three Rivers Press, 1996.

Green Schools Report Card Quiz. www.greenschools.net/form.php?modin=53.

Institute for Responsible Technology. "Creating GM-Free Schools." www.seedsofdeception.com/GMFree/TakeAction/GM-FreeSchools/index.cfm.

Oliver, Jamie. "School Food Audit." www.jamieoliver.com/foundation/jamies-food-revolution/__cms/uploads/1_Support%20Tool_Audit.pdf.

People for the Ethical Treatment of Animals. "Vegan-Friendly School Cafeteria." www.peta2.com/TAKECHARGE/pdf/VEGcafeteria300.pdf.

The Slow Cook. www.theslowcook.com.

Smith, Jeffrey M. *Seeds of Deception: Exposing Industry and Government Lies About the Safety of the Genetically Engineered Foods You're Eating*. Fairfield, Iowa: Yes! Books, 2003.

———. *Hidden Dangers in Kids' Meals*. Produced by Jeffrey M. Smith. Yes! Books, 2005. DVD, 110 minutes.

CHAPTER 2. GET CONNECTED

Friedman, Roberta R. "Community Action to Change School Food Policy: An Organizing Kit." www.betterschoolfood.org/downloads/resources/BSF_MPHA_Community_Action.pdf.

McConnell, Carmel. *Change Activist: Make Big Things Happen Fast.* New York: Basic Books, 2003.

Two Angry Moms. "Useful Links." http://angrymoms.org/links.php.

CHAPTER 3. THE WONKY CHAPTER

Environmental Working Group. Farm Subsidy Database. http://farm.ewg.org/.

Levine, Susan. *School Lunch Politics: The Surprising History of America's Favorite Welfare Program.* Princeton, N.J.: Princeton University Press, 2008.

Library of Congress. "History of School Gardens." Video. www.youtube.com/watch?v= N14bTyHH-rA.

Miner, Barbara. "Don't Bite the Hand that Feeds." *Rethinking Schools.* www.rethinkingschools. org/restrict.asp?path=archive/20_04/bite204.shtml.

Muller, Mark, and Heather Schoonover. "Food Without Thought: How U.S. Farm Policy Contributes to Obesity." Summary of the full report "Food Without Thought: How U.S. Farm Policy Contributes to Obesity." Institute for Agriculture and Trade Policy, November 2006. www.iatp.org/iatp/factsheets.cfm?accountID=258&refID=89968.

Richardson, Jill. "Are School Lunches Setting Kids Up for Obesity and Poor Nutrition?" *AlterNet*, February 2010. www.alternet.org/food/145803/are_school_lunches_setting_kids_up_for_ obesity_and_poor_nutrition.

United States Department of Agriculture, Food and Nutrition Services. Nutrition Assistance Programs. www.fns.usda.gov/fns.

CHAPTER 4. LOCAL WELLNESS POLICIES

Action for Healthy Kids. "Wellness Policy Tool." www.actionforhealthykids.org/school-programs/our-programs/wellness-policy-tool/wellness-tool-5.html.

Brown, Janet. "Model Wellness Policy Guide." Center for Ecoliteracy. 2010. www.ecoliteracy.org/ sites/default/files/uploads/cel_model_wellness_policy_guide.pdf.

Cama, Shireen, et al. "School Wellness Policy and Practice: Meeting the Needs of Low-Income Students." Food Research and Action Center, February 2006. www.frac.org/pdf/wellness_ guide2006.pdf#search=%22school%20wellness%22.

Center for Science in the Public Interest. "Healthy School Snacks." http://cspinet.org/nutrition policy/healthy_school_snacks.html.

———. "School Foods Toolkit: A Guide to Improving School Foods and Beverages." www .cspinet.org/schoolfoodkit.

———. "Sweet Deals: School Fundraising Can Be Healthy and Profitable, Says CSPI." February 2007. http://cspinet.org/new/200702141.html.

Connecticut State Department of Education. "School Wellness Policy Reports." www.sde.ct.gov/sde/cwp/view.asp?a=2626&q=322168.

Fair Trade Federation. "Fair Trade Fundraisers." www.fairtradefederation.org/ht/d/sp/i/211/pid/211.

Food Allergy and Anaphylaxis Network. "School Guidelines for Managing Students with Allergies." www.foodallergy.org/page/food-allergy—anaphylaxis-network-guidelines.

Kaselak, Lisa. *Let Them Eat Cake*. Directed by Lisa Kaselak. Fanlight Productions, 2006. DVD, 33 minutes.

National Alliance for Nutrition and Activity. "Model School Wellness Policies." www.schoolwellnesspolicies.org.

NoJunkFood.org. www.nojunkfood.org.

Physicians Committee for Responsible Medicine. "School Lunch Guide 2007." www.pcrm.org/newsletter/sep07/report_card.html and www.healthyschoollunches.org.

The Robert Wood Johnson Foundation. "Local School Wellness Policies: How Are Schools Implementing the Congressional Mandate?" June 2009. www.rwjf.org/files/research/20090708 localwellness.pdf.

Transition Towns United States. www.transitionus.org.

United States Department of Agriculture, Food and Nutrition Service. "The Local Process: How to Create and Implement a Local Wellness Policy." www.fns.usda.gov/tn/Healthy/wellness policy_steps.html.

———. "Team Nutrition Training Grants." http://teamnutrition.usda.gov/grants.html.

CHAPTER 5. TIPPING SCALES TO TIPPING POINTS

Chez Panisse Foundation. www.chezpanissefoundation.org.

Wellness in the Schools. www.wellnessintheschools.org.

s'Cool Food. www.scoolfood.org.

School Food Trust. www.schoolfoodtrust.org.uk.

CHAPTER 6. FARM TO CAFETERIA

Appalachian Sustainable Agriculture Project. "Growing Minds Farm to School Program." www .growing-minds.org.

Center for Ecoliteracy. "Rethinking School Lunch: Financial Calculator." www.ecoliteracy.org/downloads/rsl-financial-calculator.

Community Food Security Coalition. www.foodsecurity.org.

Cook for America: Where School Food Is the Solution, Not the Problem. www.cookforamerica.com.

FoodRoutes. www.foodroutes.org/farmtoschool.jsp.

The Lunch Box: Healthy Tools to Help All Schools. "Recipes." www.thelunchbox.org/menus-recipes.

National Farm to School Network. www.farmtoschool.org.

National Sustainable Agriculture Information Service. www.attra.ncat.org.

Root Cause: Advancing Innovation for Social Impact. www.rootcause.org.

School Food Focus: Transforming Food Options for Children in Urban Schools. www
.schoolfoodfocus.org.

Sustainable Food Systems. www.sustainablefoodsystems.com.

Sustainable Table: Serving Up Healthy Food Choices. www.sustainabletable.org.

United States Department of Agriculture, Food Nutrition Services. "Department of Defense
Fresh Fruit and Vegetable Program." www.fns.usda.gov/fdd/programs/dod/default.htm.

———. "Food Buying Guide for Child Nutrition Programs." www.fns.usda.gov/tn/resources/
foodbuyingguide.html.

———. "Menu Planner for Healthy School Meals." www.fns.usda.gov/tn/resources/menuplanner.html.

———, Rural Development. "Value Added Producer Grants." www.rurdev.usda.gov/rbs/coops/
tvadg.htm.

Wellness in the Schools "Cook for Kids" Program. www.wellnessintheschools.org/index.php?
option=com_content&view=article&id=3&Itemid=17.

CHAPTER 7. TEACH FOOD

GARDEN PLANNING AND LESSON PLANS

American Community Gardening Association. www.communitygarden.org.

Bell, Lucy et al. *The Year-Round Organic School Garden: A Guide to Planning, Designing and Creating an Organic School Garden*. Living Classroom Publication, 2008.

Bucklin-Sporer, Arden, and Rachel Kathleen Pringle. *How to Grow a School Garden: A Complete
Guide for Parents and Teachers*. Portland, Ore.: Timber Press, 2010.

Center for Environmental Education. Free lesson plans for all subjects, K–12 and adults. www
.ceeonline.org/greenGuide/curriculum/curriculumLibrary.aspx.

Earth Box: Homegrown Vegetables Without a Garden. www.earthbox.com.

The Growing Classroom. www.gardeningwithkids.org/11-4017.html.

Life Lab: Bring Learning to Life in the Garden. www.lifelab.org.

Princeton School Gardens. "Garden Planning & Lesson Plans." Linked to the New Jersey state
standards for K–5. www.prs.k12.nj.us/GardenCoop/GardenCoopGuideNov07.pdf.

Square Foot Gardening. www.squarefootgardening.com.

United States Department of Agriculture, Agriculture in the Classroom. www.agclassroom.org.

Waters, Alice. *Edible Schoolyard: A Universal Idea*. San Francisco: Chronicle Books, 2008.

GENERAL

Center for Ecoliteracy. www.ecoliteracy.org.

———. *Big Ideas: Linking Food, Culture, Health and the Environment*. www.ecoliteracy.org/books/
big-ideas-linking-food-culture-health-and-environment.

Connecticut State Department of Education. "Action Guide for School Nutrition and Physical Activity Policies." www.state.ct.us/sde/deps/Student/NutritionEd/index.htm.

Earth Voice Food Choice. www.earthvoicefoodchoice.com/manual.html.

Green Teacher: Education for Planet Earth. www.greenteacher.com.

Harvard School of Public Health Prevention Research Center. "Planet Health" curriculum. www.hsph.harvard.edu/research/prc/projects/planet/.

Havala, Suzanne. "Food Is Elementary: A Hands-On Curriculum For Young Students." *Vegetarian Journal*. July 2000. www.findarticles.com/p/articles/mi_m0FDE/is_4_19/ai_64391431/.

Pollan, Michael. *Food Rules: An Eater's Manual*. New York: Penguin Books, 2009.

Stone, Michael K. *Smart by Nature: Schooling for Sustainability*. Healdsburg, Calif: Watershed Media, 2009. www.ecoliteracy.org/books/smart-nature-schooling-sustainability.

REAL FOOD IS . . .

Jacobsen, Rowan. *American Terroir: Savoring the Flavors of Our Woods, Waters, and Fields*. New York: Bloomsbury, 2010.

K–6 Students, Lincoln Elementary, Mount Vernon, Washington. *Lincoln's Journey to Real Food*. Video. Farm to School "Real Food Is" Video Contest. www.farmtoschool.mirocommunity.org/video/53/lincolns-journey-to-real-food; also http://vimeo.com/10361088, 2010.

New York Sun Works: The Greenhouse Project. www.nysunworks.org.

RESEARCH ON IMPACT OF SCHOOL GARDENS

Goldberg, Jeanne P., et al. "The Effects of School Garden Experiences on Middle School–Aged Students' Knowledge, Attitudes, and Behaviors Associated with Vegetable Consumption." *Health Promotion Practice* 12 (January 2011): 36–43, first published October 21, 2009. www.urbansprouts.org/wp-content/uploads/2010/01/Ratcliffe-et-al_The-effects-of-school-garden-experiences_HPP_electronic_2009.pdf.

University of Minnesota, Children's Garden West Central Research and Outreach Center. http://childrens.wcroc.cfans.umn.edu/pages/links/researchLinks1.php.

SEEDS

Fedco Co-Op Garden Supplies (Waterville, Maine). www.fedcoseeds.com.

High Mowing Organic Seeds (Wolcott, Vermont). www.highmowingseeds.com.

Johnny's Selected Seeds (Winslow, Maine). www.johnnyseeds.com.

Seeds of Change (Santa Fe, New Mexico). www.seedsofchange.com.

Seed Savers Exchange: Passing on Our Garden Heritage (Decorah, Iowa). www.seedsavers.org.

SOIL TESTING

University of California–Davis, Postharvest Technology Research and Information Center. http://postharvest.ucdavis.edu/Produce/Storage/index.shtml.

University of Massachusetts, Soil and Plant Tissue Testing Laboratory. www.umass.edu/plsoils/
    soiltest.

CHAPTER 8. OUTSOURCED

Federal Register. "Procurement Requirements for the National School Lunch, School Break-
    fast and Special Milk Programs." www.federalregister.gov/articles/2007/10/31/E7-21420/
    procurement-requirements-for-the-national-school-lunch-school-breakfast-and-special-milk-
    programs#p-39.
Freshlunches: Making Healthy Lunches Easy. www.freshlunches.com.
National Archives and Records Administration, "Specs for Bids 7CFR210." http://ecfr.gpoaccess.
    gov/cgi/t/text/text-idx?c=ecfr&tpl=/ecfrbrowse/Title07/7cfr210_main_02.tpl.
Revolution Foods: Healthy School Lunches for All Kids. www.revfoods.com.

CHAPTER 9. SCHOOL FOOD FROM SCRATCH

Harper, Clare, Lesley Wood, and Claire Mitchell. "The Provision of School Food in Eighteen
    Countries." School Food Trust, July 2008. http://www.schoolfoodtrust.org.uk/school-cooks-
    caterers/reports/the-provision-of-school-food-in-18-countries/.
Morgan, Kevin, and Robert Sonnino. *The School Food Revolution: Public Food and the Challenge of
    Sustainable Development*. Oxford, UK: Earthscan Publications, 2010.
Poppendieck, Janet. *Free for All: Fixing School Food in America (California Studies in Food and Cul-
    ture)*. Berkeley, Calif.: University of California Press, 2010.
University of California at Berkeley, Dr. Robert C. and Veronica Atkins Center for Weight and
    Health. "Changing Students' Knowledge, Attitudes and Behavior in Relation to Food." Sep-
    tember 2010. www.chezpanissefoundation.org/uploads/file/sli_exec%20sum_100921.pdf.
"What's For School Lunch?" www.whatsforschoollunch.blogspot.com/search/label/UK.

INDEX